Biomaterials and Nanotechnology for Tissue Engineering

Biomaterials and Nanotechnology for Tissue Engineering

Edited by
Swaminathan Sethuraman
Uma Maheswari Krishnan
Anuradha Subramanian

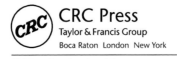

CRC Press
Taylor & Francis Group
Boca Raton London New York

CRC Press is an imprint of the
Taylor & Francis Group, an **informa** business

CRC Press
Taylor & Francis Group
6000 Broken Sound Parkway NW, Suite 300
Boca Raton, FL 33487-2742

First issued in paperback 2020

© 2017 by Taylor & Francis Group, LLC
CRC Press is an imprint of Taylor & Francis Group, an Informa business

No claim to original U.S. Government works

ISBN-13: 978-1-4987-4373-0 (hbk)
ISBN-13: 978-0-367-73672-9 (pbk)

Visit the Taylor & Francis Web site at
http://www.taylorandfrancis.com

and the CRC Press Web site at
http://www.crcpress.com

Contents

Section I   Introduction

Section II   Skeletal Tissue Engineering

Section III   Regeneration of Sensory System

Section IV   Tissue Engineering Strategies to Improve Transport, Metabolic, and Synthetic Functions

Section V   Additive Manufacturing-Based Tissue Engineering

Section VI   Translational Aspects of Tissue Engineering

Foreword

It is my pleasure to write the foreword for *Biomaterials and Nanotechnology for Tissue Engineering* for CRC Press. This book contains 14 chapters on the applications of nanotechnology in biomaterials and tissue engineering. This book aims to provide an overview of the rationale involved in the choice of materials for regeneration of different tissues and the future directions in this fascinating area.

This book begins by discussing nanotechnology approaches to tissue engineering. It then covers tissue engineering of connective tissue, such as regeneration of bone tissue, cartilage, and ligaments. This book continues with sections covering bioengineering of skin, and tissue engineering-based functional restoration of blood vessels. It then looks at the engineering of the liver and pancreas. From there, the interesting area of neural regeneration is discussed, followed by tissue engineering therapies for ocular regeneration, and then dental applications. This book concludes by examining image-guided tissue engineering, a discussion of tissue engineered medical products and finally looks at regulatory challenges and ethics.

In summary, *Biomaterials and Nanotechnology for Tissue Engineering* examines many timely topics and should be a useful book for scientists in these important areas.

Robert Langer
MIT

Preface

Advancements in nanotechnology have resulted in the emergence of engineered biomaterial constructs that have ushered in a new era of regenerative medicine in the healthcare sector. Search for ideal scaffold materials has become indispensable in regenerative medicine owing to variations between soft, hard, and interfacial tissues in addition to patient-specific requirements. Fine-tuning the physical, chemical, and biological properties of biomaterials can improve the scaffold performance since it is tailored to restore the diseased tissues. Customizing the properties of tissue constructs is essential for translation of these materials from lab to clinic to meet the growing demand for tissue-specific and patient-specific scaffolds. The current paradigm in the field of tissue engineering is to mimic the native extracellular matrix through patterning intricate hierarchical nano-dimensional features in microarchitecture by various approaches, thereby providing an ideal *milieu* to facilitate tissue progression. The advent of sophisticated technologies, such as rapid prototyping, has promoted tissue engineering as a viable treatment alternative for patients suffering from tissue and organ failure. This book consolidates the progress made in scaffold materials, tissue-specific strategies, fabrication approaches, and development of tissue-engineered medical products. A separate discussion on safety concerns on the use of nanostructured materials has also been included. Section I provides an overview on the various nanotechnology approaches adopted in tissue engineering. Tissue-specific strategies for regeneration of skeletal, skin, neural, ocular, vascular, pancreatic, and hepatic tissues have been detailed in Sections II, III, and IV. The various facets of laser-assisted bioprinting for tissue engineering have been discussed in Section V, while Section VI elaborates on translation of tissue-engineered commercial products for clinical use and also deals with the safety aspects of nanomaterials and the challenges involved.

Section I briefly outlines the various approaches such as self-assembly, electrospinning, and layer-by-layer techniques to fabricate biomimetic tissue scaffolds with hierarchical organization of nano–micro structures as well as nanodiagnostics and nanoscale drug delivery systems. The influence of surface nanotopography on the cell fate processes has also been elaborated in this section. Section II deals with the biomedical applications of natural and synthetic polymers toward skeletal tissue engineering. Regenerating bone tissue remains a challenge, as it requires appropriate mechanical properties with adequate porous vascularizable architecture in addition to osteoconductive, osteointegrative, and osteoinductive properties. This section also highlights various strategies to fabricate nanofibers and their applications in bone regeneration apart from a discussion on emerging technologies to address the limitations of current bone grafts. A description of ideal properties for cartilage tissue constructs, choice of biomaterials, and surface modifications employed in the design of cartilage scaffolds is also provided in Section II.

The current scenario in biomaterial-based tissue engineering on the regeneration of specific sensory tissues namely skin, nerve, and ocular has been discussed in Section III. Chapter 6 on skin regeneration discusses in-depth on the integration of mechanical, biochemical stimuli apart from use of novel materials of natural and synthetic origin with appropriate topography for functional regeneration of skin and its appendages. Emerging strategies such as stem cell therapy, mi-RNA delivery, melanocyte incorporated skin, photosynthetically activated wound healing, and skin-on-a-chip are also discussed. Injuries to the central nervous system and peripheral nervous system can lead to permanent disabilities. A detailed discussion highlighting recent advances in the use of biomaterials and nanotechnology for central nerve repair and peripheral nerve repair has been provided in Chapter 7. Application of tissue engineering principles in ophthalmology to overcome challenges such as graft rejection, infection, inflammation, and vision impairment has been the focus of Chapter 8. This chapter deals with a wide range of biomaterials for opthalmological applications and also on recent innovations in the regeneration of various ocular components such as cornea, retina, lachrymal gland, as well as replacement strategies for lens and vitreous fluid.

The progress in tissue engineering strategies for the repair and reconstruction of various functional tissues, such as blood vessels, pancreas, and liver involved in the transportation, metabolism, and synthesis, respectively, are elaborated in Chapters 9, 10, and 11, respectively. Developing vasculature using biomaterials and decellularized matrices and scaffold-free approaches such as cell sheet conduits, 3D bioprinting, as well as the clinical success of tissue-engineered blood vessels are outlined in this section. Engineering bioartificial pancreas using Islet cells and biomaterials, clinical trials, and current challenges in clinical applications has been described in Chapter 10. Chapter 11 in this section elaborates on the various therapeutic interventions, starting from conventional cell and biomaterial-based approaches, extracorporeal devices toward organogenesis for the treatment of acute and chronic liver diseases and failures.

The emergence of three-dimensional rapid prototyping of tissues and organs ensures the precise spatio-temporal positioning of biological and physical components. Section V discusses the rapidly evolving laser-assisted bioprinting field for tissue engineering that can potentially reconstruct the native system. The fundamentals of laser-induced forward transfer, underlying principles, and the materials employed have been elaborated along with descriptions of applications such as bioprinting of biomaterials, cells, DNA, peptides, and *in vivo* bioprinting with clinical implications.

Section VI discusses the progress of tissue-engineered medical products, which represents innovative technologies, materials, and treatments aiming to address unmet clinical needs—ranging from musculoskeletal applications to nerve and cardiovascular regeneration. Surgical repair, artificial prostheses, and mechanical devices considered "gold standard" treatments, however, fall short in total repair and long-term recovery from significant tissue/organ damage. Chapter 13 focuses on tissue devices being used today for bone, cartilage, tendon, skin, nerves, and tissue interfaces and also discusses the research being done to develop them for future applications.

Despite emerging as a strong alternative to current treatments, the complexity of tissues and organs introduce challenges for researchers and engineers to ensure that these products are safe and effective prior to clinical trials and commercialization. The Food and Drug Administration (FDA) evaluates the safety and effectiveness of medical products based on scientific and regulatory considerations assessed dependent on the product's characteristics, preclinical studies, and proposed clinical trials. Thus, product development is often a long-term, multidisciplinary effort in order to develop a proper scientific and technical database to ensure a product's complete safety and effectiveness. Several tissue-engineered medical products exist, addressing the repair and regeneration of various tissues such as cartilage (NeoCart®, CARTIPATCH®), tendon (Graftjacket®, X-Repair®), and bone (OP-1/BMP-7, IngeniOs HA®). Many more tissue-engineered medical products are under development, attempting to further expand the field to address larger, more serious, complex, and even total organ applications. This section also elaborates the health and safety implications of nanoparticles such as toxicological assessment techniques, nanoparticle dosing, and factors that influences the toxicity of nanoparticles such as material properties and host factors.

Advanced biomaterials and nanotechnology approaches for tissue engineering has convincingly progressed to commercialization of clinical products. The nanotechnology interventions and polymeric biomaterials for soft and hard tissues discussed in this book would provide an insight to the readers about the progress made in this field and also future challenges that need to be addressed by tissue engineers. This book covers the fundamentals and recent advances benefitting both the beginners and experts working in this field.

The editors express their gratitude to all the experts for their valuable contributions and sharing their expertise in the completion of this book.

S. Swaminathan, PhD
K. Uma Maheswari, PhD
S. Anuradha, PhD

Editors

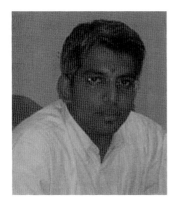

Swaminathan Sethuraman is the dean, sponsored research and director, Centre for Nanotechnology & Advanced Biomaterials (CeNTAB), School of Chemical & Biotechnology at SASTRA University, Thanjavur, Tamil Nadu, India. Dr. Sethuraman earned his PhD from the Department of Chemical Engineering at Drexel University, Philadelphia, and worked on the development of low temperature setting polymer–ceramic composite cements for bone tissue engineering. Later, he joined as a research associate in the Department of Orthopaedic Surgery at the University of Virginia, Charlottesville. He is the recipient of several awards including Innovative Young Biotechnology Award (IYBA—2006) from the Department of Biotechnology, Government of India, Material Research Society of India Medal for the year 2009 from Materials Research Society of India, and Young Career Award in Nano Science and Nanotechnology from the Department of Science and Technology, Government of India, in 2015.

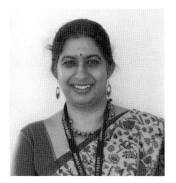

Uma Maheswari Krishnan is currently the associate dean in the School of Chemical and Biotechnology, SASTRA University, Thanjavur, Tamil Nadu, India, and Deakin Indo-Australian Chair professor. She earned her PhD in applied chemistry from Bharathiyar University, Tamil Nadu, India. Prior to research training from University of Arkansas, in 2005, she was a postdoctoral fellow at the University of Texas, in 2002. Dr. Krishnan's research interests are drug delivery, gene delivery, tissue engineering, and biosensors.

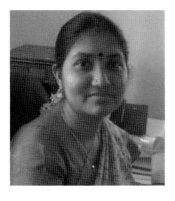

Anuradha Subramanian is an assistant professor—Research, at the Centre for Nanotechnology & Advanced Biomaterials (CeNTAB), School of Chemical and Biotechnology, SASTRA University, Thanjavur, Tamil Nadu, India. Her PhD work was on development of novel 3D nanofibrous scaffolds for neural regeneration and earned her degree from the School of Chemical and Biotechnology, SASTRA University, Thanjavur, Tamil Nadu, India. Dr. Subramanian's research interests include tissue engineering, theranostics, self-assembled nano-structures, and 3D bioprinting.

Contributors

Olajide Abiola
Institute for Regenerative Engineering
Raymond and Beverly Sackler Center for
    Biomedical, Biological, Physical and
    Engineering Sciences
Department of Orthopaedic Surgery
The University of Connecticut Health Center
Farmington, Connecticut

Joëlle Amédée-Vilamitjana
Institut National de la Sante et de la
    Recherche Medicale (INSERM)
Bioingénierie Tissulaire
Université Bordeaux
Bordeaux, France

Nandana Bhardwaj
Life Science Division
Institute of Advanced Study in Science
    and Technology (IASST)
Assam, India

Bibhas Kumar Bhunia
Department of Bioscience and
    Bioengineering
Indian Institute of Technology Guwahati
    (IITG)
Assam, India

Jean-Michel Bourget
Institut National de la Sante et de la
    Recherche Medicale (INSERM)
Bioingénierie Tissulaire
Université Bordeaux
Bordeaux, France

Sylvain Catros
Institut National de la Sante et de la
    Recherche Medicale (INSERM)
Bioingénierie Tissulaire
Université Bordeaux
Bordeaux, France

Wei Chang
Department of Chemistry, Chemical
    Biology, and Biomedical Engineering
Stevens Institute of Technology
Hoboken, New Jersey

Kaushik Chatterjee
Department of Materials Engineering
Indian Institute of Science
Karnataka, India

Clancy J. Clark
Department of Surgery, Wake Forest
    University School of Medicine
Wake Forest School of Medicine
Winston-Salem, North Carolina

Hélène Desrus
Institut National de la Sante et de la
    Recherche Medicale (INSERM)
Bioingénierie Tissulaire
Université Bordeaux
Bordeaux, France

Raphaël Devillard
Institut National de la Sante et de la
    Recherche Medicale (INSERM)
Bioingénierie Tissulaire
Université Bordeaux
Bordeaux, France

Amit Dinda
Department of Pharmacology
All India Institute of Medical Sciences
New Delhi, India

Joseph W. Freeman
Department of Biomedical Engineering
Rutgers University
Piscataway, New Jersey

Jean-Christophe Fricain
Institut National de la Sante et de la
    Recherche Medicale (INSERM)
Bioingénierie Tissulaire
Université Bordeaux
Bordeaux, France

Y. K. Gupta
Department of Pharmacology
All India Institute of Medical
    Sciences
New Delhi, India

Jérôme Kalisky
Institut National de la Sante et de la
    Recherche Medicale (INSERM)
Bioingénierie Tissulaire
Université Bordeaux
Bordeaux, France

Matthew Kandl
Department of Chemistry, Chemical
    Biology, and Biomedical
    Engineering
Stevens Institute of Technology
Hoboken, New Jersey

Olivia Kérourédan
Institut National de la Sante et de la
    Recherche Medicale (INSERM)
Bioingénierie Tissulaire
Université Bordeaux
Bordeaux, France

Karen Kong
Department of Chemistry, Chemical
    Biology, and Biomedical
    Engineering
Stevens Institute of Technology
Hoboken, New Jersey

Uma Maheswari Krishnan
Centre for Nanotechnology & Advanced
    Biomaterials (CeNTAB)
School of Chemical and Biotechnology
    (SCBT)
SASTRA University
Tamil Nadu, India

Jadi Praveen Kumar
Department of Bioscience and
    Bioengineering
Indian Institute of Technology Guwahati
    (IITG)
Assam, India

Sachin Kumar
Department of Materials Engineering
Indian Institute of Science
Karnataka, India

Sangamesh G. Kumbar
Institute for Regenerative Engineering
Raymond and Beverly Sackler Center for
    Biomedical, Biological, Physical and
    Engineering Sciences
Department of Orthopaedic Surgery
The University of Connecticut Health
    Center
Farmington, Connecticut

and

Department of Biomedical Engineering
University of Connecticut
Storrs, Connecticut

Cato T. Laurencin
Institute for Regenerative Engineering
Raymond and Beverly Sackler Center for
    Biomedical, Biological, Physical and
    Engineering Sciences
Department of Orthopaedic Surgery
and
Department of Reconstructive Sciences
The University of Connecticut Health
    Center
Farmington, Connecticut

and

Department of Chemical and Biomolecular
    Engineering
and
Department of Biomedical Engineering,
    Department of Materials Science and
    Engineering
University of Connecticut
Storrs, Connecticut

Paul Lee
Department of Chemistry, Chemical
  Biology, and Biomedical
  Engineering
Stevens Institute of Technology
Hoboken, New Jersey

Biman B. Mandal
Department of Bioscience and
  Bioengineering
Indian Institute of Technology Guwahati
  (IITG)
Assam, India

Ohan S. Manoukian
Institute for Regenerative Engineering
Raymond and Beverly Sackler Center for
  Biomedical, Biological, Physical and
  Engineering Sciences
Department of Orthopaedic Surgery
The University of Connecticut Health
  Center
Farmington, Connecticut

and

Department of Biomedical
  Engineering
University of Connecticut
Storrs, Connecticut

Shreya Mehrotra
Department of Bioscience and
  Bioengineering
Indian Institute of Technology Guwahati
  (IITG)
Assam, India

Sai Rama Krishna Meka
Department of Materials Engineering
Indian Institute of Science
Karnataka, India

Prabha D. Nair
Division of Tissue Engineering and
  Regeneration Technologies
Biomedical Technology Wing
Sree Chitra Tirunal Institute for Medical
  Sciences and Technology
Kerala, India

Jonathan Nip
Institute for Regenerative
  Engineering
Raymond and Beverly Sackler Center for
  Biomedical, Biological, Physical and
  Engineering Sciences
Department of Orthopaedic Surgery
The University of Connecticut Health
  Center
Farmington, Connecticut

Emmanuel C. Opara
Wake Forest Institute for Regenerative
  Medicine
Virginia Tech-Wake Forest School of
  Biomedical Engineering & Sciences
Wake Forest School of Medicine
Winston-Salem, North Carolina

Janani Radhakrishnan
Centre for Nanotechnology & Advanced
  Biomaterials (CeNTAB)
School of Chemical and Biotechnology
  (SCBT)
SASTRA University
Tamil Nadu, India

Rahul V. G.
Division of Tissue Engineering and
  Regeneration Technologies
Biomedical Technology Wing
Sree Chitra Tirunal Institute for Medical
  Sciences and Technology
Kerala, India

Murielle Rémy
Institut National de la Sante et de la
  Recherche Medicale (INSERM)
Bioingénierie Tissulaire
Université Bordeaux
Bordeaux, France

Rachel Rosa
Department of Chemistry, Chemical
  Biology, and Biomedical
  Engineering
Stevens Institute of Technology
Hoboken, New Jersey

Swaminathan Sethuraman
Centre for Nanotechnology & Advanced
  Biomaterials (CeNTAB)
School of Chemical and Biotechnology
  (SCBT)
SASTRA University
Tamil Nadu, India

Munish Shah
Department of Chemistry, Chemical
  Biology, and Biomedical
  Engineering
Stevens Institute of Technology
Hoboken, New Jersey

Yogendra Pratap Singh
Department of Bioscience and
  Bioengineering
Indian Institute of Technology Guwahati
  (IITG)
Assam, India

Kevin J. Smith
Department of Biomedical
  Engineering
University of Connecticut
Storrs, Connecticut

Anuradha Subramanian
Centre for Nanotechnology & Advanced
  Biomaterials (CeNTAB)
School of Chemical and Biotechnology
  (SCBT)
SASTRA University
Tamil Nadu, India

Brittany L. Taylor
Department of Biomedical Engineering
Rutgers University
Piscataway, New Jersey

Varadraj N. Vernekar
Institute for Regenerative Engineering
Raymond and Beverly Sackler Center for
  Biomedical Biological, Physical and
  Engineering Sciences
Department of Orthopaedic Surgery
The University of Connecticut Health Center
Farmington, Connecticut

Xiaojun Yu
Department of Chemistry, Chemical
  Biology, and Biomedical Engineering
Stevens Institute of Technology
Hoboken, New Jersey

Section I

Introduction

1

Nanotechnology Approaches to Regenerative Engineering

Varadraj N. Vernekar, Kevin J. Smith, and Cato T. Laurencin

CONTENTS

1.1 Introduction and Background

The deficit in organ and tissue donation is a significant unmet healthcare need worldwide. In the United States itself, the organ waiting lists have swelled disproportionately in comparison to the increase in the number of transplants (U.S. Department of Health and Human Services, 2015). Due to the acute shortage of donor organs, many die while on the waiting list. Currently, typical treatments for replacement of damaged or lost tissue are the use of autografts and allografts (Dlaska et al., 2015). Whereas these two options perform fairly well, allografts carry the risk of infections, and autografts have issues with availability and donor morbidity. To supplant these approaches, the field of biomaterials has explored alternative materials and methods to repair damaged or diseased tissue (Ratner et al., 2013). Advances in chemistry have enabled the use of metals, ceramics, and polymers, which can be tailored for specific mechanical, biological, and chemical properties; however, these options still have problems associated with foreign body response and imperfect integration into the body. These challenges associated with first-generation biomaterials have led to the generation of intelligent or stealth biomaterials that are not easily detected by the bodies' immune system or isolated by fibrous capsules. Notwithstanding these advances in biomaterials, we have still not been able to provide seamless tissue and organ replacement to effectively meet the outstanding worldwide demand. Toward that end, tissue engineering started about 30 years ago as an alternative approach to achieve replacement of damaged tissues and organs (Skalak and Fox, 1988; Nerem, 1991; Langer and Vacanti, 1993).

On the basis of the toolkits and knowledge base available from the mid-1980s, different definitions of tissue engineering have been seen. The following, perhaps, captures the main idea of tissue engineering from that time: tissue engineering is an interdisciplinary field utilizing knowledge of engineering, materials science, and the life sciences to generate structural components that can be used as biological substitutes that replace, restore, maintain, or improve damaged tissues and organs function (Langer and Vacanti, 1993). Laurencin further defined it as "the application of biological, chemical and engineering principals toward the repair, restoration, or regeneration of living tissue using biomaterials, cells, and factors alone or in combination" (Laurencin et al., 1999, p. 21). Historically, tissue engineering approaches have been categorized into three distinct classes: isolated cells, tissue-inductive materials, and cell-loaded matrices (Langer and Vacanti, 1993). The delivery of isolated cells is appealing due to its simplicity, but suffers from low cellular retention rates and is insufficient for large-scale defects. The use of tissue-inducing materials is a more promising option that encompasses aspects of controlled drug release from the biomaterial. Nevertheless, cell-loaded matrices of natural, synthetic, or composite materials are the most comprehensive and robust platform that can include the benefits of both the previous approaches and more. The objective is for the scaffold matrices to provide a physiologically relevant microenvironment to the cells seeded within them, with eventual resorption of these matrices as they get replaced by the extracellular matrix (ECM) produced by the cells. The idea underlying tissue engineering is that the scaffold-seeded cells can spontaneously reassemble into organotypic/tissue-mimetic structures, given instructive guidance and support via appropriate scaffold material, bioactive factors, and external physical stimulation, usually in some combination. Several bioresorbable materials such as poly(lactic-*co*-glycolic acid) (PLGA), spurred initially by the development of resorbable sutures, and subsequently by controlled drug release platforms have emerged as excellent candidates for this purpose, and have received FDA approval (Lee and Mooney, 2001).

Although material scientists tend to specify the 1–100 nm as the realm of nanotechnology (Nalwa, 1999; Sobolev, 2015), the size range of bioactive features that influence cellular behavior is actually in the nanometer–micrometer range. Therefore, we refer to nanotechnology as the process of manipulating components at the nanoscale in the 1 to <1000 nm (submicron range). Nanotechnology is distinguished from chemistry by its focus on nanoscale physical structures that present chemical functions rather than the chemistry itself. Nanotechnology is engaged with the processes for manufacturing and manipulating properties at the nanoscale. Nanofabrication techniques can create precise physical structures or mimic biological structures that in combination with their chemical and mechanical properties can influence specific properties of cells. Materials used to synthesize nanostructures include proteins, polymers, dendrimers, fullerenes and other carbon-based structures, lipid–water micelles, viral capsids, metals, metal oxides, and ceramics. Some target structures that nanotechnology seeks to mimic include ECM components; growth factors; signaling molecules; and subcellular organelle components such as ribosomes, proteasomes, ion channels, and transport vesicles. Using nanotechnology, biomimetic physical correlates of these entities such as monolayers, micelles, particles, fibers, and scaffolds can be fabricated with uniformity and specificity. In turn, these nanoscale features with unique and defined characteristics such as pore size, porosity, tortuosity, biocompatibility, biodegradability, and mechanical properties, can influence higher-level functions in tissue regeneration.

1.2 Tissue Engineering

Tissue engineering is a rapidly developing interdisciplinary field that seeks to repair, restore, replace, or enhance biological tissue and organs. It integrates biology, chemistry, material science, and engineering. Tissue engineering approaches are based on the principle that by incorporating biocompatible scaffolds containing specific tissue-mimetic extracellular structures, appropriate cell types, and the necessary tissue-specific signaling, trophic, and vascularization cues the cells will be maintained and regulated to spontaneously organize into higher-order functional tissues and even whole organs.

When the field of tissue engineering was emerging, the available knowledge and toolkits were not as developed and expansive as we see now. For example, material science was applied to tissue engineering, but the use of nanotechnology in tissue regeneration was not yet realized. With the insight that, beyond the microarchitecture, it is the integral nanoarchitecture and topography of the ECM that influences local cellular behavior by supporting a host of cell–ECM, cell–cell, and cell–soluble factor interactions (Taipale and Keski-Oja, 1997) there has been a consistent shift in focus from the micro- to the nanoscale. For example, with the understanding that the cellular niche is essentially a natural web of hierarchically organized nanofibers of structural proteins such as collagen and elastin, cell adhesive proteins such as laminin and fibronectin, and fillers such as the brush-like glycosaminoglycans (GAGs), the design of ECM mimicking scaffolds has shifted focus from the macro-, to the micro-, to the nanoscale, over the years.

Tissue engineering has faced the following challenges: (1) the generated scaffold platform must provide a conducive biocompatible environment for the assembly and housing of cells by promoting cell adhesion, viability, growth, proliferation, differentiation, morphogenesis, and integration; (2) engineered tissue must address wound healing; and (3) the engineered tissue is vascularized for long-term maintenance, and, if necessary, innervation. For true biomimetic tissue formation, all three of these challenges must be addressed and the new engineered tissue must fully (structurally and functionally) integrate into the body. Progress in the fulfillment of these goals has led to applications in skin (Supp and Boyce, 2005), cartilage (Freed et al., 1997), bladder (Oberpenning et al., 1999), bone (Thesleff et al., 2011), cornea (Shah et al., 2008), and blood vessels (L'heureux et al., 1998), but we have still not seen as many regulatory authority-cleared commercially available tissue-engineered products in the market. Furthermore, the third challenge is still significantly unmet, and; therefore, the early developments have been in tissues that are either poorly vascularized natively or show very high-intrinsic regenerative potential. Perhaps, the incorporation of techniques and knowledge from the rising fields of nanotechnology, stem cell science, and developmental biology need to be incorporated into the shifting paradigm of tissue regeneration to overcome the challenges that traditional tissue engineering has faced so far.

1.3 Regenerative Engineering

Advances in materials science have allowed us to harness nanotechnology as a tool for engineering tissues, which was not the case when the field of tissue engineering began roughly 30 years ago. Alongside our deepening understanding of biology, our understanding of biological chemistry has advanced to the point that in many cases we now precisely understand the molecular level interactions governing cellular behavior. We have realized that static and dynamic cues from the extracellular space are, in fact, key to influencing cellular behavior in a spatiotemporal manner, and therefore, can assist in the larger goal of tissue regeneration. Multiple signaling pathways are transmitted from the extracellular environment at the nanoscale via different transducing agents through the cell membrane, cytoskeleton, organelles, and cytosol, to the cell nucleus, eventually resulting in the production of new proteins. In turn, these generated proteins determine cellular destiny. Likewise, with advances in chemistry and processing techniques, materials science has developed in precision from the millimeter, to the micrometer, to the nanometer range at the molecular level itself, giving birth to the field of nanotechnology. Since we now know that nanoscale cues determine the behavior of cells and thereby control their destiny, nanotechnology holds tremendous potential in the manipulation of cellular behavior for engineering tissue regeneration.

Over the last 15 years, we now have a deeper understanding of both adult and embryonic stem cells, and have even developed induced pluripotent stem cells, developing new knowledge about tissue genesis from stem cells and related effective tools in our toolkit to regenerate tissue. Furthermore, although we have barely scratched the surface, our understanding of the developmental biology of limb regeneration in the salamander and the newt has brought new insights into the process of wound repair and regeneration.

With these new developments in mind, the shifting paradigm of tissue engineering can be more accurately described as "regenerative engineering" (Laurencin and Khan, 2013). Laurencin recently defined this new field as the integration of tissue engineering with advanced material science, stem cell science, and areas of developmental biology for the regeneration of complex tissues, organs, and organ systems (Reichert et al., 2011). Whereas tissue engineering brought together the fields of engineering and science in general, regenerative engineering will specifically converge the fields of tissue engineering, advance materials, stem cell science, and developmental biology toward the goal of tissue regeneration.

1.3.1 Nanotechnology Applications in Regenerative Engineering

Nanotechnology is enabling medicine through advances in diagnostics and therapeutics, biomaterials and drug delivery, and regenerative engineering. Cellular and tissue environments usually have individual components in the five to several hundreds of nanometers in size range. It envisages that these individual nanocomponents when combined, sort of like a "lego" puzzle following specific "rules," into a superstructure along with cells will give rise to tissues with unique properties. Advances in nanotechnology have started to fill this nanoscale design need in tissue engineering by enabling the fabrication of nanoarchitectural structural mimics of the ECM, the creation of nanotopographical surfaces, and nanoencapsulated drug release systems with high spatiotemporal control (Goldberg et al., 2007). Although these embodiments are pushing the boundaries at controlling and instructing cellular behavior, the challenge still remains in augmenting the properties of these structural mimics with the essential functional complexity of the composite material that is the ECM, toward truly emulating it, and successfully regenerating tissues and organs. In the following subsections we discuss some of the applications of nanotechnology in regenerative engineering toward addressing these challenges.

1.3.1.1 Nanofabricated Topography

ECM structural features such as fibers and pores, with characteristic dimensions in the length-scale of cellular protrusions, may influence contact guidance mechanisms by which cells migrate through three-dimensional (3D) extracellular environments (Abraham et al., 1999; Lutolf and Hubbell, 2005). As a first step to assess the influence of nanoscale environments in controlling cell function and fate, cell-contacting substrates have been engineered to present different nanoscale topographies through a combination of geometry and patterns (Shi et al., 2010). For example, applying lithographic techniques, nanopatterns such as grooves, posts, and pits can be created (Norman and Desai, 2006; Bettinger et al., 2009). Likewise, micelle lithography, anodization, and electrospinning methods can be applied to fabricate nanoscale spheres, tubes, and fibers (Xu et al., 2004; Park et al., 2007; Huang et al., 2009). Furthermore, polymer demixing, phase separation, electrospinning, colloidal lithography, chemical etching, self-assembly methods can be applied to fabricate unordered nanotopographies (Norman and Desai, 2006). Using these different nanotopographies different cellular processes such as cell morphological changes (Xu et al., 2004; Yim et al., 2007; Kim et al., 2010), alignment (Xu et al., 2004; Yim et al., 2007; Kim et al., 2010), signaling (Ranzinger et al., 2009; Kim et al., 2010), adhesion (Xu et al., 2004; Yim et al., 2007; Kim et al., 2010), migration (Xu et al., 2004), proliferation (Yim et al., 2007), and differentiation (Dalby et al., 2007; Yim et al., 2007; Oh et al., 2009) can be manipulated. Furthermore, instructive biorecognition can be provided to the different nanotopographies through the incorporation of bioactive ECM molecules such as collagen-I, III, IV, laminin, fibronectin; bioactive peptides such as RGD (oligopeptide arginine–glycine–aspartic acid), IKVAV (oligopeptide isoleucine–lysine–valine–alanine–valine), and YIGSR (oligo peptide tyrosine–isoleucine–glycine–serine–arginine); and growth factors by using various surface modification techniques (Kumar, 2005). Our emerging understanding of how cells respond to different nanofeatures in their immediate vicinity will determine future combinations of nanotopography and cell types to achieve desirable outcomes in regenerative engineering.

1.3.1.2 Nanofabricated Scaffolds

Simultaneously as our understanding of cell–nanotopography interactions has advanced, so has the development of 3D nanofeatured scaffolds for housing the cells. The basic feature of 3D nanoscaled scaffolds—the nanofiber—seeks to mimic the physical structure of protein nanofibers in the ECM. The high surface area to volume ratio, porosity, and spatial interconnectivity that all types of nanofibrous structures present can promote tissue regeneration by maximizing cell–ECM interactions; the transport of trophic factors, oxygen, nutrients, carbon dioxide, and waste; cell migration; and vascularization.

The primary methods to fabricate nanofibrous structures are electrospinning, which creates both aligned and randomly distributed fibers; self-assembly, which perhaps most closely emulates natural ECM nanofibrous assembly; and phase transition, which allows for the fabrication of sponge-like structures out of a fibrous network (Shi et al., 2010). These techniques use different types of polymeric, nanocomposite, and carbon nanotube-based materials (Murugan and Ramakrishna, 2005; Edwards et al., 2009).

Due of the close connection between the cellular cytoskeleton and the ECM via different types of junctions and ligand–receptor interactions, cells can sense and respond particularly to the mechanical properties of their environment. Consequently, beyond the biochemical properties, the biophysical properties of the ECM exert a major influence on various cellular functions such as adhesion, migration, proliferation, development, and differentiation. Therefore, control over cell-housing scaffolding structure properties is important. Of particular importance are the properties of surface chemistry, topography, and mechanical properties. Surface chemistry entails surface functionality, charge, hydrophobicity, hydrophilicity, and adhesiveness. Topography entails features size, aspect ratio, geometry, spacing, roughness, porosity, and tortuosity. Finally, mechanical properties include properties such as elasticity, fatigue strength, etc. Nanotechnology can be used to tune all of these properties. For example, by fine tuning the elasticity of a matrix used to house cells the differentiation of stem cells to different lineages was demonstrated (Engler et al., 2006). Manipulating such properties can enable implants to be seeded with cell precursors that will naturally develop into the desired cells and tissues over time, which is of particular relevance when using stem cells in regenerative engineering.

Toward incorporating multiple desirable properties into scaffolds, Burdick and coworkers recently developed a nanofibrous hydrogel that uses spatially patterned chemical cues to create selective cell development patterns within a scaffold (Wade et al., 2015). This sort of nanoscale control is enticing because it provides a methodology to selectively influence different types of cells including stem cells within a single scaffold based on their location in the scaffold. Some of the prominent nanofabrication techniques used for regenerative engineering applications are discussed next.

1. *Self-Assembly*: Molecular self-assembly approaches the engineering of tissue scaffolding materials by emulating natural ECM both structurally and functionally and promoting cell–matrix interactions. Spontaneous self-assemblies of amphiphilic peptides results from the additive action of weak and noncovalent interactions of individual nanofibrous components to generate higher-order structures such as tubules, micelles, and gels, all of which can be used as structural components to build ECM-like scaffolds (Zhang and Zhao, 2004). These peptidal assemblies can have fiber diameters as small as 10 nm, and scaffold pore sizes between 5 and 200 nm, significantly smaller than those produced by electrospinning (Zhang, 2003). 3D interwoven nanofiber-based hydrogels formed using self-assembling peptides such as the RADA (oligo peptide with repeating sequence arginine–alanine–aspartic acid–alanine) peptides offer an elegant solution as an injectable drug delivery and regenerative engineering system (Koutsopoulos and Zhang, 2012). Other widely investigated ECM-derived self-assembling polypeptides used to synthesize injectable hydrogel scaffolds include elastin- and collagen-based proteins, as well as fibrin and silk proteins. The advantage of using the hydrogel approach is that the delivery of the cell-loaded scaffold can be done minimally invasively into irregularly shaped wound sites that they can eventually conform to and set upon phase transition. Moreover, these hydrogel scaffolds can shorten operating times, minimize postoperative pain and scar tissue, potentially reducing cost. Furthermore, these self-assembling peptides show good biocompatibility, minimal immune responses, degrade into amino acids that are readily metabolized *in vivo*, and therefore, provide a resorbable scaffold that is advantageous for both drug delivery and regenerative engineering applications (Koutsopoulos and Zhang, 2012).

2. *Electrospinning*: Although the first patent on electrospinning was granted over 80 years ago, application of this technique to regenerative engineering has increased dramatically only in the last 15 years since the pioneering work by Laurencin and coworkers (Li et al., 2002; Laurencin and Ko, 2004). Electrospinning is the extraction of polymeric nanofibers from an evaporating polymeric solution emanating from a needle jet under a high-voltage electrical field that leads to the deposition of ECM-like nanofibrous structures on a target electrode plate. Electrospinning produces nonwoven nanofibrous meshes that exhibit physical structures similar to that of the fibrous protein-based architecture in native ECM. Although the diameters of the

electrospun fibers are usually at the upper limits of the 50–500 nm range that is seen in natural ECM, by tuning the various fabrication process parameters, physical properties such as average fiber diameter, pore size, tensile strength, and drug-release characteristics of these nanofibrous meshes can be optimized for specific design goals (Goldberg et al., 2007). One of the challenges that all scaffold designs face, particularly electrospun fibrous scaffolds, is control over uniformly seeding adequate number of cells into the scaffold. Recent developments include a methodology to incorporate cells within electrospun scaffolds that typically exhibit poor cell infiltration capabilities; thus, providing a solution to this problem (Sampson et al., 2014). Likewise, polymeric electrospun nanofibers intrinsically lack biochemical recognition cues; therefore, they require the immobilization of tissue-conducive cell-responsive domains (Kim and Mooney, 1998; Lutolf and Hubbell, 2005).

3. *Layer-by-Layer (LBL) Fabrication*: LBL fabrication is a method that produces electrostatically stabilized multiple polyelectrolyte layers with nanometer scale precision. This nanofabrication method is advantageous for its tunability, drug delivery properties, and biocompatibility. The use of LBL coatings can assist in mitigating an immune response and facilitate wound healing through drug delivery (Tang et al., 2006). Self-degradable polyelectrolytes such as polyglutamic acid have been used to generate degradable LBL materials that are independent of qualifying factors such as enzymatic degradation, ionic strength, or electrical stimulation (Tang et al., 2006). Such LBL deposition methods can also be used to fine tune the surface properties of polymeric scaffolds fabricated by other methods (Hammond, 2004).

4. *Bioanalyte-Sensitive Polymeric Hydrogel Synthesis*: This method is more linker-chemistry than nanotechnology; however, we have included it as it provides nanoscale control for both regenerative engineering and drug delivery applications in regenerative engineering. A wide variety of biohybrid hydrogels has been developed for these applications. These include the incorporation into the hydrogels of highly specific and high-affinity proteins and peptides that are enzymatically cleavable, serve as cell adhesion molecules, or get released as signals to trigger a biological process, which is key for the success of the engineered scaffold tissue such as vascularization (Mann et al., 2001; Burdick and Anseth, 2002; Lutolf and Hubbell, 2005; Phelps et al., 2010). A popular base polymer used for such hydrogel synthesis, followed by specific bioanalyte "decoration," is polyethylene glycol (PEG), known for its high hydrophilicity, very low protein adsorption, and general bioinert "stealth" characteristics.

1.3.1.3 Nanoscale Drug Delivery

Localized delivery of multiple factors, controlled for parameters such as release rate, sequence, pattern, period, bioavailability, pharmacodynamics, and cell-specific targeting within 3D scaffolds is key to dynamically instructing cells toward tissue regeneration in a highly controlled manner (Richardson et al., 2001). This level of control is achieved by controlling the size and geometry of drug carriers using nanotechnology. An outstanding challenge for the long-term viability of tissue-engineered scaffolds is vascularization, which is necessary for the transport of key nutrients and oxygen and removal of wastes. It is well known that the release of angiogenic and vasculogenic factors such as vascular endothelial growth factor can promote vascularization. However, indiscriminate release of angiogenic factors is associated with multiple risks factors; therefore, the release has to be controlled, localized, and sustained over a specified period. Likewise, specific considerations apply to biologically instructive factors other than growth factors, such as proteins, nucleic acids, deoxyribonucleic acid (DNA), small-interfering ribonucleic acid (siRNA), aptamers, etc., which need to be released into engineered scaffolds as well, depending on the application.

To achieve controlled release, several fabrication approaches have been investigated such as the encapsulation of these biological factors by physical blending or chemical conjugation offering different levels of success (Thanou and Duncan, 2003; Jiang et al., 2004). Nanofabrication provides an addition to this toolkit to fine tune drug release characteristics (Zhang and Uludağ, 2009). Polymeric nanoparticle-based drug delivery is one of the well-researched subcategories for drug delivery due to the high level of control over polymers and the ease of fabrication. Other nanosystems that can be employed for drug delivery in regenerative engineering include lipid–water micelles, dendrimer, fullerenes and other carbon-based structures, and inorganic nanomaterials. Some of these nanocarriers enable coencapsulation of multiple drugs and control individual agent release in a temporal fashion (Sengupta et al., 2005). Others enable triggering of drug release in response to environmental stimuli such as pH, temperature, light, drugs, etc. (Caldorera-Moore and Peppas, 2009); these type of "intelligent" systems can be designed to specifically sense and respond directly to pathophysiological conditions. Tuning the nanofabrication process parameters, material formulations, drug loading, biocompatibility, and degradation characteristics can help achieve the desired localized delivery of multiple factors that are controlled for key release parameters within 3D scaffolds.

More drug candidates for regenerative engineering beyond growth factors and nucleic acids include hormones, secondary messenger molecules, adhesion molecules, chemokines, cytokines, small molecule drugs, etc. The application of nanotechnology to several of these candidates has extended the drug half-life *in vivo*; improved hydrophobic drug solubility; selectively sequestered, controlled, and tuned simultaneous hydrophilic and hydrophilic drug release; and reduced potential immunogenicity, drug toxicity, administration frequency, etc. For example, biological molecules can be conjugated with PEG to form PEGylated molecules, which improve their stability and retention times *in vivo*, in addition to providing them with "stealth" properties avoiding activating the immune system (Veronese and Mero, 2008). Nanoscale drug delivery methods can be subdivided into four primary categories (Hughes, 2005).

1. *Polymeric Nanoparticle-Based*: This type of drug delivery can be conducted with a number of different polymers allowing greater control over material and release properties. Polymeric nanoparticles can be synthesized from a variety of polymers such as polyesters, polyethers, polyphosphazenes that offer excellent control of properties such as release rate, degradation rate, etc. (Ma, 2008). One such application includes the use of PLGA to form nanoparticles densely loaded with siRNA for sustained gene silencing (Woodrow et al., 2009), which has applications in the coordinated steps of cell transformation in regenerative engineering.

2. *Carbon Based*: This type of drug delivery employs higher-order structures of carbon such as carbon nanotubes and fullerenes, which are readily internalized into cells because of their very small size, and therefore, provide an efficacious platform for drug delivery. Furthermore, carbon nanotubes provide very high aspect ratio and surface area for functionalization with small molecules or proteins-based drugs. Beyond drug delivery, carbon nanotubes is an important regenerative engineering nanomaterial that can be applied to diagnostics (cell tracking and sensing microenvironments), delivering transfection agents, and creating tissue structural

scaffolding with novel properties such as electrical conductivity that may aid in directing cell outcome (Harrison and Atala, 2007). However, concerns about the long-term biocompatibility of these nonbiodegradable carbon-based nanomaterials, related to oxidative stress, inflammation, and genetic damage, have not been fully addressed in a systematic manner (Kunzmann et al., 2011; Novoselov et al., 2012).

3. *Metal Based*: This type of drug delivery is through hollow metal nanoshell particles. Such group of nanoparticles can be particularly useful if they also carry distinctive magnetic properties and other tunable characteristics. Advances in fabrication techniques of metallic nanoparticles enable the attachment of various ligands or coatings to the generated nanoparticles. These ligands or coatings can serve many purposes, such as protective coatings to prevent degradation, barrier coatings to mitigate immune response, therapeutic drugs for drug delivery, and fluorophores for ease of imaging (Sun et al., 2008).

4. *Nanofiber Based*: Drug delivery can also be achieved from drug-loaded nanofibers prepared by electrospinning or self-assembly techniques (Sun et al., 2003; Hosseinkhani et al., 2006). The subsequent drug release from nanofiber-based drug delivery scaffolds can be tuned to obtain a linear release rate, ideal for therapeutic applications, by the use of nanofibers with core–shell structures with internally core-loaded drugs (Sun et al., 2003). The drug release kinetics can be further fine tuned by changing the porosity and thickness of the nanofiber shell.

1.3.1.4 Nanodiagnostics

Nanotechnology has provided alternative approaches such as magnetic nanoparticles (Riehemann et al., 2009), quantum dots (Dubertret et al., 2002), gold nanoparticles (Chanda et al., 2010), and carbon nanotubes (De La Zerda et al., 2008) to track cell fate in engineered scaffolds and monitor the progress of tissue formation in a noninvasive manner *in vivo*. Cell tracking *in vivo* is important; for example, in the delivery of stem cells through an engineered scaffold it is important to verify that the stem cells target the desired area and verify the therapeutic effects attributed to the stem cells.

By using internalized superparamagnetic iron oxide (SPIO) nanoparticles, researchers can track the commonly used mesenchymal stem cells (MSCs). The magnetic nanoparticles are then imaged using magnetic resonance imaging (MRI), providing information about the placement of individual cells. This is useful for determining migration of cells, penetration into a scaffold, and other vital outcomes in tissue-engineered solutions.

A second stem cell labeling method that utilizes nanotechnology is quantum dot labeling. Quantum dots are nanocrystals with tunable excitation and emission properties. Quantum dots are internalized in stem cells through peptides, such as RGD, TAT (oligo peptide glycine–arginine–lysine–lysine–arginine–arginine–glutamine–arginine–arginine–arginine–proline–glutamine), or cholera toxin (Chen et al., 2014). The use of quantum dots is advantageous because the optical imaging that is used for detection is both more widespread and less expensive than MRI imaging used for the SPIO nanoparticles (Engler et al., 2006).

Furthermore, nanotechnology applications in diagnostics can be combined with therapeutic drug delivery in a site-specific fashion; this has led to the emerging field of theranostics (Debbage and Jaschke, 2008). This technology enables the examination of the site of drug delivery to inform the commensurate and simultaneous release of drugs, and can help in ensuring effective coordination of the various engineered regenerative steps in a well-orchestrated manner.

1.4 Concluding Remarks

Regenerative engineering aims at true recreation of biological tissues. Nanotechnology is the process of manipulating components at the nanoscale. The potential for the use of nanotechnology in regenerative engineering and related drug delivery and diagnostics applications is currently under extensive investigation. There are several exciting possibilities such as the combination of nanotechnologies with other technologies to potentiate outcomes that cannot be accomplished by any individual technology alone. For example, the incorporation of nanostructures into microfabricated engineered scaffolds could enable better control of cell function via cell–nanotopography interactions (Dvir et al., 2011).

Yet, the unique structural organization, biochemical composition, and viscoelastic characteristics of different tissue-types present nontrivial challenges for their regeneration using a "one-design-fits-all" approach. Furthermore, there will be hurdles to cross before clinical translation of these emerging complex scaffolds technologies; for example, long-term biocompatibility and biodegradation, industrialized fabrication and processing, sterilization procedures without affecting the nanomicrostructures and compromising the activity of the proteins therein, controlled and uniform cell seeding within these scaffolds and subsequent bioreactor processing, and the entire clinical logistics involved would need to be figured out on a case-by-case basis. The complexity of the task to accurately recapitulate the spatial and temporal components of the extracellular environment, from the micro- and nanoscale structure of ECM to the presentation of cell adhesion molecules, growth factors, and cytokines, is a major challenge faced by regenerative engineering.

As our understanding of the nanoscale structural, compositional, and mechanical rules of hierarchical organization of tissues and organs and the cell–material interface from the molecular to the macroscale advances, advancing nanotechnology will push the field of biomaterials toward the rational design and development of complex and smart materials that will interact with cells in unprecedented ways and be instructive in directing tissue regeneration. For example, nanotechnological tools for guiding cells in a controlled manner to desired locations within advanced engineered scaffolds will be useful for engineering complex multicellular tissues.

Many other interesting areas also stand to benefit from these development at the intersection of nanotechnology and regenerative engineering such as biomaterials- (Bae et al. 2014), organ-on-a-chip- (Huh et al., 2010), cell sheet- (Elloumi-Hannachi et al., 2010), and stem cell- (Liu et al., 2015) engineering. The cumulative achievement of these endeavors will impact not only regenerative medicine, but other fields in medicine and beyond as well.

References

Abraham, V.C., Krishnamurthi, V., Taylor, D.L., Lanni, F. 1999. The actin-based nanomachine at the leading edge of migrating cells. *Biophys J.* 77: 1721–1732.

Bae, H., Chu, H., Edalat, F. et al. 2014. Development of functional biomaterials with micro- and nanoscale technologies for tissue engineering and drug delivery applications. *J Tissue Eng Regen Med.* 8: 1–14.

Bettinger, C.J., Langer, R., Borenstein, J.T. 2009. Engineering substrate topography at the micro- and nanoscale to control cell function. *Angew Chem Int Ed Engl.* 48: 5406–5415.

Burdick, J.A., Anseth, K.S. 2002. Photoencapsulation of osteoblasts in injectable RGD-modified PEG hydrogels for bone tissue engineering. *Biomaterials.* 23: 4315–4323.

Caldorera-Moore, M., Peppas, N.A. 2009. Micro- and nanotechnologies for intelligent and responsive biomaterial-based medical systems. *Adv Drug Deliv Rev.* 61: 1391–1401.

Chanda, N., Kattumuri, V., Shukla, R. et al. 2010. Bombesin functionalized gold nanoparticles show *in vitro* and *in vivo* cancer receptor specificity. *Proc Natl Acad Sci USA.* 107: 8760–8765.

Chen, G., Tian, F., Zhang, Y., Zhang, Y., Li, C., Wang, Q. 2014. Tracking of transplanted human mesenchymal stem cells in living mice using near-infrared Ag_2S quantum dots. *Adv Funct Mater.* 24: 2481–2488.

Dalby, M.J., Gadegaard, N., Tare, R. et al. 2007. The control of human mesenchymal cell differentiation using nanoscale symmetry and disorder. *Nat Mater.* 6: 997–1003.

Debbage, P., Jaschke, W. 2008. Molecular imaging with nanoparticles: Giant roles for dwarf actors. *Histochem Cell Biol.* 130: 845–875.

De la Zerda, A., Zavaleta, C., Keren, S. et al. 2008. Carbon nanotubes as photoacoustic molecular imaging agents in living mice. *Nat Nanotechnol.* 3: 557–562.

Dlaska, C.E., Andersson, G., Brittberg, M., Suedkamp, N.P., Raschke, M.J., Schuetz, M.A. 2015. Clinical translation in tissue engineering—The surgeon's view. *Curr Mol Bio Rep.* 1: 61–70.

Dubertret, B., Skourides, P., Norris, D.J., Noireaux, V., Brivanlou, A.H., Libchaber, A. 2002. *In vivo* imaging of quantum dots encapsulated in phospholipid micelles. *Science.* 298: 1759–1762.

Dvir, T., Timko, B.P., Kohane, D.S., Langer, R. 2011. Nanotechnological strategies for engineering complex tissues. *Nat Nanotechnol.* 6: 13–22.

Edwards, S.L., Werkmeister, J.A., Ramshaw, J.A. 2009. Carbon nanotubes in scaffolds for tissue engineering. *Expert Rev Med Devices.* 6: 499–505.

Elloumi-Hannachi, I., Yamato, M., Okano, T. 2010. Cell sheet engineering: A unique nanotechnology for scaffold-free tissue reconstruction with clinical applications in regenerative medicine. *J Intern Med.* 267: 54–70.

Engler, A.J., Sen, S., Sweeney, H.L., Discher, D.E. 2006. Matrix elasticity directs stem cell lineage specification. *Cell.* 126: 677–689.

Freed, L.E., Langer, R., Martin, I., Pellis, N.R., Vunjak-Novakovic, G. 1997. Tissue engineering of cartilage in space. *Proc Natl Acad Sci USA.* 94: 13885–13890.

Goldberg, M., Langer, R., Jia, X. 2007. Nanostructured materials for applications in drug delivery and tissue engineering. *J Biomater Sci.* 8: 241–268.

Hammond, P.T. 2004. Form and function in multilayer assembly: New applications at the nanoscale. *Adv Mater.* 16: 1271–1293.

Harrison, B.S., Atala, A. 2007. Carbon nanotube applications for tissue engineering. *Biomaterials.* 28: 344–353.

Hosseinkhani, H., Hosseinkhani, M., Khademhosseini, A., Kobayashi, H., Tabata, Y. 2006. Enhanced angiogenesis through controlled release of basic fibroblast growth factor from peptide amphiphile for tissue regeneration. *Biomaterials.* 27: 5836–5844.

Huang, J., Grater, S.V., Corbellini, F. et al. 2009. Impact of order and disorder in RGD nanopatterns on cell adhesion. *Nano Lett.* 9: 1111–1116.

Hughes, G.A. 2005. Nanostructure-mediated drug delivery. *Nanomedicine.* 1: 22–30.

Huh, D., Matthews, B.D., Mammoto, A., Montoya-Zavala, M., Hsin, H.Y., Ingber, D.E. 2010. Reconstituting organ-level lung functions on a chip. *Science.* 328: 1662–1668.

Jiang, H., Fang, D., Hsiao, B., Chu, B., Chen, W. 2004. Preparation and characterization of ibuprofen-loaded poly (lactide-co-glycolide)/poly (ethylene glycol)-g-chitosan electrospun membranes. *J Biomater Sci.* 15: 279–296.

Kim, B.S., Mooney, D.J. 1998. Development of biocompatible synthetic extracellular matrices for tissue engineering. *Trends Biotechnol.* 16: 224–230.

Kim, D.H., Lipke, E.A., Kim, P. et al. 2010. Nanoscale cues regulate the structure and function of macroscopic cardiac tissue constructs. *Proc Natl Acad Sci.* 107: 565–570.

Koutsopoulos, S., Zhang, S. 2012. Two-layered injectable self-assembling peptide scaffold hydrogels for long-term sustained release of human antibodies. *J Control Release.* 160: 451–458.

Kumar, C.S.S.R. 2005. *Biofunctionalization of Nanomaterials.* Weinheim: Wiley-VCH.

Kunzmann, A., Andersson, B., Thurnherr, T., Krug, H., Scheynius, A., Fadeel, B. 2011. Toxicology of engineered nanomaterials: Focus on biocompatibility, biodistribution and biodegradation. *Biochim Biophys Acta.* 1810: 361–373.

Langer, R., Vacanti, J.P. 1993. Tissue engineering. *Science.* 260: 920–926.

Laurencin, C.T., Ambrosio, A.M., Borden, M.D., Cooper J.A. Jr. 1999. Tissue engineering: Orthopedic applications. *Ann Rev Biomed Eng.* 1: 19–46.

Laurencin, C.T., Khan, Y. 2013. *Regenerative Engineering.* Boca Raton: CRC Press.

Laurencin, C.T., Ko, F.K. 2004. Hybrid nanofibril matrices for use as tissue engineering devices. Google Patents. US 20030050711 A1.

Lee, K.Y., Mooney, D.J. 2001. Hydrogels for tissue engineering. *Chem Rev.* 101: 1869–1880.

L'Heureux, N., Pâquet, S., Labbé, R., Germain, L., Auger, F.A. 1998. A completely biological tissue-engineered human blood vessel. *FASEB J.* 12: 47–56.

Li, W.J., Laurencin, C.T., Caterson, E.J., Tuan, R.S., Ko, F.K. 2002. Electrospun nanofibrous structure: A novel scaffold for tissue engineering. *J Biomed Mater Res.* 60: 613–621.

Liu, H., Zhang, Z., Seong Toh, W., Ng, K.W., Sant, S., Salgado, A. 2015. Stem cells: Microenvironment, micro/nanotechnology, and application. *Stem Cells Int.* 2015: 398510.

Lutolf, M.P., Hubbell, J.A. 2005. Synthetic biomaterials as instructive extracellular microenvironments for morphogenesis in tissue engineering. *Nat Biotech.* 23 (1): 47–55.

Ma, P.X. 2008. Biomimetic materials for tissue engineering. *Adv Drug Deliv Rev.* 60: 184–198.

Mann, B.K., Gobin, A.S., Tsai, A.T., Schmedlen, R.H., West, J.L. 2001. Smooth muscle cell growth in photopolymerized hydrogels with cell adhesive and proteolytically degradable domains: Synthetic ECM analogs for tissue engineering. *Biomaterials.* 22: 3045–3051.

Murugan, R., Ramakrishna, S. 2005. Development of nanocomposites for bone grafting. *Compos Sci Technol.* 65: 2385–2406.

Nalwa, H.S. 1999. *Handbook of Nanostructured Materials and Nanotechnology.* Vol. 3. Cambridge: Academic Press.

Nerem, R.M. 1991. Cellular engineering. *Ann Biomed Eng.* 19: 529–545.

Norman, J.J., Desai, T.A. 2006. Methods for fabrication of nanoscale topography for tissue engineering scaffolds. *Ann Biomed Eng.* 34: 89–101.

Novoselov, K.S., Fal'Ko, V.I., Colombo, L., Gellert, P.R., Schwab, M.G., Kim, K. 2012. A roadmap for grapheme. *Nature.* 490: 192–200.

Oberpenning, F., Meng, J., Yoo, J.J., Atala, A. 1999. De novo reconstitution of a functional mammalian urinary bladder by tissue engineering. *Nat Biotechnol.* 17: 149–155.

Oh, S., Brammer, K.S., Li, Y.S. et al. 2009. Stem cell fate dictated solely by altered nanotube dimension. *Proc Natl Acad Sci USA.* 106: 2130–2135.

Park, J., Bauer, S., von der Mark, K., Schmuki, P. 2007. Nanosize and vitality: TiO_2 nanotube diameter directs cell fate. *Nano Lett.* 7: 1686–1691.

Phelps, E.A., Landázuri, N., Thulé, P.M., Taylor, W.R., García, A.J. 2010. Bioartificial matrices for therapeutic vascularization. *Proc Natl Acad Sci USA.* 107: 3323–3328.

Ranzinger, J., Krippner-Heidenreich, A., Haraszti, T. et al. 2009. Nanoscale arrangement of apoptotic ligands reveals a demand for a minimal lateral distance for efficient death receptor activation. *Nano Lett.* 9: 4240–4245.

Ratner, B.D, Hoffman, A.S., Schoen, F.J., Lemons, J.E. 2013. *Introduction-Biomaterials Science: An Evolving, Multidisciplinary Endeavor.* Academic Press Elsevier Inc.: Waltham, MA, USA.

Reichert, W.M., Ratner, B.D., Anderson, J. et al. 2011. 2010 Panel on the biomaterials grand challenges. *J Biomed Mater Res A.* 96: 275–1287.

Richardson, T.P., Peters, M.C., Ennett, A.B., Mooney, D.J. 2001. Polymeric system for dual growth factor delivery. *Nat Biotechnol.* 19: 1029–1034.

Riehemann, K., Schneider, S.W., Luger, T.A., Godin, B., Ferrari, M., Fuchs, H. 2009. Nanomedicine—Challenge and perspectives. *Angew Chem Int Ed Engl.* 48: 872–897.

Sampson, S.L., Saraiva, L., Gustafsson, K., Jayasinghe, S.N., Robertson, B.D. 2014. Cell electrospinning: An *in vitro* and *in vivo* study. *Small.* 10: 78–82.

Sengupta, S., Eavarone, D., Capila, I. et al. 2005. Temporal targeting of tumour cells and neovasculature with a nanoscale delivery system. *Nature.* 436: 568–572.

Shah, A., Brugnano, J., Sun, S., Vase, A., Orwin, E. 2008. The development of a tissue-engineered cornea: Biomaterials and culture methods. *Pediatr Res.* 63: 535–544.

Shi, J., Votruba, A.R., Farokhzad, O.C., Langer, R. 2010. Nanotechnology in drug delivery and tissue engineering: From discovery to applications. *Nano Lett.* 10: 3223–3230.

Skalak, R., Fox, C.F. (ed.) 1988. Tissue engineering. In *Proceedings of a workshop*, Granlibakken, Lake Tahoe, California.

Sobolev, K. 2015. Nanotechnology and nanoengineering of construction materials. In *Nanotechnology in Construction.* New York City: Springer, 3–13.

Sun, C., Lee, J.S., Zhang, M. 2008. Magnetic nanoparticles in MR imaging and drug delivery. *Adv Drug Deliv Rev.* 60: 1252–1265.

Sun, Z., Zussman, E., Yarin, A.L., Wendorff, J.H., Greiner, A. 2003. Compound core–shell polymer nanofibers by co-electrospinning. *Adv Mater.* 15: 1929–1932.

Supp, D.M., Boyce, S.T. 2005. Engineered skin substitutes: Practices and potentials. *Clin Dermatol.* 23: 403–412.

Taipale, J., Keski-Oja, J. 1997. Growth factors in the extracellular matrix. *FASEB J.* 11: 51–59.

Tang, Z., Wang, Y., Podsiadlo, P., Kotov, N.A. 2006. Biomedical applications of layer-by-layer assembly: From biomimetics to tissue engineering. *Adv Mater.* 18: 3203.

Thanou, M., Duncan, R. 2003. Polymer–protein and polymer–drug conjugates in cancer therapy. *Curr Opin Investig Drugs.* 4: 701–709.

Thesleff, T., Lehtimäki, K., Niskakangas, T. et al. 2011. Cranioplasty with adipose-derived stem cells and biomaterial: A novel method for cranial reconstruction. *Neurosurgery.* 68: 1535–1540.

U.S. Department of Health and Human Services, OPTN/SRTR. 2013. Annual data report: Introduction. 2015. *Am J Transplant.* 15: 8–10.

Veronese, F.M., Mero, A. 2008. The impact of PEGylation on biological therapies. *BioDrugs.* 22: 315–329.

Wade, R.J., Bassin, E.J., Gramlich, W.M., Burdick, J.A. 2015. Nanofibrous hydrogels with spatially patterned biochemical signals to control cell behavior. *Adv Mater.* 27: 1356–1362.

Woodrow, K.A., Cu, Y., Booth, C.J., Saucier-Sawyer, J.K., Wood, M.J., Saltzman, W.M. 2009. Intravaginal gene silencing using biodegradable polymer nanoparticles densely loaded with small-interfering RNA. *Nat Mater.* 8: 526–533.

Xu, C.Y., Inai, R., Kotaki, M., Ramakrishna, S. 2004. Aligned biodegradable nanofibrous structure: A potential scaffold for blood vessel engineering. *Biomaterials.* 25: 877–886.

Yim, E.K., Pang, S.W., Leong, K.W. 2007. Synthetic nanostructures inducing differentiation of human mesenchymal stem cells into neuronal lineage. *Exp Cell Res.* 313: 1820–1829.

Zhang, S. 2003. Fabrication of novel biomaterials through molecular self-assembly. *Nat Biotechnol.* 21: 1171–1178.

Zhang, S., Uludağ, H. 2009. Nanoparticulate systems for growth factor delivery. *Pharm Res.* 26: 1561–1580.

Zhang, S., Zhao, X. 2004. Design of molecular biological materials using peptide motifs. *J Mater Chem.* 14: 2082–2086.

2

Nanofibers Design for Guided Cellular Behavior

Anuradha Subramanian and Swaminathan Sethuraman

CONTENTS

2.1 Introduction

Native tissue has hierarchically ordered dynamic nanostructured extracellular matrix (ECM) components that regulate cellular behavior such as polarity, adhesion, proliferation, migration, orientation, and differentiation (Kozel et al., 2006). ECM has been proposed to be an excellent cellular glue comprising a complex and dynamic network of fibrous proteins, majorly collagen and elastin in the viscous microenvironment of glycoaminoglycans, glycoproteins, proteoglycans, and several soluble growth factors. Fibrous collagen and elastin in the ECM provides tensile strength and extensibility to the tissues thereby enabling them to resist the plastic deformation and rupture, and endure mechanical loading. In addition to scaffolding, ECM also coordinates cellular function through physical and mechanical stimulus. This chapter explains the role of fibrous ECM components on the regulation of cellular fate in tissues to understand the rationale of nanofiber geometry on control of cell behavior and how the nanofiber–ECM analog helps to organize the cellular function and tissue progression for tissue engineering applications.

2.2 Fibrous ECM Components

Majority of the ECM components such as collagen, elastin, fibronectin, and laminin are fibrous in nature contributing to structural and adhesive support for tissue progression

(Muiznieks and Keeley, 2013). This section outlines the role of supramolecular assembly of ECM proteins toward the mechanical and biological properties of the tissues. Collagen is the chief fibrous protein present in the ECM with a broad range of functions such as structural support, adhesive function, cell migration, angiogenesis, tissue morphogenesis, and organogenesis (Gosline et al., 2002). Collagens are classified based on the function and domain homology, which includes fibril-forming collagen, fibril-associated collagen, network-forming collagen, transmembrane collagens, endostatin-producing collagen, anchoring fibrils, and beaded filament-forming collagen (Kadler et al., 2007). Of the various types of collagens, fibrillar collagen (type I, II, III, V, and XI) is the principal form assembled into collagen fibrils of 10–300 nm in diameter (Kadler et al., 2007). Fibril-associated collagens such as type IX and XII helps the collagen fibrils to link one another and also to other ECM components (Mayne and Burgeson, 1987). In network-forming collagens (type IV and VII), type VII tends to assemble into specialized structures called anchoring fibrils, which helps to attach the basal lamina of epithelial to connective tissue (Than et al., 2002). Mature basal laminae are mainly made up of type IV, organized into mesh-like sheets contributing to the barrier function and mechanical support for adjacent cells (Alberts et al., 1994). Establishment of covalent cross-links between the lysine residues of collagen molecules determines the tensile strength of fibrils (Kadler et al., 1996).

Elastic fibers are another class of fibrous proteins present in the ECM providing mechanical strength especially elasticity to the tissues. Tissues such as blood vessels, skin, lungs, and other dynamic connective tissues require resilience that helps to recoil at the end of the transient stretch (Sage, 1982). Elastic fibers comprise inner core cross-linked elastin surrounded by microfibrillar layer (Faury, 2001). Microfibrils consist of many proteins such as fibrillin, fibulin, and microfibril-associated glycoproteins and provides a structural and organizational support for the assembly of elastins (Midwood and Schwarzbauer, 2002). In addition, the stretching ability of elastin is mainly controlled by the tight association of collagen fibrils.

Fibronectin protein exists in fibrous form possessing binding site for collagen in its N-terminal end and two other binding sites in C-terminal region for both glycosaminoglycans and integrins (Tarone et al., 1982). This fibronectin fibrils offer elasticity and contribute to the major adhesive function of ECM apart from maintaining the hemostasis and tissue organization (Abu-Lail et al., 2006). Further, fibronectin binds to cell-surface integrins such as integrin α5β1, α4β1, and αvβ3, which are connected to the cytoskeleton and maintain cell phenotype through the organization of intracellular actin filaments (Singh and Schwarzbauer, 2012). Laminin is one of the ubiquitous ECM fibrous proteins present in the basement membrane assisting cell adhesion, migration, proliferation, and differentiation in many tissues. Cell-surface receptors such as integrins, dystroglycan, and syndecan promote the self-association of laminin into the independent polymeric fibrous networks (Neal et al., 2009).

Thus, the fibrous architecture of major ECM proteins demonstrate the scaffolding function by providing excellent mechanical strength at the tissue level. Apart from the presence of biological recognition motif, this geometry also promotes physical cell–ECM communication through integrin–actin networks, thereby controlling the cell fate based on the extracellular environment. Hence, biomaterial scaffolds with nanofiber geometry receives considerable attention in tissue engineering applications.

2.3 Nanofiber Geometry as ECM Analog

Cells can control growth and differentiation in response to external stimuli based on their ability to sense the nano- and microgeometries from the environment. Nanofiber

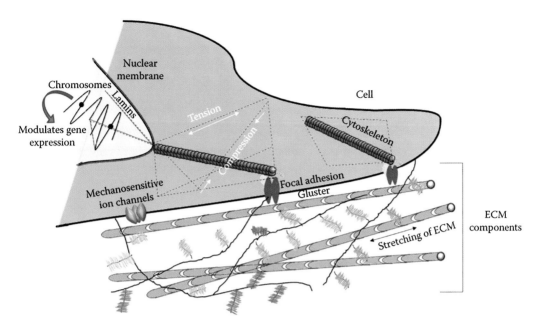

FIGURE 2.1
Major events in the focal adhesion-mediated signal transduction.

geometry mediates cell adhesion through the spatial distribution of focal contacts (Singhvi et al., 1994; Curtis and Wilkinson, 1997). This integrin-mediated cell–substrate adhesion has been found to control cell morphology, polarization, viability, proliferation, and differentiation through the regulation of intracellular signals named focal adhesion-mediated signal transduction (Figure 2.1). Factors such as fiber morphology, diameter, orientation, and spacing between the fibers play a vital role in the guidance of cellular responses (Wang and Nain, 2014). This section describes the influence of fibrous architecture toward cell fate.

2.4 Role of Nanofibers on the Guidance of Cell Behavior

2.4.1 Cell Polarity

Cell polarization is a key process in maintaining the specific cellular shapes and structures and in mediating the specialized cellular functions. Biomaterial topography has altered the polarization of embryonic hippocampal neurons, thereby supporting the axonal outgrowth. It was observed that the biomaterial surface features smaller than the soma had shown twofold increase in the polarization of neurons than on the smoother substrate (Gomez et al., 2007). Similarly, electrospun poly(lactic-*co*-glycolic acid) (PLGA) substrate improved the neuronal polarization up to 30%–50% than the casted films, thus, confirming the influence of subcellular features on neurons (Lee et al., 2010). Variation in polarization may be due to the topography-enabled reorganization of focal adhesion clusters, which may directly alter both cytoskeleton proteins as well as gene expressions. Dorsal root ganglia (DRG) neurons cultured on the Poly L-lactic acid (PLLA) fibers enhanced the neurite orientation and extension, which may be attributed to the presence of lesser angle between the fibers facilitating the neurite extension toward the fiber direction (Corey et al., 2007). Gertz et al. (2010) elucidated the acceleration of polarity in motor neurons when cultured on the PLLA nanofibers than the film and glass controls.

Directional secretion of secretory cells such as salivary gland acinar and ductile cells demands the apicobasal polarity that was maintained by both tight junctions and adherens junctions through the assembly of various proteins such as claudins, occludin, and ZO-1 (Baker, 2010). PLGA nanofibrous (NF) scaffold was found to promote the apicobasal polarity of mouse ductal submandibular epithelial cell line (SIMS cells) and rat parotid acinar epithelial cell line (SMGC10 cells) through the determination of apical localization of tight junction-scaffolding protein (ZO-1) as compared to film (Cantara et al., 2012).

2.4.2 Cell Adhesion and Shape

Geometry of fiber assembly controls the shape of cell, based on the organization of cytoskeleton proteins on the substrate (Zhu et al., 2010). Morphology and spreading of cell has been found to be affected greatly by fiber diameter and spacing between the fibers (Chew et al., 2008). Higher number of rat Schwann cells were adhered on both PLGA random and aligned electrospun fibers after 3, 6, and 12 h of seeding than PLGA films (Radhakrishnan et al., 2015). Human aortic endothelial cells cultured on electrospun polycaprolactone/collagen scaffold of various fiber diameters (500 nm, 1 µm, 2 µm, and 5 µm) has been observed to show various focal adhesion points and cytoskeletal organization, which directly influences the shape of the endothelial cells. As 500 nm facilitated the occurrence of multiple focal points, the cytoskeleton organization was found to be extended in the cells (Khang, 2012). Increasing the fiber diameter from 0.14 to 0.76 µm increased the cell area and aspect ratio, however, there was no significant change observed in the morphology of fibroblast cultured on 3.6 µm fibers with respect to spin-coated PLGA substrates (Bashur et al., 2006). In a similar fashion, projected cell area of MC3T3–E1 preosteoblast was reduced significantly on fibers with diameter of 0.14 and 2.1 µm than the smooth surfaces (Badami et al., 2006).

Nanofiber architecture induced the expression of integrin–beta 1 adhesion molecule in human umbilical vein endothelial cells (HUVEC) and outgrowth endothelial cells (OEC) compared to microfibrous silk fibroin nets (Bondar et al., 2007). Cells were found to exhibit different geometry such as flat, spindle, parallel, and polygonal on flat, suspended arrays of aligned fibers with two different interfiber lateral distances (>20 µm and <20 µm) and double-layered intersecting fibers, respectively (Sheets et al., 2013). Wang et al., demonstrated that the increase of divergent angle in the suspended nanofibers increases the shape index of the C2C12 mouse myoblasts while maintaining the cell area constant as cell–fiber adhesion points directly affect the focal adhesion arrangement. The change in the cellular geometry further alters the shape of the nucleus, thereby affecting the gene expression and functional protein synthesis (Wang and Nain, 2014). Similarly, fibers of carbon with <100 nm dimension have promoted the higher alkaline phosphatase (ALP) activity and deposition of extracellular calcium compared to the fibers of >100 nm (Elias et al., 2002). Sugar-based ligand such as galactose, fructose, and lactose facilitate the adhesion of primary hepatocytes through asialoglycoprotein-mediated interaction and restore the hepatocyte phenotype for longer period of culture (Vasanthan et al., 2012). Cells cultured on substrates supporting cell spreading promote osteogenic differentiation, while substrates that restrict cell spreading support adipogenic differentiation (McBeath et al., 2004). Receptor-mediated interaction with ECM proteins determines the shape of cells in

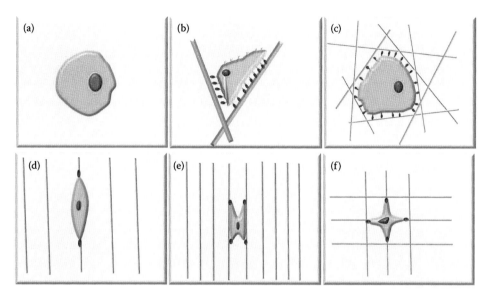

FIGURE 2.2
Illustrating the influence of scaffold topography on cell shape. Morphology of cell cultured on (a) film, (b) microfibers, (c) random nanofibers, (d) aligned nanofibers with large spacing, (e) aligned nanofibers with narrow spacing, and (f) intersected nanofibers.

the tissue. Similarly, topography of the ECM analog decides the cell phenotype based on the cell–scaffold interactions. Figure 2.2 illustrates the role of scaffold architecture on the control of cell shape.

Cells cultured on film attains weakly spread and round morphology as it lacks submicron structures as well as roughness as shown in Figure 2.2a. On microfibrous substrate, cells can spread across the microfibers to bridge the larger pores, adopting irregular shape with poorly spread morphology via the development of focal adhesion clusters all over the cell boundary (Figure 2.2b). Submicron features in the nanofibers can promote more roughness and high surface to volume ratio and accommodate more number of cells as compared to microfibers. Cells adopt flattened morphology on exposure to larger number of fibers, which in turn creates multiple adhesion points and improves cell spreading (Figure 2.2c). However, orientation of fibers can align the cells toward its direction as in Figure 2.2d and e because of the establishment of ordered focal contacts toward the fiber. Further, spacing between the fibers determines cell geometry through the variation in the arrangement of focal adhesion clusters. Cells exists in spindle morphology when cultured on the oriented fibers with the spacing larger than the cell size (Figure 2.2d) due to the recruitment of two focal adhesion points on each ends. Conversely, parallel-shaped conformation was observed when the cells were cultured on uniaxially aligned fibers with lesser spacing. This is because the cells can span across the oriented fibers and construct four focal contact points (Figure 2.2e). Intersected fibers could change the cell morphology as polygonal by creating four or more focal contacts (Figure 2.2f).

2.4.3 Cell Proliferation

High surface-area-to-volume ratio of NF substrates can accommodate more number of cells as well as protein absorption, thereby effectively modulating cell behavior as well as proliferation with respect to the solvent-casted films (Leong et al., 2009). Coating of nanofibers onto the porous spiral-shaped scaffolds by solvent casting and salt-leaching process enhanced the rat Schwann cell proliferation in both dynamic and static culture conditions as compared to uncoated porous spiral-shaped scaffolds (Valmikinathan et al., 2011). Chitosan nanofibers enhanced both mouse and human osteoblast proliferation by stimulating deoxyribonucleic acid (DNA) replication via osteopontin (OPN) gene expression than the chitosan films (Ho et al., 2014). Similarly, nanofibers of both carbon nanotubes/polyurethane composites and polyurethane promoted endothelial cell proliferation than smooth films (Han et al., 2008). Thin coating of hydroxyl apatite in poly-ε-caprolactone (PCL)/polyvinyl alcohol nanofibers enhanced the proliferation and differentiation potential of mesenchymal stem cells (MSCs) toward osteoblasts (Proseck et al., 2012). PCL/chitosan-electrospun scaffolds demonstrated the bipolar elongations with optimal proliferation of rat Schwann cells than PCL scaffolds (Prabhakaran et al., 2008). Fibrinogen-electrospun scaffolds of less than 200 nm exhibited better endothelial cell adhesion and found to guide the cell behavior than the preadsorbed fibrinogen on flat substrates (Gugutkov et al., 2013). Hepatocyte growth was pronounced on porous PCL nanofibers with respect to nonporous PCL nanofibers (Lubasová et al., 2010; Lubasová and Martinova, 2011). Electrospun PCL scaffolds promoted the reversal of reduced proliferation phenotype in genetically edited cells, which was completely absent when cultured on polylysine or fibronectin-coated dish surfaces (Borjigin et al., 2012). Designer peptide NF scaffolds significantly enhanced the proliferation of MC3T3–E1 cells as compared to pure RAD16 (Horii et al., 2007).

Although the effect of NF topography and its dimension is more potent on the regulation of cell proliferation, there are few reports demonstrating the variation in topography influence with respect to the cell type as well as biomaterials. Based on the cell type, nanofibers have been demonstrated to enhance, hinder, or does not show any impact on cell proliferation with respect to flat substrates. This variation may be due to the inclination of different cell types toward the specific topography. Xu et al. (2004) reported that the proliferation and function of endothelial cells were promoted on casted films than the poly(L-lactic acid) nanofibers, while the vascular smooth muscle cells prefer fibrous topography better than the flat substrates. Moroni et al. (2006) characterized the effect of fiber diameter on human mesenchymal stem cell (hMSC) proliferation and proved that the diameter of smooth fibers closer to the cell dimension compromised the fiber curvature, thereby facilitating the optimal cell seeding and proliferation. Density of osteoprogenitor cells has been found to increase significantly with increasing fiber diameter (Badami et al., 2006).

2.4.4 Cell Migration

Nanotopography has been found to modify cell geometry, which in turn influences the migration speed of the cells. Sharma et al. (2013) proved the role of structural stiffness of fibers on the regulation of cell migration. Cells were found to migrate faster on fibers with lower stiffness. Jain et al. (2014) had investigated the role of aligned polycaprolactone nanofibers on the migration of brain tumor cells toward an extracortical cyclopamine-conjugated collagen-based hydrogel and reduced the tumor volume significantly when compared to smooth fibers. Biophysical parameters of ECM analog such as stiffness, topography, and orientation affect the arrangement of focal adhesion complex, thereby influencing the migration potential. Migration dynamics mainly depend on the cell shape with respect to the topography. Spindle-shaped C2C12 mouse myoblast on the single fiber promotes significantly higher migration at the rate of 52 ± 11 μm h^{-1} as compared to flat-shaped cells (35 ± 7 μm h^{-1}) cultured on flat polystyrene sheets. This may be attributed to the intrinsic stretching of the spindle-shaped cells and F-actin polymerization toward the

fiber direction, which facilitates cellular polarization, thereby increasing migration potential. Further, migration speed of the myoblast has been found to be reduced drastically
from parallel-shaped cells to polygonal-shaped cells, which clearly indicate the presence
of multiple adhesion clusters displaying numerous directional freedom for the cells, which
in turn reduce the cell migration (Sheets et al., 2013). Patel et al. (2007) have observed significantly fivefold higher number of fibroblasts migrating toward the wound area in an *in
vitro* wound-healing model on the fibers oriented perpendicular to the defect axis than the
fibers aligned either in the parallel or random directions. These research outcomes clearly
explain the role of scaffold topography, cell geometry, and arrangement of focal adhesion
clusters on the determination of the cell migration speed.

2.4.5 Cell Orientation

Components of the ECM are synthesized and secreted by cells (Castaldo et al., 2013).
Orientation and organization of fibrillar ECM components are strongly influenced by the
biological functions and mechanical requirements of the tissues (Muiznieks and Keeley,
2013). For instance, mesh-like assembly of collagen type IV in basement membrane anchors
the epithelial cells to underlying connective tissues. Though the collagen type I are the
major fibrous proteins in most of the connective tissues such as bone, tendon, and skin, the
parallel orientation of collagen toward the long axis of tendon and isotropic networks of
collagen bundles in the skin contribute to the unidirectional tensile strength withstanding
multidirectional forces, respectively (Ottani et al., 2001; Silver et al., 2003). Likewise, assembly of elastin in ligaments is arranged parallel to the direction of stretching (Ronchetti et al.,
1998). Hence, supramolecular assembly of fibrous proteins in the ECM is based on the tissue
types, which are subjected to the direction of mechanical force and amplitude. Cells were
aligned along the fiber direction on aligned fibers, while irregular distribution of cells was
observed on the randomly arranged fibers as it fails to align the focal points (Figure 2.3).

Schwann cells on the aligned fibrous topography established the focal contacts along
its length, which was confirmed by the anti-vinculin staining (green fluorescence) as in
Figure 2.4.

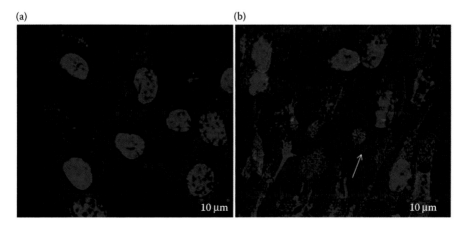

FIGURE 2.3
Confocal fluorescence micrographs of smooth muscle cells on (a) random and (b) aligned nanofibers (blue indicates nuclei staining; red, cytoskeleton staining; and arrow, fiber direction).

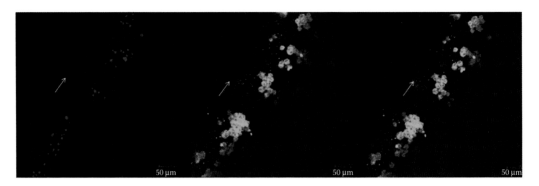

FIGURE 2.4
Laser scanning confocal fluorescence images of nuclei and focal adhesion of Schwann cells on aligned electrospun scaffolds after third day (blue indicates nuclei staining using Hoechst; green, focal contacts using antivinculin staining; and arrow, direction of fibers).

Aligned nanofiber topography has promoted cell extension and orientation toward the fiber direction, while clustering of cells with low elongation factor was observed on the fibers arranged randomly (Subramanian et al., 2012a,b). Nanofiber architectures function as artificial axons, thereby promoting the myelin-associated gene expressions in Schwann cells as compared to films (Radhakrishnan et al., 2015).

2.4.6 Cell Differentiation and ECM Production

ECM production as well as its orientation is determined chiefly by the cell shape as well as cell orientation (Engelmayr et al., 2006; Moroni et al., 2006). Nanotopography and diameter of the fibrous scaffolds could influence the cell spreading or aggregation and alter the ECM production. For instance, chondrocytes have been programmed to retain the round phenotype by inducing aggregation, which subsequently produce higher content of collagen II and glycosaminoglycans (Woodfield et al., 2006). However, osteoblasts have been found to promote the ECM production when they are in spreaded morphology (Boyan et al., 2003).

In native tissues, cell–ECM interactions exert mechanical tension to actin cytoskeleton, which in turn control cells of different phases such as growth and differentiation by altering the cell shape. In a similar fashion, cells change its shape and cytoskeleton properties based on the scaffold geometry and confer the mechanical forces directly to the nucleus, thereby modifying the nuclear shape resulting in the alteration of gene and protein expression (Guilak et al., 2009). As the intermediate filaments of cytoskeleton linked with the lamin filaments of nucleoskeleton are connected with telomeric ends of interphase chromosomes, tension in the cytoskeleton has been directly transformed to the chromosomes and affects the gene expression (Dahl and Kalinowski, 2011). Nanofiber architecture of poly(caprolactone-*co*-[ethyl ethylene phosphate]) has reduced the glial scar by stimulating gene silencing and apoptosis of primary rat cortical astrocytes than solvent-cast films for central nervous system (CNS) regeneration (Cao et al., 2012). Endothelial cells cultured on NF scaffolds demonstrated antithrombogenic activity by releasing lesser amount of tissue factor as compared to smooth films of polyurethane (Han et al., 2008). Aligned PCL nanofibers have upregulated the myelination markers such as myelin-associated glycoprotein (MAG), myelin-specific gene (P0), and downregulated the expression of immature Schwann cell markers than the two-dimensional PCL films (Chew et al., 2008).

TABLE 2.1

Role of Nanofiber Topography on the Cellular Differentiation

Biomaterials in Fibrous Scaffolds	Cell Source	Expression of Biomarkers	References
PCL	hMSCs	Osteogenesis: runt-related transcription factor (RUNX2); osteocalcin (OCN); ALP	Chang et al. (2013)
3D PLLA	Human bone marrow MSCs	Myogenic differentiation: myosin heavy chain (MHC); a-smooth muscle actin (aSMA); calponin	Tian et al. (2010)
Peptide-functionalized polyhydroxyalkanoate	Schwann cell line RT4-D6P2T	Myelination: peripheral myelin protein 22 (PMP22); neutrophins: glial cell-derived neutrophic factor (GDNF); brain-derived neutrophic factor (BDNF); ciliary neurotrophic factor (CNTF); nerve growth factor (NGF)	Masaeli et al. (2014)
Self-assembling peptide-enriched electrospun PCL	Human osteoblasts cells	Osteogenesis: human osteopontin (hOPN); human bone sialoprotein (hBSP); human alkaline phosphatase (hALP)	Danesin et al. (2012)
Chitosan	Mesenchymal cell line (D1 ORL UVA) derived from multipotent mouse bone marrow stromal precursor	Chondrogenesis: aggrecan; collagen II; collagen X	Ragetly et al. (2010)
Solid-walled PLLA	Amniotic fluid-derived stem cells (AFSCs)	Osteogenesis: BMP-7; osterix (OSX); RUNX2; OCN; ALP; OPN	Sun et al. (2010)
Polyelectrolyte complexation of chitosan and alginate	hMSCs	In specific differentiation media osteogenesis: collagen I; OCN; OPN; osteonectin Chondrogenesis: aggrecan; SOX9; collagen II & X	Yim et al. (2006)
PLLA, PCL	Human-induced pluripotent stem cell-derived MSCs	Tenogenesis: tendon/ligament-associated marker -tenomodulin (TNMD)	Czaplewski et al. (2014)

(Continued)

TABLE 2.1 (*Continued*)

Role of Nanofiber Topography on the Cellular Differentiation

Biomaterials in Fibrous Scaffolds	Cell Source	Expression of Biomarkers	References
3D polyethylene terephthalate (PET)	Human amniotic fluid stem cells	In specific differentiation media osteogenesis: RUNX2; OPN adipogenesis: adipose fatty acid-binding protein (aP2); peroxisome; proliferative activated receptor-γ (PPAR-γ); lipoprotein lipase (LPL)	Liu et al. (2014)
3D porous NF PLLA	Human bone marrow-derived MSCs	Chondrogenesis: collagen II; aggrecan	Hu et al. (2009)
RGD-modified chitosan–alginate polyelectrolyte complex (PEC)	Differentiated human bone marrow-derived MSCs	Transdifferentiation to hepatocyte-like cells: human cytokeratin 18 (CK18); albumin; hepatocyte nuclear factor-4 alpha (HNF-4a)	Tai et al. (2010)
PLLA	Human dental pulp stem cells	Odontogenic differentiation: ALP; dentin matrix protein-1 (DMP-1); dentin sialophosphoprotein (DSSP); OCN	Wang et al. (2010)
Chitosan–PCL	Neuron-like PC-12 cells	Neurite extension: β-tubulin; differentiation and neurite growth: neurofilament-200 (NF-200)	Cooper et al. (2011)
Hydrogel of NIPAAM/AAc/HEMA-oHB6 (86/4/10) and polyurethane-blended fibrous matrix	Cardiosphere-derived cells	Cardiac differentiation: cardiac troponin T (cTnT); calcium channel (CACNA1c); cardiac myosin heavy chain (MYH6)	Xu et al. (2014)

Orientation of nanofibers instructs the human tendon stem/progenitor cell (hTSPC) to teno-lineage through integrin- and myosin-mediated mechanotransduction even in the presence of osteogenic medium (Yin et al., 2010). In addition, integrin-based adhesion promotes sequential chemical events such as activation of myosin light chain kinase (MLCK), contraction of stress fibers, activation of focal adhesion kinase, and also change in the calcium flux and G-protein events in cells (Wozniak et al., 2004). Self-assembling peptide nanofiber scaffolds made of RADA16-I coupled with short biological recognition motif has pronounced effect on the differentiation of osteoprogenitor cells by influencing ALP and osteocalcin secretion than pure RAD16 (Horii et al., 2007). Recently, multilayered scaffolds have received much attention for tissue engineering applications. Scaffolds made of PLA–PLGA comprising inner aligned fibrous layer and outer random fibrous layer with rolipram promotes axonal growth and angiogenesis by decreasing the scar tissue and chondroitin sulfate in lesion (Zhu et al., 2010). Table 2.1 shows the role of nanofiber topography on the cellular differentiation through the upregulation of specific genetic markers.

2.5 Conclusion

Irrespective of the synthesis methods, ECM-resembling architecture of NF geometry has many advantages such as higher porosity, high surface-area-to-volume ratio, biodegradablility, programmable mechanical strength, and biocompatibility. This fibrous geometry and its dimension determine the morphology of cells through the integrin-based adhesion. The arrangement of focal adhesion clusters at the cell–fiber interaction sites generate tension in the cytoskeleton of cells, which in turn translate the tension to lamins of nucleoskeleton, thereby altering the expression of genes by mechanical force-induced signal transduction. In addition, cell–fiber interaction promotes respective ECM production by establishing the cell–cell communication. Moreover, nanofiber topography provides complex mechanical signals that initiate sequential biochemical events via opening of mechanosensitive ion channels and the stimulation of secondary messengers, which ultimately regulates cell fate such as adhesion, polarization, viability, growth, and differentiation. Thus, the influence of nanofiber topography on the cell behavior has been well established for various types of tissue progressions.

References

Abu-Lail, N. I., Ohashi, T., Clark, R. L., Erickson, H. P., Zauscher, S. 2006. Understanding the elasticity of fibronectin fibrils: Unfolding strengths of FN-III and GFP domains measured by single molecule force spectroscopy. *Matrix Biol.* 25: 175–184.

Alberts, B., Johnson, A., Lewis, J., Raff, M., Roberts, K., Watson, J. D. 1994. *Molecular Biology of the Cell.* Garland Publishing Inc., New York.

Badami, A. S., Kreke, M. R., Thompson, M. S., Riffle, J. S., Goldstein, A. S. 2006. Effect of fiber diameter on spreading, proliferation, and differentiation of osteoblastic cells on electrospun poly(lactic acid) substrates. *Biomaterials.* 27: 596–606.

Baker, O. J. 2010. Tight junctions in salivary epithelium. *J Biomed Biotechnol.* 2010: 278–291.

Bashur, C. A., Dahlgren, L. A., Goldstein, A. S. 2006. Effect of fiber diameter and orientation on fibroblast morphology and proliferation on electrospun poly(D,L-lactic-*co*-glycolic acid) meshes. *Biomaterials.* 27: 5681–5688.

Bondar, B., Fuchs, S., Motta, A., Migliaresi, C., Kirkpatrick, C. J. 2007. Functionality of endothelial cells on silk fibroin nets: Comparative study of micro- and nanometric fibre size. *Biomaterials.* 29: 561–572.

Borjigin, M., Strouse, B., Niamat, R. A., Bialk, P., Eskridge, C., Xie, J., Kmiec, E. B. 2012. Proliferation of genetically modified human cells on electrospun nanofiber scaffolds. *Mol Ther Nucleic Acids.* 1: e59.

Boyan, B. D., Lossdorfer, S., Wang, L., Zhao, G., Lohmann, C. H., Cochran, D. L., Schwartz, Z. 2003. Osteoblasts generate an osteogenic microenvironment when grown on surfaces with rough microtopographies. *Eur Cell Mater.* 6: 22–27.

Cantara, S. I., Soscia, D. A., Sequeira, S., Jean-Gillies, R., Castracane, J., Larsen, M. 2012. Selective functionalization of nanofiber scaffolds to regulate salivary gland epithelial cell proliferation and polarity. *Biomaterials.* 33: 8372–8382.

Cao, H., Marcy, G., Goh, E. L., Wang, F., Wang, J., Chew, S. Y. 2012. The effects of nanofiber topography on astrocyte behavior and gene silencing efficiency. *Macromol Biosci.* 12: 666–674.

Castaldo, C., Meglio, F. D., Miraglia, R., Sacco, A. M., Romano, V., Bancone, C., Corte, A. D., Montagnani, S., Nurzynska, D. 2013. Cardiac fibroblast-derived extracellular matrix (biomatrix) as a model for the studies of cardiac primitive cell biological properties in normal and pathological adult human heart. *Biomed Res Int.* 2013: 352370.

Chang, J. C., Fujita, S., Tonami, H., Kato, K., Iwata, H., Hsu, S. H. 2013. Cell orientation and regulation of cell–cell communication in human mesenchymal stem cells on different patterns of electrospun fibers. *Biomed Mater.* 8: 055002.

Chew, S. Y., Mi, R., Hoke, A., Leong, K. W. 2008. The effect of the alignment of electrospun fibrous scaffolds on Schwann cell maturation. *Biomaterials.* 29: 653–661.

Cooper, A., Bhattarai, N., Zhang, M. 2011. Fabrication and cellular compatibility of aligned chitosan–PCL fibers for nerve tissue regeneration. *Carbohydr Polym.* 85: 149–156.

Corey, J. M., Lin, D. Y., Mycek, K. B., Chen, Q., Samuel, S., Feldman, E. L., Martin, D. C. 2007. Aligned electrospun nanofibers specify the direction of dorsal root ganglia neurite growth. *J Biomed Mater Res A.* 83: 636–645.

Curtis, A., Wilkinson, C. 1997. Review: Topographical control of cells. *Biomaterials* 18: 1573–1583.

Czaplewski, S. K., Tsai, T. L., Duenwald-Kuehl, S. E., Vanderby, R., Li, W. J. 2014. Tenogenic differentiation of human induced pluripotent stem cell-derived mesenchymal stem cells dictated by properties of braided submicron fibrous scaffolds. *Biomaterials.* 35: 6907–6917.

Dahl, K. N., Kalinowski, A. 2011. Nucleoskeleton mechanics at a glance. *J Cell Sci.* 124: 675–678.

Danesin, R., Brun, P., Roso, M. et al. 2012. Self-assembling peptide-enriched electrospun polycaprolactone scaffolds promote the h-osteoblast adhesion and modulate differentiation-associated gene expression. *Bone.* 51: 851–859.

Elias, K. L., Price, R. L., Webster, T. J. 2002. Enhanced functions of osteoblasts on nanometer diameter carbon fibers. *Biomaterials.* 23: 3279–3287.

Engelmayr Jr, G. C., Papworth, G. D., Watkins, S. C., Mayer Jr, J. E., Sacks, M. S. 2006. Guidance of engineered tissue collagen orientation by large-scale scaffold microstructures. *J Biomech.* 39: 1819–1831.

Faury, G. 2001. Function–structure relationship of elastic arteries in evolution: From microfibrils to elastin and elastic fibres. *Pathol Biol (Paris).* 49: 310–325.

Gertz, C. C., Leach, M. K., Birrell, L. K., Martin, D. C., Feldman, E. L., Corey, J. M. 2010. Accelerated neuritogenesis and maturation of primary spinal motor neurons in response to nanofibers. *Dev Neurobiol.* 70: 589–603.

Gomez, N., Lu, Y., Chen, S., Schmidt, C. E. 2007. Immobilized nerve growth factor and microtopography have distinct effects on polarization versus axon elongation in hippocampal cells in culture. *Biomaterials.* 28: 271–284.

Gosline, J., Lillie, M., Carrington, E., Guerette, P., Ortlepp, C., Savage, K. 2002. Elastic proteins: Biological roles and mechanical properties. *Philos Trans R Soc Lond B Biol Sci.* 357: 121–132.

Gugutkov, D., Gustavsson, J., Ginebra, M. P., Altankov, G. 2013. Fibrinogen nanofibers for guiding endothelial cell behavior. *Biomater. Sci.* 1: 1065–1073.

Guilak, F., Cohn, D. M., Estes, B. T., Gimble, J. M., Liedtke, W., Chen, C. S. 2009. Control of stem cell fate by physical interactions with the extracellular matrix. *Cell Stem Cell.* 5: 17–26.

Han, Z. Z., Kong, H., Meng, J., Wang, C. Y., Xie, S. S., Xu, H. Y. 2008. Biological responses of endothelial cells to aligned nanofibers of MWNT/PU by electrospinning. *7th Asian-Pacific Conference on Medical and Biological Engineering, IFMBE Proceedings* 19: 194–197.

Ho, M. H., Liao, M. H., Lin, Y. L., Lai, C. H., Lin, P. I., Chen, R. M. 2014. Improving effects of chitosan nanofiber scaffolds on osteoblast proliferation and maturation. *Int J Nanomed.* 9: 4293–4304.

Horii, A., Wang, X., Gelain, F., Zhang, S. 2007. Biological designer self-assembling peptide nanofiber scaffolds significantly enhance osteoblast proliferation, differentiation and 3-D migration. *PLoS One.* 2(2): e190.

Hu, J., Feng, K., Liu, X., Ma, P. X. 2009. Chondrogenic and osteogenic differentiations of human bone marrow-derived mesenchymal stem cells on a nanofibrous scaffold with designed pore network. *Biomaterials.* 30: 5061–5067.

Jain, A., Betancur, M., Patel, G. D., Valmikinathan, C. M., Mukhatyar, V. J., Vakharia, A., Pai, S. B., Brahma, B., MacDonald, T. J., Bellamkonda, R. V. 2014. Guiding intracortical brain tumour cells to an extracortical cytotoxic hydrogel using aligned polymeric nanofibers. *Nat Mater.* 13: 308–316.

Kadler, K. E., Baldock, C., Bella, J., Boot-Handford, R. P. 2007. Collagen at a glance. *J Cell Sci.* 120: 1955–1958.

Kadler, K. E., Holmes, D. F., Trotter, J. A., Chapman, J. A. 1996. Collagen fibril formation. *Biochem J.* 316: 1–11.

Khang, G. 2012. *Hand Book of Intelligent Scaffolds for Tissue Engineering and Regenerative Medicine.* Pan Stanford Publishing Pte. Ltd., USA.

Kozel, B. A., Rongish, B. J., Czirok, A., Zach, J., Little, C. D., Davis, E. C., Knutsen, R. H., Wagenseil, J. E., Levy, M. A., Mecham, R. P. 2006. Elastic fiber formation: A dynamic view of extracellular matrix assembly using timer reporters. *J Cell Physiol.* 207: 87–96.

Lee, J. Y., Bashur, C. A., Gomez, N., Goldstein, A. S., Schmidt, C. E. 2010. Enhanced polarization of embryonic hippocampal neurons on micron scale electrospun fibers. *J Biomed Mater Res A.* 92: 1398–1406.

Leong, M. F., Chian, K. S., Mhaisalkar, P. S., Ong, W. F., Ratner, B. D. 2009. Effect of electrospun poly(D,L-lactide) fibrous scaffold with nanoporous surface on attachment of porcine esophageal epithelial cells and protein adsorption. *J Biomed Mater Res A.* 89: 1040–1048.

Liu, M., Li, Y., Yang, S. 2014. Expansion of human amniotic fluid stem cells in 3-dimensional fibrous scaffolds in a stirred bioreactor. *Biochem Eng J.* 82: 71–80.

Lubasová, D., Martinova, L. 2011. Controlled morphology of porous polyvinyl butyral nanofibers. *J Nanomater.* 2011: 292516.

Lubasová, D., Martinová, L., Mareková, D., Kostecká, P. 2010. *Cell Growth on Porous and Non-Porous Polycaprolactone Nanofibers.* Presented Nanocon 2010, Olomouc, Czech Republic, EU.

Masaeli, E., Wieringa, P. A., Morshed, M., Nasr-Esfahani, M. H., Sadri, S., Blitterswijk, C. A., Moroni, L. 2014. Peptide functionalized polyhydroxyalkanoate nanofibrous scaffolds enhance Schwann cells activity. *Nanomedicine.* 10: 1559–1569.

Mayne, R., Burgeson, R. 1987. *Structure and Function of Collagen Types.* Academic Press, Inc, Orlando, FL.

McBeath, R., Pirone, D. M., Nelson, C. M., Bhadriraju, K., Chen, C. S. 2004. Cell shape, cytoskeletal tension, and RhoA regulate stem cell lineage commitment. *Dev Cell.* 6: 483–495.

Midwood, K. S., Schwarzbauer, J. E. 2002. Elastic fibers: Building bridges between cells and their matrix. *Curr Biol.* 12: R279–R281.

Moroni, L., Licht, R., Boer, J., Wijn, J. R., Blitterswijk, C. A. 2006. Fiber diameter and texture of electrospun PEOT/PBT scaffolds influence human mesenchymal stem cell proliferation and morphology, and the release of incorporated compounds. *Biomaterials.* 27: 4911–4922.

Muiznieks, L. D., Keeley, F. W. 2013. Molecular assembly and mechanical properties of the extracel-
    lular matrix: A fibrous protein perspective. *Biochim Biophys Acta*. 1832: 866–875.
Neal, R. A., McClugage, S. G., Link, M. C., Sefcik, L. S., Ogle, R. C., Botchwey, E. A. 2009. Laminin
    nanofiber meshes that mimic morphological properties and bioactivity of basement mem-
    branes. *Tissue Eng C: Meth*. 15: 11–21.
Ottani, V., Raspanti, M., Ruggeri, A. 2001. Collagen structure and functional implications. *Micron*.
    32: 251–260.
Patel, S., Kurpinski, K., Quigley, R. et al. 2007. Bioactive nanofibers: Synergistic effects of nanotopog-
    raphy and chemical signaling on cell guidance. *Nano Lett*. 7: 2122–2128.
Prabhakaran, M. P., Venugopal, J. R., Chyan, T. T. et al. 2008. Electrospun biocomposite nanofibrous
    scaffolds for neural tissue engineering. *Tissue Eng A*. 14: 1787–1797.
Proseck, E., Buzgo, M., Rampichov, M. et al. 2012. Thin-layer hydroxyapatite deposition on a nano-
    fiber surface stimulates mesenchymal stem cell proliferation and their differentiation into
    osteoblasts. *J Biomed Biotechnol*. 2012: 428503.
Radhakrishnan, J., Kuppuswamy, A. A., Sethuraman, S., Subramanian, A. 2015. Topographic cue
    from electrospun scaffolds regulate myelin-related gene expressions in schwann cells. *J.
    Biomed. Nanotechnol*. 11: 512–521.
Ragetly, G., Griffon, D. J., Chung, Y. S. 2010. The effect of type II collagen coating of chitosan fibrous
    scaffolds on mesenchymal stem cell adhesion and chondrogenesis. *Acta Biomater*. 6: 3988–3997.
Ronchetti, I. P., Alessandrini, A., Contri, M. B. et al. 1998. Study of elastic fiber organization by scan-
    ning force microscopy, *Matrix Biol*. 17: 75–83.
Sage, H. 1982. Structure–function relationship in the evolution of elastin. *J. Invest. Dermatol*. 79:
    146s–153s.
Sharma, P., Sheets, K., Elankumaran, S., Nain, A. S. 2013. The mechanistic influence of aligned nano-
    fibers on cell shape, migration and blebbing dynamics of glioma cells. *Integr Biol*. 5: 1036–1044.
Sheets, K., Wunsch, S., Ng, C., Nain, A. S. 2013. Shape-dependent cell migration and focal adhesion
    organization on suspended and aligned nanofiber scaffolds. *Acta Biomater*. 9: 7169–7177.
Silver, F. H., Freeman, J. W., Seehra, G. P. 2003. Collagen self-assembly and the development of ten-
    don mechanical properties. *J Biomech*. 36: 1529–1553.
Singh, P., Schwarzbauer, J. E. 2012. Fibronectin and stem cell differentiation–lessons from chondro-
    genesis. *J Cell Sci*. 125: 3703–3712.
Singhvi, R., Stephanopoulos, G., Wang, D. I. C. 1994. Effects of substratum morphology on cell physi-
    ology. *Biotechnol Bioeng*. 43: 764–771.
Subramanian, A., Krishnan, U. M., Sethuraman, S. 2012a. Axially aligned electrically conducting
    biodegradable nanofibers for neural regeneration. *J Mater Sci Mater Med*. 23: 1797–1809.
Subramanian, A., Krishnan, U. M., Sethuraman, S. 2012b. Fabrication, characterization and *in vitro* eval-
    uation of aligned PLGA–PCL nanofibers for neural regeneration. *Ann Biomed Eng*. 40: 2098–2110.
Sun, H., Feng, K., Hu, J., Soker, S., Atala, A., Ma, P. X. 2010. Osteogenic differentiation of human
    amniotic fluid-derived stem cells induced by bone morphogenetic protein-7 and enhanced by
    nanofibrous scaffolds. *Biomaterials*. 31: 1133–1139.
Tai, B. C., Du, C., Gao, S., Wan, A. C., Ying, J. Y. 2010. The use of a polyelectrolyte fibrous scaffold to
    deliver differentiated hMSCs to the liver. *Biomaterials*. 31: 48–57.
Tarone, G., Galetto, G., Prat, M., Comoglio, M. 1982. Cell surface molecules and fibronectin-mediated
    cell adhesion: Effect of proteolytic digestion of membrane proteins. *J Cell Biol*. 94: 179–186.
Than, M. E., Henrich, S., Huber, R. et al. 2002. The 1.9-A crystal structure of the noncollagenous
    (NC1) domain of human placenta collagen IV shows stabilization via a novel type of covalent
    Met-Lys cross-link. *Proc Natl Acad Sci USA*. 99: 6607–6612.
Tian, H., Bharadwaj, S., Liu, Y. et al. 2010. Myogenic differentiation of human bone marrow mesen-
    chymal stem cells on a 3D nano fibrous scaffold for bladder tissue engineering. *Biomaterials*.
    31: 870–877.
Valmikinathan, C. M., Hoffman, J., Yu, X. 2011. Impact of scaffold micro and macro architecture
    on Schwann cell proliferation under dynamic conditions in a rotating wall vessel bioreactor.
    Mater Sci Eng C: Mater Biol Appl. 31: 22–29.

Vasanthan, K. S., Subramanian, A., Krishnan, U. M., Sethuraman, S. 2012. Role of biomaterials, therapeutic molecules and cells for hepatic tissue engineering. *Biotechnol Adv.* 30: 742–752.

Wang, J., Liu, X., Jin, X. et al. 2010. The odontogenic differentiation of human dental pulp stem cells on nanofibrous poly(L-lactic acid) scaffolds *in vitro* and *in vivo*. *Acta Biomater.* 6: 3856–3863.

Wang, J., Nain, A. S. 2014. Suspended micro/nanofiber hierarchical biological scaffolds fabricated using non-electrospinning STEP technique. *Langmuir.* 30: 13641–13649.

Woodfield, T. B., Miot, S., Martin, I., Blitterswijk, C. A., Riesle, J. 2006. The regulation of expanded human nasal chondrocyte re-differentiation capacity by substrate composition and gas plasma surface modification. *Biomaterials.* 27: 1043–1053.

Wozniak, M. A., Modzelewska, K., Kwong, L., Keely, P. J. 2004. Focal adhesion regulation of cell behavior. *Biochimica et Biophysica Acta.* 1692: 103–119.

Xu, C., Yang, F., Wang, S., Ramakrishna, S. 2004. *In vitro* study of human vascular endothelial cell function on materials with various surface roughness. *J Biomed Mater Res A.* 71: 154–161.

Xu, Y., Patnaik, S., Guo, X. et al. 2014. Cardiac differentiation of cardiosphere-derived cells in scaffolds mimicking morphology of the cardiac extracellular matrix. *Acta Biomater.* 10: 3449–3462.

Yim, E. K., Wan, A. C., Le Visage, C., Liao, I. C., Leong, K. W. 2006. Proliferation and differentiation of human mesenchymal stem cell encapsulated in polyelectrolyte complexation fibrous scaffold. *Biomaterials.* 27: 6111–6122.

Yin, Z., Chen, X., Chen, J. L. et al. 2010. The regulation of tendon stem cell differentiation by the alignment of nanofibers. *Biomaterials.* 31: 2163–2175.

Zhu, Y., Wang, A., Shen, W. et al. 2010. Nanofibrous patches for spinal cord regeneration. *Adv Funct Mater.* 20: 1433–1440.

Section II

Skeletal Tissue Engineering

3

Nanofibrous Scaffolds for the Regeneration of Bone Tissue

Sai Rama Krishna Meka, Sachin Kumar, and Kaushik Chatterjee

CONTENTS

3.1 Introduction

Bone pathology leads to serious challenges for an individual's physical activity and survival. Large bone defects in most cases become irreversible. The regenerative capacity of most tissues, including the bone, decelerates with age and its associated pathological conditions. Surgical and therapeutic interventions are practiced as alternatives to natural healing and repair. In particular, for bone repair, substitutes such as grafts (autograft or allograft) and permanent implants are the conventional approaches. Common risks involve multiple surgeries, immune rejection, failure due to nonintegration, and subsequent side effects.

The growing demand for improved and lasting solutions to bone pathologies necessitates engineering a bone-like tissue substitute. Ideally, the properties of the scaffold must closely mimic that of the bone to support regeneration and subsequent integration with the surrounding tissue through the normal healing process. Bone tissue engineering is aimed at accelerating the healing process and imparting the regenerative capacity through a variety of bone-like three-dimensional (3D) scaffolds, when combined with ideal biomaterial properties, bone stimulants, and bone precursor cells. Among many types of scaffolds relevant to bone tissue engineering, nanofibrous scaffolds are particularly promising and thus are being widely investigated.

Nanofibrous scaffolds mimic the architecture of the extracellular matrix (ECM) of native bone tissues that facilitates bone regeneration. ECM of bone tissue comprises both organic (collagenous and noncollagenous proteins) and inorganic (calcium phosphate/mineral crystals). The collagenous nanofibers (50–500 nm in diameter) that are the major components of the organic phase give resilience, whereas the inorganic component imparts stiffness to the bone tissue (Bandyopadhyay-Ghosh, 2008). The electrospinning technique is widely used to prepare such nanofibrous scaffolds for bone tissue engineering. In this chapter, we review the basic principles of electrospinning to prepare the nanofibrous scaffolds and also the recent advances in the technique to generate more complex 3D scaffolds for efficient tissue generation. We also highlight the variety of nanofibrous architecture and material compositions that have been successfully fabricated.

3.2 Fabrication Methods for Preparing Nanofibers

Electrospinning is a simple and cost-efficient technique that has emerged as a popular technique to produce nanostructured fibers for a variety of biomedical applications including drug delivery and tissue scaffolds. With the ease of handling and the ability to tune parameters, electrospun fibers of desired fiber diameters ranging from tens of nanometers to several micrometers can be prepared. The basic electrospinning setup is as shown in Figure 3.1a. The principle of electrospinning technique involves the application of an electric field to overcome the surface tension of the ejecting polymer solution such that a thin liquid jet ejects to form the fibrous network onto a collector as the solvent evaporates. This process is primarily governed by three sets of parameters as follows: (i) intrinsic properties of the polymer solution such as the polymer molecular weight (Koski et al., 2004), concentration (Yang et al., 2004), conductivity (Huang et al., 2006), surface tension (Thompson et al., 2007), and its viscosity (Koski et al., 2004), etc.; (ii) working conditions such as flow

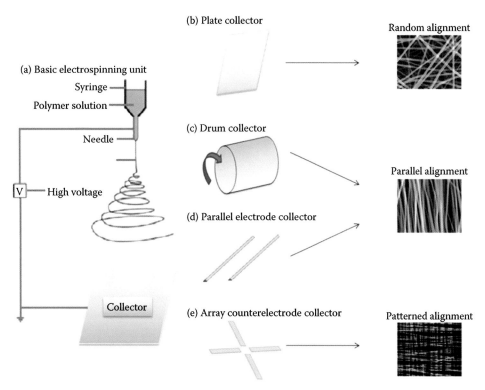

FIGURE 3.1
Schematic illustration of electrospinning process to obtain nanofibers of different alignments. (a) Design of basic electrospinning unit. (b) Random aligned nanofibers obtained through plate collector. (c,d) Parallel aligned nanofibers obtained through drum and parallel electrode collector. (e) Patterned aligned nanofibers obtained through array counter electrode as collector.

rate (Zuo et al., 2005), voltage (Deitzel et al., 2001), working distance between the needle/spinneret and the collector (Zuo et al., 2005), and the choice of the collector (Li et al., 2004); and (iii) environmental conditions such as temperature (Mit-uppatham et al., 2004) and humidity (Casper et al., 2004). These parameters can be tuned to generate a wide variety of fibrous networks with desired physicochemical properties that find use in biomedical applications such as tissue regeneration and drug delivery. In this section, we discuss the conventional design of an electrospinning apparatus and some recent advancement in its design to achieve complex nanostructured fibers for tissue engineering. We also highlight the associated advantages and drawbacks of these designs and the scaffolds obtained as summarized in Table 3.1.

3.2.1 Two Dimensional or Thin Nanofibrous Mats

Two-dimensional (2D)-thin nanofibrous mats can be obtained using a basic electrospinning apparatus with a flat collector (Figure 3.1). The mats collected on a flat collector exhibit random alignment with continuous fibers of desired diameter. The fiber morphology can be varied by either modifying the design of the collector or the spinneret. The fiber mat is thin and typically the cell migration into the mat is minimal such that these mats may be considered as pseudo-3D or essentially 2D-nanofibrous scaffolds.

TABLE 3.1

Strategies Adapted to Electrospinning to Obtain 3D-Nanofibrous Scaffolds

Technique	Advantages	Disadvantages	References
Postelectrospinning modifications	Prepare desired patterns	Time consuming, large gaps between adjacent mats	Nam et al. (2007), Leung et al. (2012), Shim et al. (2010), Wang et al. (2008), Wang et al. (2010), Soliman et al. (2010), Pham et al. (2006), Madurantakam et al. (2013), Kidoaki et al. (2005), Erisken et al. (2008), Beachley et al. (2014), Smit et al. (2005), Teo et al. (2007), Yousefzadeh et al. (2012)
Multilayering	Control on thickness porosity and number of layers spun	Time consuming	Wang et al. (2010), Soliman et al. (2010), Pham et al. (2006), Madurantakam et al. (2013), Kidoaki et al. (2005)
Collection process liquid-assisted collection	Larger pore size could be obtained	Additional molding and freezing process required	Erisken et al. (2008), Beachley et al. (2014), Smit et al. (2005), Teo et al. (2007), Yousefzadeh et al. (2012)
Template-assisted collection	Control over patterns, porosity, thickness, and mechanical properties	Prerequisite of templates	Teo et al. (2007), Hong et al. (2011), Ki et al. (2007), Martins et al. (2009)
Textile technology	Large-scale production, different architectures, high mechanical strength	Complexity in the integration of textile processing	Beachley et al. (2014), Park et al. (2008), Schneider et al. (2009), Vaquette and Cooper-White (2011), Blair (2015), Zhou and Gong (2008), Joseph et al. (2015), Ali et al. (2011), Ali et al. (2012)

3.2.1.1 Collectors for Random and Aligned Nanofibers

Flat metal collectors yield continuous random nanofibrous mats (Figure 3.1b). The nanotopography of random nanofiber-induced responses in human mesenchymal stromal cells (hMSCs), similar to osteogenic supplements, led to osteogenic differentiation (Liu et al., 2013). The control of the cell shape due to the nanofibrous structure is believed to play an important role (Kumar et al., 2011). A rotating drum or parallel electrode collecting system is used to prepare parallel aligned fibers (Figure 3.1c and d) and array of counterelectrodes (Figure 3.1e) to prepare patterned aligned fibers (Liao et al., 2012). Controlled cellular orientation can be obtained by aligning fibrous substrates, which can be used to direct the attachment, morphology, mobility, and proliferation of the stem cells and also to direct their fate (Kolambkar et al., 2013; Lee et al., 2013).

Recently, Liu et al. reported that the randomly oriented poly(caprolactone) (PCL) nanofibers promoted osteogenic differentiation of hMSCs than the parallely aligned fibrous substrates (Liu et al., 2013). In addition, Kolambkar et al. reported that aligned nanofiber substrates prepared from PCL and surfaces coated with type-I collagen-mimetic peptide (GFOGER motif) did not influence osteogenic differentiation besides displaying enhanced cell migration along the direction of fiber orientation compared to random fibers. They concluded that the lower alkaline phosphatase (ALP) activity and mineral deposition on the aligned fibers could be due to enhanced hMSC migration (Kolambkar et al., 2013).

However, Lee et al. demonstrated that the aligned nanofiber mesh provided spatial guidance for hMSC migration *in vitro* as well as bone formation *in vivo* (Lee et al., 2013).

3.2.1.2 Spinneret Designs for Core–Sheath Nanofibers

As tissue scaffolds, electrospun polymer nanofibers not only provide support for cell attachment, but can also be used for the release of incorporated drugs to stimulate tissue formation. The properties of the fiber mats such as morphology and polymer composition can be varied to tailor the release profiles of the encapsulated drugs (Li et al., 2010; Su et al., 2012). To overcome limitations such as burst release and ensure the stability of labile biomolecules and drugs during the electrospinning process, core–shell nanofibrous structures were developed using various designs of the spinnerets as shown in Figure 3.2a. In addition, it has been proposed that the tailored release of a combination of multiple drugs and growth factors can offer an efficient therapeutic strategy for the treatment of disease and tissue regeneration simultaneously (Su et al., 2012). Thus, coaxial spinnerets have been designed to obtain core–shell polymer bilayered nanofibers carrying individual therapeutic molecules in the separate layers of the core and the outer sheath of fibers (Yu et al., 2015). Therapeutic molecules can also be coelectrospun in a core–shell format along with the mineral components such as silica particles for enhancing the mechanical properties of the fiber matrix and for sustained release of drugs to promote generation (Kang et al., 2015).

Su et al. prepared core–shell structures of poly(L-lactide-*co*-caprolactone) (PLLACL)-collagen fibers to demonstrate the controlled and tailored release of bone morphogenic protein-2 (BMP-2) and dexamethasone when compared to their release from blended electrospun fibers (Su et al., 2012). Further, this controlled release of growth factors from core–shell structures enhanced osteogenic differentiation of hMSCs. Recently, Kang et al.

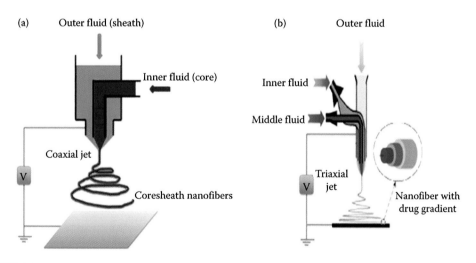

FIGURE 3.2

Schematic illustration of spinneret designs to obtain different layered morphology within a nanofiber for tailored drug release. (a) Coaxial spinneret. (Reproduced from Li, F., Song, Y., Zhao, Y. 2010. Core–shell nanofibers: Nano channel and capsule by coaxial electrospinning. In *Nanofibers*, ed., Kumar A., InTech Open Access Publisher. With permission.) (b) Triaxial spinneret. (Reprinted with permission from Yu, D. G., Li, X., Wang, X., Yang, J., Bligh, S. A., Williams, G. R. 2015. Nanofibers fabricated using triaxial electrospinning as zero order drug delivery systems. *ACS Appl Mater Interfaces*. 7: 18891–18897. Copyright 2015. American Chemical Society.)

developed core–shell structures with poly(ethylene oxide) (PEO) as the core and PCL as the sheath in which the dual growth factors, fibroblast growth factor-18 (FGF-18), an osteogenic enhancer encapsulated in mesoporous bioactive glass nanospheres and fibroblast growth factor-2 (FGF-2), an angiogenic stimulator were incorporated into the PEO core. Such a system ensures the sequential release of fast-releasing FGF-2 and slow-releasing FGF-18 from the nanospheres, thus, enhancing the bone formation in rat calvarial defects (Kang et al., 2015). More recently, trilayered ethyl cellulose nanofibers were obtained through triaxial electrospinning using a novel triaxial spinneret (Figure 3.2b) to encapsulate ketoprofen with increasing concentration from the outer to the inner layer. Yu summarized that such a design helps in obtaining nanofibers with sophisticated structural features and ensures the linear release pattern of the drug (Yu et al., 2015).

Other notable spinneret designs include multiple jets/spinnerets (also discussed in Section 3.2.2.2) for coelectrospinning/simultaneous electrospinning from two or more spinnerets to increase the pore size (Tian et al., 2014) or simultaneous electrospinning and electrospraying from two different spinnerets (Francis et al., 2010) to improve the bioactivity of the fibrous substrates. Francis et al. reported that the simultaneous electrospinning of gelatin nanofibers with electrospraying of hydroxyapatite (HA) nanoparticles enhanced human fetal osteoblast proliferation and mineralization when compared to gelatin/HA fibrous substrates (Francis et al., 2010).

3.2.1.3 Postelectrospinning Surface Modifications

Coelectrospinning or electrospinning of polymer solution mixed with various nanoparticles is a common process to improve biomechanical properties of nanofibers. However, the ceramic particles loaded in the polymer fibers might not be completely exposed to the surface of the composite scaffolds where cells come in contact. The increase in nanoparticulate concentration could improve the outcome, but restricts the electrospinnability. To improve the surface properties of the nanofibers to stimulate desired cellular responses such as cell attachment, mineralization, and subsequent tissue formation, several mineralized bone-forming nanofibrous substrates were reported. In particular, postelectrospinning processing methods such as incubation or soaking of electrospun scaffolds in calcium phosphate solutions (Ravichandran et al., 2012), simulated body fluid (SBF) (C. He et al., 2014), and electrodeposition (C. He et al., 2014) were developed.

Initial studies were conducted by simple incubation of electrospun scaffolds in calcium phosphate solutions for substantial precipitation of bone-like minerals to obtain the osteophilic microenvironment showing improved osteogenic and mineralization profiles of bone precursor cells (Ravichandran et al., 2012; Meng et al., 2013). Recently, Singh et al. (2015) demonstrated novel multifunctional nanobiomatrix platform for bone regeneration and as a delivery vehicle. Here, sol–gel approach was adopted to coat the electrospun PCL nanofibers with mesoporous silica (PCL–MS) where the MS shell provides a bioactive interface covering the PCL surface with increased wettability and subsequent bone-like mineral formation upon incubation with body-simulated medium. Further, these composite fibers performed better biomechanical properties with improved osteogenic differentiation of rat mesenchymal stem cells (rMSCs). Similar postelectrospinning modification technique was reported by Ha et al. (2013), where the blend solution of polyvinyl acetate (PVAc) and isocyanato propyl dimethyl silyl cyclohexyl polyhedral oligosilsesquioxane (POSS macromer) was electrospun. Silicification of the mats was done subsequently by soaking in hydrolyzed silane solution. This composite scaffold provided improved mechanical and mineralization properties.

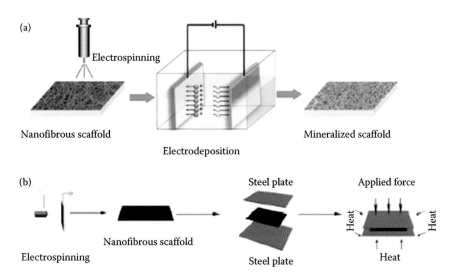

FIGURE 3.3
Schematic illustration of postelectrospinning modifications for 2D-nanofibrous mats. (a) Electrodeposition postelectrospinning. (Reprinted from *Acta Biomater.*, 10, He, C., Jin, X., Ma, P. X., Calcium phosphate deposition rate, structure and osteoconductivity on electrospun poly (L-lactic acid) matrix using electrodeposition or simulated body fluid incubation, 419–427, Copyright (2014), with permission from Elsevier.) (b) Heat and compression molding process on nanofibrous scaffolds. (Reprinted from *Mater Sci Eng B.*, 176, Cao, D., Fu, Z., Li, C., Heat and compression molded electrospun poly(L-lactide) membranes: Preparation and characterization, 900–905, Copyright 2011, with permission from Elsevier.)

In addition, electrodeposition postelectrospinning as shown in Figure 3.3a was reported (Ravichandran et al., 2012). Here, He et al. (2013) compared the mineralization rate by MC3T3 cells between surface mineralized composite nanofibrous mats prepared by either electrodeposition of calcium and phosphate precursor solutions or soaking in SBF. The electrodeposited mineralized scaffolds showed two to three orders of magnitude mineralization faster than the SBF method with reduction in mineralization time from 2 weeks to 1 hour. In a different postelectrospin modification, surface entrapment and surface entrapment-graft techniques are used where, poly(lactide-*co*-glycolide) (PLGA) nanofibrous mats were soaked either in gelatin or sodium alginate/gelatin solutions, which improved hydrophilicity as well as the tensile strength (Meng et al., 2012).

Further, to improve tensile strength of electrospun membranes, Cao et al. (2011) proposed heat-assisted compression of poly-L-lactide (PLLA)-electrospun mats as shown in Figure 3.3b. This approach helps to crystallize in alpha form and introduce strong fiber-to-fiber linkages (Cao et al., 2011). Besides surface modification, increase in pore size is important for cell infiltration and further tissue ingrowth by coelectrospinning with sacrificial/ water-soluble polymers (Whited et al., 2011; Phipps et al., 2012). In a study conducted by Phipps et al. (2012), a water-soluble sacrificial polymer PEO was mixed with the PCL/collagen/HA for coelectrospinning. This blend has shown to improve pore size after washing in water with subsequent greater cell infiltration shown in mouse calvaria/scaffold after 8 days of culture (Phipps et al., 2012).

3.2.2 3D Thick and Macroporous Nanofibrous Structures

Although 2D-thin nanofibrous structures are obtained with a basic electrospinning setup, these fibrous mats lack sufficient mechanical integrity for use as implants in hard tissue regeneration and the pore size is not optimal for cellular infiltration and vascularization—important events in bone tissue regeneration (Nam et al., 2007). To overcome these limitations, several novel strategies have been developed and adapted in the electrospinning setup. These designs could further be categorized under four sections namely, postelectrospinning modifications, multilayered electrospinning, template- or liquid-assisted collectors, and textile engineering as summarized in Table 2.1.

3.2.2.1 Postelectrospinning Processing

3D scaffolds are prepared from thin electrospun fibrous mats by postprocessing, such as folding (Leung et al., 2012), rolling (Shim et al., 2009), or mechanical expansion (Shim et al., 2010) of fiber mats to obtain scaffolds of desired shapes with variable thickness. However, 3D-macrostructured scaffolds obtained by folding of many aligned nanofiber sheets leads to large gaps between the folds and thus the cell attachment is seen only on the 2D surface. It fails to form bridges between folds making the process inefficient to prepare thicker scaffolds (Leung et al., 2012). The rolled macrostructures were first developed with double-layered chitosan nano/microfibers (Wang et al., 2008). Here, chitosan nanofibers were electrospun on the surface of previously spun microfibers and, finally, the double-layered fibrous meshes were rolled to develop a cylindrical shape.

Mechanical expansion of as-spun PLLA microfibers lead to thick 3D-microporous structures, which was shown to enhance osteoblast proliferation and cell infiltration when compared to 2D fibrous mats. These modified structures were further demonstrated for enhanced bone formation *in vivo* in rat calvarial defects (Shim et al., 2010). However, such expansion has not been adapted for nanofibrous mats, but could offer a clue in expanding submicron fibrous mats. In a recent study, Wang and Yu developed integrated scaffolds where spiral PCL nanofibrous scaffolds were inserted into sintered PLGA tubular microstructures as shown in Figure 3.4a. These integrated scaffolds were shown to have good porosity and compressive strength, which augmented osteoblast proliferation, cellular infiltration, and matrix mineralization when compared to sintered PLGA tubular

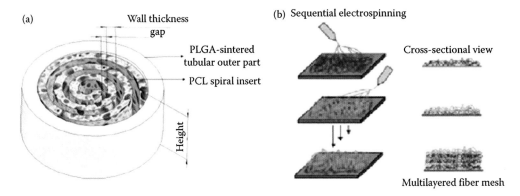

FIGURE 3.4
Schematic illustration of 3D-nanofibrous scaffold formation through (a) spiral PCL nanofibrous mats integrated into PLGA-sintered tubular structures. (Reprinted from *Acta Biomater.*, 6, Wang, J., Yu, X., Preparation, characterization and *in vitro* analysis of novel structured nanofibrous scaffolds for bone tissue engineering, 3004–3012, Copyright 2010, with permission from Elsevier.) (b) Multilayering through sequential electrospinning. (Reprinted from *Biomaterials*, 26, Kidoaki, S., Kwon, I. K., Matsuda, T., Mesoscopic spatial designs of nano- and microfiber meshes for tissue-engineering matrix and scaffold based on newly devised multilayering and mixing electrospinning techniques, 37–46, Copyright 2005, with permission from Elsevier.)

structures (Wang and Yu, 2010). The postelectrospinning modification process being slow and inefficient render them unsuitable for large-scale production. Thus, new strategies to prepare 3D substrates suited for fast and large-scale production are being explored.

3.2.2.2 Multilayered Electrospinning

Relative to many advanced 3D designs, multilayered electrospinning is a slow and complex process involving the use of mixed/coelectrospinning (Soliman et al., 2010) and sequential electrospinning (Kidoaki et al., 2005; Pham et al., 2006; Madurantakam et al., 2013) as depicted in Figure 3.4b. However, the significant advantage of multilayering is the precise control over fiber diameter, porosity, thickness, and number of layers, all of which significantly influence cell behavior. Erisken et al. demonstrated the fabrication of functionally graded nonwoven meshes of PCL incorporated with tricalcium phosphate (TCP) nanoparticles using a new hybrid twin-screw extrusion/electrospinning (TSEE) process (Erisken et al., 2008). Further, this hybrid mesh is proposed to mimic the bone–cartilage interface. Most recently, Beachley et al. designed a collecting device that uses electrostatic forces to deposit aligned nanofibers between two computer-controlled parallel mobile tracks. This mobile collector allows for continuous distribution and assembly of aligned and crisscrossed nanofiber arrays into composite sheets with tunable fiber density (Beachley et al., 2014).

3.2.2.3 Macrostructures Obtained by Specific Collection Technique

To enable rapid and large-scale production of 3D-nanofibrous scaffolds with macrostructures several designs have been proposed in the collection process, which include liquid-assisted collection and template-assisted collection. Water-based liquid-assisted collection process as shown in Figure 3.5a is used to collect aligned micro/nanoelectrospun fiber arrays with the help of a water reservoir collector or a water vortex (Smit et al., 2005; Teo et al., 2007; Yousefzadeh et al., 2012). Hierarchically organized PCL 3D-nanofibrous meshes were fabricated using a water vortex in which the PCL 3D meshes were collected and placed in a mold (Teo et al., 2008). These were either dried at room temperature or freeze dried. The freeze-dried meshes showed visible porous structure when compared to compact structure without pores obtained by drying.

Water can be replaced with low surface tension solvents such as methanol or ethanol where thick 3D-fibrous structures of PCL, silk fibroin, and PLGA were deposited into liquid bath following which fluffy stacks electrospun fibers get accumulated (Ki et al., 2007; Hong and Kim, 2011). Finally, foamed-3D structures were formed with subsequent freezing at low temperatures, which has pores larger than 2D fibrous structures as shown in Figure 3.5b making them attractive for tissue regeneration. The drawback of this process is the need of an additional setup for molding and freezing process. Template-assisted collection includes microfibrous templates (Martins et al., 2009), mechanical templates (Zhang and Chang, 2008), and patterned templates (Wang et al., 2009). Microfibers prepared by either prototyping (Martins et al., 2009) or melt spinning (Martins et al., 2009) act as fibrous templates on which the nanofibers are electrospun to form nano/microfibrous structures (Park et al., 2008) as shown in Figure 3.5c through e.

Zhang et al. introduced 3D mechanical collectors to collect nanofibers with 3D macrostructures using manipulation of electric field and electric forces (Zhang and Chang, 2008). This technique is helpful in fabricating micro/macrotubes of different morphologies and interconnections. Schneider et al. fabricated cotton-wool-like nanocomposites by using a rotating drum collector and evaluated its performance as bone substitute material *in vitro* and *in vivo* (Schneider et al., 2009). Patterned templates comprise tailored collectors usually

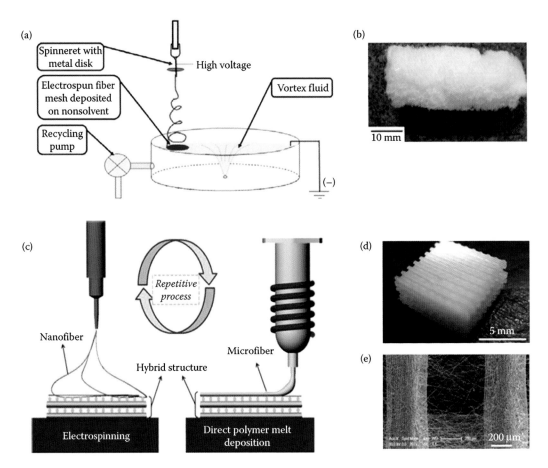

FIGURE 3.5
Schematic illustration of collector designs. (a) Water/liquid vortex-assisted collector. (From Yousefzadeh, M. et al. 2012. *J Eng Fibr Fabr.* 7. With permission.) (b) Freeze-dried PCL 3D mesh with visible pores collected from liquid vortex. (From Teo, W. et al. 2008. *Curr Nanosci.* 4: 361–369. With permission.) (c) Hybrid scaffolds containing microfibers and nanofiber matrices built through electrospinning over microfibers as template prepared through melt deposition. (d) Photograph of the overall 3D woodpile structure with dimensions of 9 mm × 9 mm × 3.5 mm. (e) Magnified SEM image of the hybrid basic unit layer composed of microfibers and the electrospun nanofibers matrix. (Reprinted from *Acta Biomater*, 4, Park, S. H. et al. Development of dual scale scaffolds via direct polymer melt deposition and electrospinning for applications in tissue regeneration, 1198–1207, Copyright 2008, with permission from Elsevier.)

of meshes of different orientations to increase pore size for cell penetration, thickness, and mechanical properties (Wang et al., 2009; Vaquette and Cooper-White, 2011).

3.2.2.4 Textile Technology

The major drawback in many designs of the electrospinning unit is that the nanofibers obtained are nonwoven meshes/fluffy mass of small size or of weak strength. This could restrain their final application in tissue engineering (Blair, 2015). Integrating industrial processing or textile technology through various collector designs to the electrospinning setup would benefit in efficient yarning and further processing to braided, knitted, and woven textile constructs with controlled architecture and high mechanical strength (Zhou

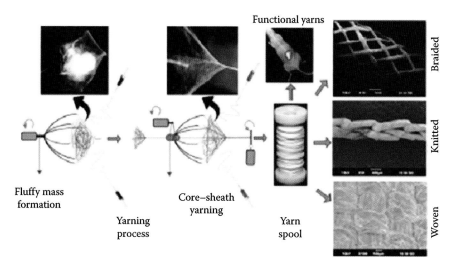

FIGURE 3.6
Schematic illustration of integrating substrate-less electrospinning with textile technology. (Reprinted with permission from Joseph, J., Nair, S. V., Menon, D. Integrating substrate-less electrospinning with textile technology for creating biodegradable 3D structures. *Nano Lett.* 15, 5420–5426. Copyright 2015 American Chemical Society.)

and Gong, 2008; Ali et al., 2011; Joseph et al., 2015). Thus, the fabricated nano/microtextiles could be employed in various biomedical and tissue engineering applications (Zhou and Gong, 2008; Ali et al., 2011). This process is an adaptation from the conventional textile processing where the continuous yarns were drawn and further weaved from fluffy cotton. Successful yarning is obtained by electrospinning deposition onto specialized collectors such as liquid targets (Teo et al., 2007), funnel targets (Ali et al., 2012; J. X. He et al., 2014), and dual ring electrodes (M. Li et al., 2008). More recently, Joseph et al. developed a new open collector design, which permitted substrate-less formation of fluffy mass at a single plane upon electrospinning. This allowed for rapid formation of continuous high-strength drug/dye-loaded core–sheath yarns with controlled architecture (Joseph et al., 2015) as shown in Figure 3.6. Here, they demonstrated the integration of substrate-less electrospinning with textile processing for creating biodegradable 3D structures for biomedical applications.

In addition, Cai et al. have developed 3D-macroporous scaffolds from aligned electro-spun PLLA/PCL nanofibrous yarns, processed through sequential yarning and honey-combing assembling at 65°C. Here, they demonstrated its potential use for bone tissue regeneration by evaluating its performance *in vitro* and *in vivo*. *In vitro* studies showed enhanced proliferation and penetration of human embryonic stem-cell-derived mesen-chymal stem cells with detectable mineralization. Furthermore, studies with rabbit tibia bone-defect model showed that this novel scaffold allowed bony tissue formation around the scaffold as well as inside the scaffold at 3 weeks and 6 weeks *in vivo* (Cai et al., 2012).

3.3 Polymers for Electrospinning

The inherent ability of electrospinning techniques to generate nanofiber scaffold resem-bling native ECM has opened new frontier in tissue engineering. For electrospinning, polymeric materials are used to prepare polymeric nanofibers scaffold. Over the years, polymer-derived scaffolds are gaining importance in tissue engineering, which include natural and synthetic polymers and their blends as compiled in Figure 3.7.

3.3.1 Natural Biopolymers for Bone Tissue Engineering

Polymeric scaffolds prepared from naturally derived polymers have shown great potential in tissue engineering applications including bone regeneration. The major advantage is that the scaffold presents a cellular microenvironment that closely mimics the ECM. Biopolymers present in the ECM-derived scaffolds have been shown to influence cellular morphology and functions (Sellaro et al., 2007; Zvibel et al., 2013). In bone tissue engineering, researchers are working on creating biological substitute biomaterials to repair bone tissue defects (Burg et al., 2000; Mallick, 2014). Naturally derived biopolymers set the baseline and also provide critical clues for upgrading and developing new biomaterials with desired functionality. The natural biomedical biopolymers comprise polysaccharide biopolymers (cellulose, chitosan, chitin, and alginate) and protein-based biopolymers (collagen, gelatin, elastin, and silk). These biopolymers are derived from animal- and plant-based sources. Among natural biopolymers collagen, gelatin, chitosan, elastin, silk fibroin, and keratin are some of the most commonly used for bone tissue engineering.

Collagen, a biopolymer, is the most abundant constituent of ECM for both hard and soft tissues in the human body. Collagen provides mechanical stability to the ECM network and also regulates cellular responses through biochemical signals (Badylak et al., 2009). There are more than 20 different forms of collagen present in nature. Most of them are

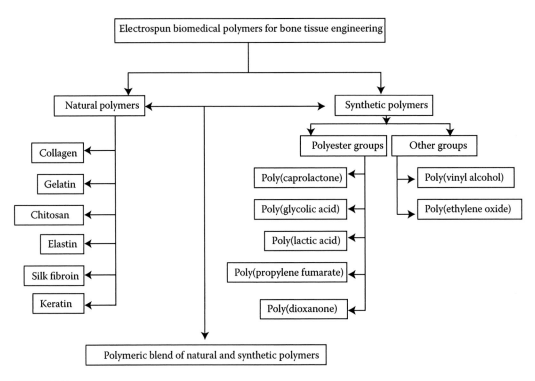

FIGURE 3.7
List of most frequently used natural and synthetic biomedical polymers for bone tissue engineering.

found as fibrillar network structures supporting different tissue architectures and their integrity. Collagen with its several key advantages such as good cytocompatibilty, hydrophilic nature, biodegradability, and limited antigenecity is extensively utilized for tissue engineering (Chevallay and Herbage, 2000; Boccafoschi et al., 2005). Collagen-based biomaterials have shown to evoke little foreign reaction with no fibrous encapsulation (Lee et al., 2001; Seal et al., 2001). Researchers have demonstrated that the electrospun nanofibers of collagen can closely mimic the structure of the natural ECM (Matthews et al., 2002).

1. *Gelatin* is derived from collagen by hydrolysis. Besides being a derivative of collagen, it is soluble in water and many polar solvents thereby making it an attractive biopolymer for biological application. Gelatin exhibits properties such as high biodegradability, no antigenecity, and most importantly it is cost efficient (Zhang et al., 2009). Gelatin also exhibits hemostatic property; it activates coagulation cascade on in contact with blood and facilitates wound healing (Kim et al., 2009). Collagen-derived gelatin nanofibers are often used to prepare scaffolds for bone tissue regeneration (Sisson et al., 2010). Some of its limitations are its gelling property at room temperature and very rapid degradation rates. Thus, gelatin is cross-linked to improve its structural stability and degradability. During cross-linking it is critical to select a chemical cross-linker with minimal cytotoxicity.

2. *Chitosan* is a linear polysaccharide derived from chitin found in shells of crustaceans such as crabs, shrimps, lobsters, etc. Chitosan is a cationic biopolymer with high charge density on its surface. The large positive charge density on chitosan has encouraged researchers to use chitosan as a nongene-transfection system (Borchard, 2001; Mansouri et al., 2004). The intrinsic bactericidal property of chitosan provides an additional advantage to chitosan for use in tissue engineering. Chitosan as a broad spectrum biopolymer promotes osteoblast growth and mineralization, and thus chitosan-based nanofibers have been used for bone regeneration (Klokkevold et al., 1996; I.-Y. Kim et al., 2008; Y. Zhang et al., 2008).

3. *Elastin* is a protein-based biopolymer usually insoluble in aqueous and organic solvents, which limits their processability; however, hydrolysis of elastin can overcome these limitations. Elastin is a constituent of natural ECM providing elasticity to tissues and organs, in particular as a significant component of the walls of blood arteries and veins, skin, and intestines (Rodgers and Weiss, 2005). Nanofibers of elastin were envisaged to provide properties similar to that of tissues. Elastin is shown to regulate cell adhesion, morphology, signaling, and physiology (Duca et al., 2004). It is reported to be an excellent biomaterial for tissues such as skin and arteries (Klein et al., 2001; Boland et al., 2004; Daamen et al., 2007). One major problem with elastin fibers is calcification under physiological conditions. Elastin serves as a nucleation site for mineralization (Paule et al., 1992). Researchers have utilized the calcification property of elastin for bone tissue engineering (Amruthwar and Janorkar, 2013).

4. *Silk fibroin* is obtained from aqueous rejuvenated silkworm silk solution. Silk being semicrystalline biopolymer with high mechanical strength has been used in textile industry, but silk has gained tremendous attention as a biomaterial for tissue engineering application in recent years. Electrospun silk fibroin nanofibers can support growth, proliferation, and differentiation of cells. Due to high biocompatibility, biodegradability, and good mechanical properties, electrospun silk fibroin

is considered as potential biopolymers for bone tissue engineering (Jin et al., 2004; Kim et al., 2005).

5. *Keratin is* the most abundant protein biopolymer found in the animal kingdom. It is a major component of hair, nails, horns, and feathers. As a result, keratin can be easily and economically sourced. Keratin forms intermolecular disulfide bonds with its surrounding chains, which provides high strength to keratin fibers. Keratin being an insoluble biopolymer is very difficult to process as a biomaterial. Researchers have tried different methods to prepare soluble keratin by alkaline and acid treatments. As keratin is a structural protein of skin, keratin scaffolds are shown to help in proliferation and differentiation of keratinocytes (Van Dyke, 2012a,b). Recently, researchers have started to exploit keratin-based scaffolds for bone tissue engineering (Blanchard et al., 1999; Van Dyke, 2014).

3.3.1.1 Application of Electrospun Natural Biopolymers in Bone Tissue Engineering

In tissue engineering, designing biomaterials that can recapitulate the structural and biological properties of the ECM is a challenge. Natural ECM helps cells to attach and organize on the ECM fiber mesh. ECM-derived biopolymers are considered to be key modulators for cellular attachment, proliferation, and differentiation (Lu et al., 2004). Figure 3.8 schematically represents cell adhesion on natural biopolymer-derived nanofibers facilitated by transmembrane interaction through binding of focal adhesion (integrin) to the natural adhesive proteins on electrospun biopolymer fibers.

During cell growth on biopolymer nanofiber, cells interact with nanofiber mat in a manner similar to that seen for interactions with native ECM which mediate cell attachment, morphology, migration, growth, and differentiation (Petreaca and Martins-Green, 2013). The presence of cell-recognizing motifs and proteins on many of the biopolymer-derived

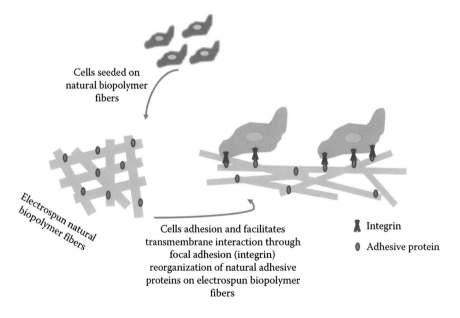

FIGURE 3.8
Schematic illustration of cell adhesion on natural biopolymer-derived nanofibers facilitated by transmembrane interactions.

nanofibers facilitates transmembrane interactions through focal adhesions. These interactions help in transferring signals from the biomaterial surface across the cell membrane to the cytoplasm and then into cell nucleus in turn influencing cell functions (Badylak et al., 2009). Furthermore, electrospun thin porous films on the surface of hard bioimplant offered an active interface between the implant and the host tissue. The presence of polymeric fiber on the hard implant surface also tends to reduce mismatch of stiffness at the material–tissue interface (Buchko et al., 2001).

For electrospun biopolymer-based scaffolds, processing conditions, mechanical and surface properties, fiber diameter, porosity, and degradability are critical to guide cell response (Mano et al., 2007). Figure 3.9 schematically shows how the scaffold fiber diameter (macro and nanosize) influences cells morphology and their interaction with fibers. Combination of macro- and nanofibers significantly enhances cell behavior due to unique macro–nanopattern morphology of the scaffold.

MG63 osteoblasts cultured on gelatin-electrospun fiber having different fiber diameter showed different responses. Osteoblasts showed better migration and penetrated into the electrospun matrix with larger diameter while more differentiation was observed on scaffolds with smaller fiber diameter. Hence, this study suggested cells have the ability to perceive variation in fiber diameter and differences in pore size to modify their response (Sisson et al., 2010). Stem cells have shown better osteogenic differentiation on silk-based scaffolds in comparison to collagen. High strength, slow degradation with Arg-Gly-Asp (RGD) sites of silk scaffolds favored stem cell differentiation toward osteogenic lineage

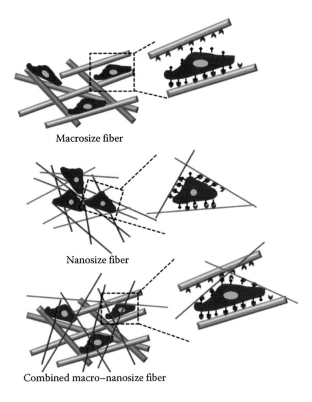

Macrosize fiber

Nanosize fiber

Combined macro–nanosize fiber

FIGURE 3.9
Schematic illustration of electrospun fiber with different fiber diameter (macro and nanosize) and their biological response.

(Meinel et al., 2004). *In vivo* use of electrospun silk fiber matrix for periodontal regeneration has shown an early bony union across the defect site. After a few months, the bone defect was completely healed by the formation of a new bone (Kim et al., 2005). In an interesting approach, Tuzlakoglu et al. presented a new scaffold architecture combining the effects of macro- and nanofibers on osteoblast bioactivity. Macro–nanointegrated electrospun fiber influenced bone cell morphology and cytoskeleton organization. High biomineralization was seen on the nano/microcombined electrospun fibers. The unique macro–nanopatterned morphology of the scaffold guided cell behavior on the scaffold (Tuzlakoglu et al., 2005).

Another interesting approach is to use two different biopolymers simultaneously to prepare nanofibers. Figure 3.10 shows schematic of electrospun fibers obtained by blending two different natural polymers A and B. Blending allows for the combination of useful properties of individual biopolymers to confer distinctive and unique combination of improved mechanical, chemical, and biological properties to the resultant blend with improved biological properties such as enhanced cell attachment as shown in the schematic.

Studies have been reported on blends of collagen with glycosaminoglycans and chitosan for tissue engineering applications (Zhong et al., 2005; Chen et al., 2010). Blend of chitin and silk fibroin fibers showed excellent cell adhesion and growth suggesting potential ability for bone tissue engineering (Yoo et al., 2008). Chitosan biopolymer shows high degree of swelling, which weakens the polymer. Chemical bonding of chitosan with alginate improves strength and also promotes osteoblast proliferation and differentiation (Li and Zhang, 2005).

Electrospun biopolymer nanofibers have low mechanical property and tend to lose structural stability upon hydration. To overcome this limitation an effective approach is to cross-link using chemical cross-linkers. Glutaraldehyde cross-linked collagen electrospun fibers have shown to have improved mechanical properties matching that of synthetic polymer products (Sell et al., 2010). Similarly, collagen fiber cross-linked by physical methods such as ultraviolet (UV) irradiation and dehydrothermal (DHT) treatment showed improvement in mechanical properties. UV-treated fiber had greater ultimate tensile

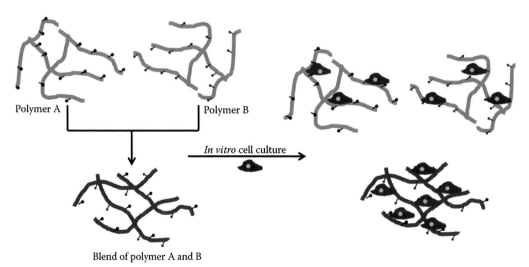

Polymer A   Polymer B

In vitro cell culture

Blend of polymer A and B

FIGURE 3.10
Schematic illustration of electrospun fibers obtained by blending two different natural polymers A and B and blending effect on cell proliferation.

strength and modulus value than DHT-treated samples (Weadock et al., 1995). 1-ethyl-3-(3-dimethylaminopropyl) carbodiimide hydrochloride (EDC) cross-linked collagen fibers exhibited improved mechanical strength with enhanced osteogenic differentiation (Mano et al., 2007). Biocompatibility of cross-link with 1,6-diisohexanecyanate (HMDI) and noncross-linked elastin fibers were studied. Cells on cross-linked fibers showed similar behavior to that of noncross-linked fibers, suggesting that cross-linking can improve physical and mechanical properties of the fibers without compromising the biological performance (Nivison-Smith et al., 2010). For gelatin nanofibers, postfabrication cross-linking is widely applied to improve the mechanical and degradation properties (Panzavolta et al., 2011). There are some reports showing cross-linked biopolymers exhibiting poor bioactivity and hydrophilicity with enhanced cytotoxicity (Zhang et al., 2006). Rigid cross-linked fibers can also prevent infiltration of cells into fibrous scaffolds (Shalumon et al., 2009).

In bone tissue engineering, growth factors such as BMP that regulate bone differentiation are widely used to further improve the performance of fibrous scaffolds (Harris et al., 1994; Cheng et al., 2003). Fibers incorporating biomolecules are able to support cell growth and guide cell differentiation for mineral deposition. These biomolecules are susceptible to denaturation during processing that involves organic solvents, which limits incorporation of biomolecules within nanofibers. Since most biopolymers are water soluble, it is a significant advantage over synthetic polymers for delivery of biomolecules. Li et al. successfully incorporated BMP-2 in electrospun silk fibroin nanofibers for bone tissue engineering (C. Li et al., 2006). The release of the incorporated BMP-2 upregulated osteogenic genes and promoted biomineralization on the nanofiber scaffolds.

Natural biopolymers have poor mechanical properties and under physiological conditions fail to retain long-term structural stability. Most of the natural ECM-derived biopolymers require chemical or physical cross-linking to avoid dissolution of electrospun fibers under hydrated environment (Li et al., 2005). Extracted natural polymers from animal or plant source are of high cost and their purity is questionable. As they are labile, natural polymers can be difficult to process into desired shapes. Another limitation with biopolymers is that surface sterilization is difficult as they are prone to denaturation and cross-linking on exposure to UV.

3.3.2 Synthetic Polymers for Bone Tissue Engineering

Synthetic polymers are inexpensive and produced on a large scale with reproducible physical, chemical, and mechanical properties under controlled environment. Electrospun nanofibers from synthetic polymer can be used to provide biomimetic environment that provides topographical cues similar to that of the native ECM. Synthetic polymer nanofibers generally process high mechanical, well-controlled microstructure and controlled degradation properties. In bone tissue engineering most frequently utilized synthetic polymers are poly(lactic acid) (PLA), PCL, poly(glycolic acid) (PGA), poly(propylene fumarate) (PPF), and their copolymers as shown in Figure 3.7. These polymers belong to the family of linear aliphatic polyester. These polyesters degrade through hydrolytic cleavage of the ester bond. Degradation products from the polyester are nontoxic and are removed by the metabolic pathways of the body. Synthetic biodegradable polyester polymer scaffolds are overtaking natural biopolymer scaffolds for tissue engineering. Slow degradation and their intrinsic structural stability in hydrated environment make polyester attractive for preparing tissue scaffolds. With significant advances in chemical modification of these polyesters, many of their limitations can be overcome to prepare scaffolds with tailored properties.

1. *Poly(caprolactone)* (PCL) is among the most popular synthetic polymers used in resorbable medical applications due to its biocompatibility and slow degradation without the formation of toxic by-products. PCL is a semicrystalline, hydrophobic polymer with a low melting point around 60°C. The low melting point and good solubility in most of the organic solvents make PCL an excellent blending material with other synthetic and natural polymers (Woodruff and Hutmacher, 2010). PCL is an attractive synthetic polymer for long-term implant and controlled drug-release applications owing to the slow degradation behavior. In a core–shell design, PCL is often used as the strong and stable polymer outer layer protecting the soft polymer core and controlling the slow release of therapeutic agents.

2. *Poly(glycolic acid)* (PGA) is a biodegradable thermoset polyester. PGA being relatively hydrophilic among these polyesters degrades rapidly in a hydrated environment. PGA-based polymeric materials are most often used for the synthesis of absorbable sutures and tissue engineering scaffolds (Middleton and Tipton, 2000). Scaffolds of PGA tend to lose mechanical and structural stability within 3–4 weeks which is attributed to the fast hydrolytic degradation. The degraded product glycolic acid is nontoxic as it enters the tricarboxylic acid cycle and is excreted as water and carbon dioxide. PGA has been used in controlled drug delivery and food packing applications.

3. *Poly(lactic acid)* (PLA) is a synthetic biopolymer obtained from an agricultural source. PLA degrades into nontoxic components and has excellent cytocompatibility. Food and Drug Administration (FDA) has approved the use of PLA for degradable surgical sutures (Okamoto and John, 2013). Although PLA is similar to PGA, an extra methyl group imparts increased hydrophobicity and slows degradation. Since PLA has high mechanical strength and degrades gradually *in vivo*, PLA is often used as a structural implant material. PLA-based implants exhibit effective load transfer to the bones (Nazre and Lin, 1994). PLA shows better heat resistance ability and can withstand temperatures up to 110°C (Fiore et al., 2010). PLA and its copolymers are extensively used for bone tissue engineering. PLA also serves as an ideal feedstock material for 3D printers for making 3D tissue scaffold, which have been attracting tremendous attention in recent years.

4. *Poly(lactide-co-glycolide)* (PLGA) is a copolymer of PLA and PGA. PLGA shows low degradation rate in comparison to pure PGA and is less brittle compared to PLA. Thus, PLGA synchronizes the properties of the two pure polymers, which helps in providing stable support to the cells. US FDA has approved the use of PLGA as a biomaterial for tissue engineering applications.

5. *Poly(propylene fumarate)* (PPF) polymer is an unsaturated polyester. The presence of the double bond in PPF provides high mechanical strength to the polymer. PPF is considered as an important biodegradable polymer for bone and dental tissue engineering. It has been used as an injectable material for bone tissue engineering applications also (Lewandrowski et al., 2000). The presence of the double bond can be used for cross-linking of PPF with other polymers. PPF is being used in the preparation of 3D scaffolds by stereolithography (Lee et al., 2006,2007).

6. *Poly(dioxanone)* (PDO) is a semicrystalline synthetic polymer with excellent mechanical, slow degradation, and shape memory properties (Boland et al., 2005). Initially, PDO was used as surgical sutures. However, over the years researchers

have started to use PDO for drug delivery and tissue engineering (Middleton and Tipton, 2000).

7. *Poly(vinyl alcohol)* (PVA) is a water-soluble and semicrystalline synthetic polymer. It is a linear polymer that can be easily synthesized. PVA is used in varieties of industrial applications such as textiles, automobiles, electronics, and medical industries. PVA has excellent oxygen and aroma barrier properties along with film-forming ability and is thus an excellent packaging material. PVA shows good mechanical degradability and biocompatibility properties. Researchers have shown the potential of PVA in tissue engineering. Semicrystalline and hydrophilic nature of PVA has been utilized to prepare hydrogels for tissue engineering (Hassan and Peppas, 2000).

8. *Poly(ethylene oxide)* (PEO), also known as poly(ethylene glycol) (PEG), is a water-soluble polymer. PEO has found wide use in applications such as pharmaceuticals, mining, paper, and cleaning products in addition to biotechnology. PEO has been used to create high-osmotic pressure in biochemistry and biomembrane experiments. PEO is also used for deoxyribonucleic acid (DNA) isolation and protein crystallization. Over the years, PEO has been gaining interest in gene delivery applications as well (Kreppel and Kochanek, 2008). Being hydrophilic and nontoxic in nature, PEO-based biomaterials have shown promise in tissue engineering applications (Jagur-Grodzinski, 2006).

3.3.2.1 Application of Electrospun Synthetic Polymers in Bone Tissue Engineering

For bone tissue engineering, osteoblasts prefer strong electrospun fibers along with macropores for their proliferation and infiltration inside the scaffold (Tuzlakoglu et al., 2005). PCL macroporous electrospun fibers have been extensively used in bone regeneration (Yoshimoto et al., 2003). In another interesting study, Nam et al. added sodium chloride particles during PCL electrospinning and the porogen salt particles from fibers were subsequently dissolved in water to form macropores for cellular ingrowth (Nam et al., 2007). Cells cultured on these scaffolds showed up to 4 mm ingrowth with high-cellular coverage. Thus, design of nanofibers with macropore size distribution is important because osteoblasts and bone marrow-derived stem cells have shown great affinity for microporous scaffolds (Nam et al., 2007). Synthetic polymers exhibit a hydrophobic surface and lack cell-binding motifs for cell adhesion. Figure 3.11 shows schematics of different techniques used for surface modification of synthetic electrospun fibers.

Surface modification of synthetic polymers improves protein adsorption and cell adhesion. PLGA polymer nanofiber surface modified with Gly-Arg-Gly-Asp-Tyr (GRGDY) peptide showed significantly enhanced cell adhesion and proliferation (Kim and Park, 2006). Poly(lactide-*co*-caprolactone) (PLCL) nanofibers treated with alkaline NaOH solution showed the presence of numerous groups such as carboxyl and hydroxyl exposed on the nanofiber surface, which not only influences initial behavior such as attachment, spreading, and migration, but also provides a hydrophilic surface for further chemical modification (Kim et al., 2010). Another simple approach is to modify synthetic polymer surface by physical irradiation techniques. Surface modification by irradiation generates chemical functional groups at the surface without affecting bulk chemistry of the polymer. Bacakova et al. have demonstrated that oxygen plasma-treated fibers showed significant increase on oxygen containing functional groups on the fiber surface. Fiber surface had more attached cell, which may be attributed to improved surface wettability by oxygen

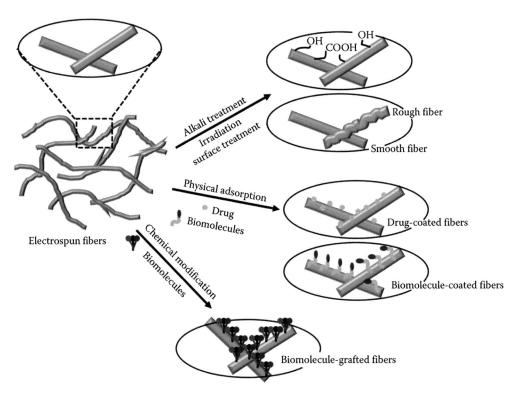

FIGURE 3.11
Schematic illustration of different techniques used for surface modification of synthetic electrospun polymers to improve bioactivity.

plasma treatment (M. Bacakova et al., 2014). In a similar study, PLLA nanofibers treated with oxygen plasma yielded carboxyl groups on the fiber surface. Thereafter, the carboxyl groups were used to graft gelatin on the PLLA fibers. Gelatin-grafted PLLA fiber showed tight attachment and enhanced differentiation of chondrocytes on the fiber matrix. *In vivo* subcutaneous implantation of gelatin-grafted PLLA fibers showed formation of ectopic cartilage tissue after 28 days (Chen and Su, 2011).

Cui et al. modified poly(D,L-lactide) (PDLLA) fiber surface with chemical functional groups such as hydroxyl, carboxyl, and amino groups, while varying their density on fiber surface (Cui et al., 2010a). The presence of functional moieties favored HA nucleation and growth on PDLLA fiber matrix. Different sizes of mineralized HA crystals were observed based on the presence of the different chemical groups on the PDLLA fibers. Figure 3.12 shows the schematics and SEM micrographs of mineralization on carboxylated electrospun PLA fiber in SBF (Cui et al., 2010a).

Fiber matrix with a mineralized surface has been shown to accelerate cell growth and differentiation. Mineralized surface showed strong affinity for cell-adhesive proteins, which favor cell adhesion to the surface (Kretlow and Mikos, 2007; Kim et al., 2008). After attachment, cells on the mineralized surface started to synthesize ECM with more bone proteins such as collagen, osteocalcin, and alkaline phosphate (Kretlow and Mikos, 2007). Hence, these studies elucidate the importance of functional groups and charge density on nanofibers mediating cell interactions and behavior.

Hydrophobic synthetic polymers are extensively used for the incorporation of hydrophobic drugs (Verreck et al., 2003). However, the incorporation of hydrophilic

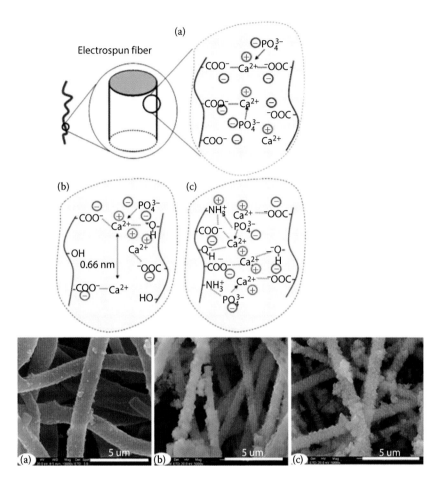

FIGURE 3.12
Hydroxyapatite nucleation on carboxylated electrospun PLA fiber in SBF with carboxyl group densities of 0.32 (a), 0.55 (b), and 0.94 nmol/cm^2 (c) after incubation in SBF for 7 days. (Reprinted from *Biomaterials*, 31, Cui, W. et al., Hydroxyapatite nucleation and growth mechanism on electrospun fibers functionalized with different chemical groups and their combinations, 4620–4629, Copyright 2010a with permission from Elsevier.)

biomacromolecules and growth factors in the synthetic hydrophobic fibers can be challenging. Incorporation within the polymer nanofibers or the surface coating of proteins, growth factors, and drugs may provide improved biological and therapeutic response. As a result, researchers have exploited PEO-based electrospun nanofibers for delivering biomacromolecules to cells (Casper et al., 2005). Srouji et al. showed the use of PEO nanofibers for incorporation of BMP-2 using core–shell design for bone regeneration (Srouji et al., 2010). Researchers have also used PEO in combination with other synthetic polymers for incorporation of biomacromolecules such as DNA in nanofibers. DNA-incorporated fibers showed large release of the DNA content for transfecting osteoblasts (Luu et al., 2003).

The major drawback with as-synthesized synthetic polymers is that most of them have hydrophobic and bioinert surface, which lack cell recognizable and physiological parameters for modulating cell behavior. Although one can modify synthetic polymers to display the specific physical and surface chemical properties, they still show limited biological properties in comparison to natural polymers. Synthetic polymers have also shown the presence of chemical initiators or impurities, which can adversely affect cell behavior (Freitag, 2003). Hence, in order to overcome the problems of natural and synthetic polymers, an effective approach would be the blending of natural and synthetic polymers.

3.3.3 Polymer Blend for Bone Tissue Engineering

Natural and synthetic polymers offer different advantages and suffer from limitations such that individually they cannot fulfill all the desired properties for preparation of nanofibrous scaffolds for bone tissue engineering. Nanofibrous mats prepared from their blend can provide scaffolds with suitable bioactive hydrophilic and mechanically strong surface optimal for cell attachment and proliferation. These new biosynthetic polymeric materials prepared by blending two or more natural and synthetic polymers have been gaining increased interest in biomedical field (Sionkowska, 2011). Kim et al. have shown that blending of gelatin in PLA nanofibers improves surface wettability, cellular affinity, and osteoblast proliferation compared to pure PLA fibers (Kim et al., 2008). Gelatin has also been blended with PCL to prepare bioactive scaffolds (Zhang et al., 2005). Blending of gelatin with synthetic polymers avoids the necessary postfabrication cross-linking. PCL has blended with various natural polymers including collagen, elastin, chitosan, and keratin (Sell et al., 2010; Roozbahani et al., 2013; Edwards et al., 2015). Blends obtained from the coelectrospinning of synthetic biodegradable polymer PLGA and two natural proteins gelatin and α-elastin exhibited swelling property upon hydration without undergoing any structural disintegration (M. Li et al., 2006). Blending synthetic polymers enhances stability of natural polymers in aqueous environment exclusive of any chemical or physical cross-linking (M. Li et al., 2006). Blending of PVA in collagen showed improved mechanical properties, which were further enhanced with glutaraldehyde cross-linking. Chemical cross-linking of PVA/collagen blend provided structural stability, which prevented dissolution in contact with biological fluids. Such strong and stable blend is a promising structural biomaterial (Giusti et al., 1994).

Control of the polymeric ratio in the blend can be used to tune the desired properties of the electrospun fibers such as the fiber diameter, porosity, roughness, and fiber structure, which significantly control cell attachment, growth, and cell infiltration. Blends with aligned nanofibrous morphology provide high surface area with directionally oriented fibers, which guides cell morphology and migration along the desired direction (Bhattarai et al., 2004). In bone tissue engineering, aligned electrospun fibers attract special attention due to the orientation-dependent mechanical properties that are similar to the bone tissue. Figure 3.13 shows the schematics of the response of cells on random and aligned electrospun fibers. Cells show aligned morphology along the fiber direction in contrast to randomly distributed cells on nonaligned electrospun fibers leading to increased differentiation and mineralization.

Work by Meng et al. showed that random and aligned nanofibers prepared from blending of synthetic PLGA copolymer with the natural polymer gelatin resulted in improved surface wettability of the blended nanofiber scaffolds due to the presence of hydrophilic gelatin moieties (Z. Meng et al., 2010). Additionally, the random-blended fiber mat with high porosity showed capillary effect leading to better water adsorption (M. Li et al., 2008). Osteoblast growth was favored on PLGA/gelatin electrospun fibers in comparison to PLGA electrospun fibers. High osteoblast growth along the oriented fibers of the aligned PLGA/gelatin electrospun fibers was better suited for bone tissue engineering.

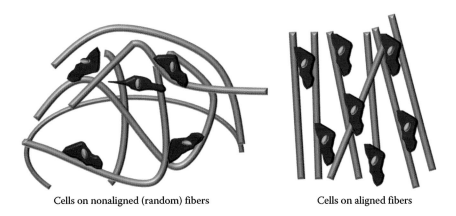

Cells on nonaligned (random) fibers   Cells on aligned fibers

FIGURE 3.13
Schematic illustration of the response of cells on random and aligned blended electrospun fibers.

Scientists have also explored the ability to prepare blend nanofibers to deliver proteins, drugs, and growth factors for bone regeneration (Sill and von Recum, 2008; Mickova et al., 2012). As discussed earlier, one of the effective ways to incorporate sensitive biomolecules or drugs in nanofiber blends is through a core–shell design (Figure 3.2). For the delivery of labile drugs and biomolecules, a major challenge is to protect them from the harsh environments such as organic solvents used for the fabrication. Encapsulating drugs, proteins, and growth factors in polymer fiber and covering with another stable polymer sheath is envisaged to be an effective strategy to deliver therapeutic agents for bone regeneration. Thus, to avoid denaturation, the drug and biomolecules are usually added to the water-soluble core of natural biopolymer in combination with a stronger and more stable synthetic polymer that forms the outer layer (Cui et al., 2010b). Core–shell model with soft natural polymer fiber core having osteogenic drug protected by strong synthetic fiber not only enhances cell response, but significantly sustains structural integrity and mechanical strength.

Although the physicochemical and mechanical properties of synthetic polymer fibers can be modulated easily, customizing biochemical properties of fibers can be challenging. Among many other approaches to improve biochemical properties of synthetic scaffold, one interesting strategy is the addition of bioactive ECM-derived particles into the synthetic fibers (Meng et al., 2007). Recently, Gibson et al. has shown an interesting study where decellularized extracellular matrix (DECM) particles were reinforced in synthetic PCL polymer nanofibers and the bioactivity on stem cells was studied. Nanofiber scaffolds having bone and cartilage DECM nanoparticles showed enhanced osteogenic differentiation of stem cells leading to high mineral deposition on nanofiber matrix. In contrast, scaffolds DECM from the spleen and lung resulted in decrease in mineralization. These findings suggest that the source of ECM particles have significant effect on stem cell behavior (Gibson et al., 2014). Cells have been shown to behave differently on different ECM-derived scaffolds and this is mainly governed by biochemical, structural, and architectural features of the respective ECM (Crapo et al., 2012; Gibson et al., 2014).

3.3.4 Ceramic Nanoparticles-Reinforced Nanofiber for Bone Tissue Engineering

ECM of bone tissues is composed primarily of an organic polymeric matrix reinforced with inorganic nanomaterials. Thus, scaffold designs increasingly involve the use of electrospun polymeric nanofibers embedded with nanoceramics to mimic the hierarchical structure of the natural ECM for bone regeneration (Bishop et al., 2006; Wutticharoenmongkol et al., 2006; Thomas et al., 2007). Peng et al. showed that the PLLA nanofibers incorporating HA mimic the natural microstructure of the bone ECM. The biological activity of both random and aligned fibers of PLLA/HA were evaluated *in vitro* using rat osteosarcoma ROS17/2.8 cells. The presence of microsized HA particles on fiber surface promoted strong cell adhesion and osteogenic differentiation (Peng et al., 2011). In another study, a combination of HA and β-TCP was used to fabricate the bioactive electrospun PCL composite fibers. Previous reports have shown that the use of HA/TCP biphasic particles result in greater bone regeneration compared to either HA or TCP alone (Arinzeh et al., 2005; Ng et al., 2008). PCL fibers with well-dispersed HA/TCP particles supported MSC growth and the cells started to deposit ECM on the composite fiber but not on the neat PCL fibers (Patlolla et al., 2010). The presence of other forms of calcium phosphate as well as bioactive bioglass and bioceramic particles is shown to impart osteoconductive and osteoinductive properties to polymeric scaffolds resulting in significant increase in cell proliferation, osteogenic differentiation, and mineralization on the scaffolds (Lu et al., 2003; Wang, 2003; Ramalingam et al., 2013). Addition of dicalcium silicate (Ca_2S) nanoparticles in PLLA electrospun fiber provided bioactivity to PLLA–Ca_2S fibers by inducing HA formation on the fiber surface when immersed in SBF. Osteoblasts cultured on PLLA–Ca_2S fiber mesh showed well-spread morphology. Osteoblast cells showed enhanced ALP activity on PLLA–Ca_2S fiber indicating increased bioactivity and osteogenic differentiation ability of the PLLA–Ca_2S fibers (Dong et al., 2014).

The use of magnetic nanoparticles (MNPs) is also a popular strategy for designing magnetic nanofibrous scaffolds for bone tissue engineering applications (Wei et al., 2011). The unique ability of MNPs to regulate osteoinduction without external magnetic force has attracted intense research in bone tissue engineering (Wu et al., 2010). Singh et al. demonstrated the use of electrospun PCL scaffolds incorporating MNPs for bone regeneration purpose (Singh et al., 2014). First, MNPs were citrated and dispersed in PCL fiber matrix. The presence of MNPs improved surface wettability and hydrolytic degradation of the PCL fibers and promoted the formation of the apatite layer in SBF. These magnetic composite fibers promoted osteoblast proliferation and osteogenic differentiation *in vitro*. Remodeling of radial segmental defects in a rat model confirmed the bone regeneration ability of the PCL–MNP nanofibrous scaffolds *in vivo* (Singh et al., 2014). In another similar study, magnetic nanofibers of chitosan (CS)/poly vinyl alcohol (PVA) were fabricated by incorporation of Fe_3O_4 nanoparticles. The bioactivity of CS/PVA/Fe_3O_4 magnetic fiber was evaluated using MG63 human osteoblast-like cells. Osteoblasts cells showed good adhesion and proliferation on magnetic biodegradable nanofibrous membranes suggesting that the magnetic composite fibers can facilitate bone regeneration (Wei et al., 2011).

Piezoelectric nature of bone encouraged research studies to use piezoelectric ceramic nanoparticles for bone tissue engineering. Piezoelectric ceramic nanoparticles with good biocompatibility and piezoelectric property of these nanoparticles help in bone regeneration (Park et al., 1981). Recently, Bagchi et al. studied the effect of different piezoelectric ceramics such as barium titanate, calcium titanate, and strontium titanate nanoparticles incorporated in PCL electrospun fibers on osteoblast proliferation and differentiation. Addition of piezoelectric ceramic nanoparticles imparted piezoelectric property to PCL fiber, which resulted in improved biological response. Electrospun PCL fibers with piezoelectric ceramic nanoparticles showed enhanced osteoblasts growth and high-osteogenic genes expression in comparison to neat PCL fibers (Bagchi et al., 2014).

3.3.5 Carbonaceous Nanoparticles-Reinforced Nanofiber for Bone Tissue Engineering

Although ceramic nanoparticles impart bioactivity to polymeric nanofibers, they make the fibers brittle. A large amount of ceramic nanoparticles is often required to elicit significant biological activity, which in turn limits electrospinnability of the polymer. As a result, researchers are investigating the use of carbonaceous nanoparticles for synthesizing polymer composite nanofibers for bone tissue engineering. In the past decades, carbonaceous nanoparticles have gained rapid attention in the biomedical field (Hopley et al., 2014). Among the various carbon-based nanoparticles, carbon nanotube (CNT), graphene, and nanodiamond (ND) are the most extensively studied to prepare electrospun composite fibers for bone tissue engineering.

1. *CNTs* are cylindrically rolled structures of carbon-based graphene sheets with tunable physical properties such as aspect ratio, diameter, and chirality (Saito et al., 1998). Among CNTs, single-walled carbon nanotubes (SWNTs) and multi-walled carbon nanotubes (MWNTs) are most often used. CNTs possess high electrical and thermal conductivity attributed to the carbon–carbon linkage through sp^2 hybridization (Nardecchia et al., 2013).

2. *Graphene* is a 2D thin layer of sp^2 hybridized carbon atoms. Graphene possesses high mechanical, optical, thermal, and electrical properties (Afanasov et al., 2009). Given the large surface area of graphene, a low fraction of graphene in the polymer matrix can more effectively enhance the mechanical and electrical properties over other carbonaceous nanoparticles (Rao et al., 2010).

3. *Nanodiamonds* are carbon-based nanoparticles synthesized mainly by detonation. NDs are mainly composed of carbon–diamond core and periphery having traces of functional groups such as hydroxyl, carboxyl, and amine (Mochalin et al., 2012). NDs are a relatively new class of carbonaceous materials that are also gaining attention in biomedical applications.

There have been many reports indicating cytotoxicity of carbonaceous particles when cells were exposed to the suspended particles. Nanoparticles with high-aspect ratio and high-surface area tend to agglomerate faster in suspension and settle in the form of agglomerates on the cell surface. Agglomerated nanoparticles on the cell surface limit supply of nutrients generating stress ultimately causing cell death (Y. Zhang et al., 2010). Furthermore, the chemistry, size, shape, and concentration of the suspended carbonaceous particles determine their interactions with the cell and subsequent cytotoxicity (Y. Zhang et al., 2010; X. Zhang et al., 2012). The synthesis and processing techniques to produce carbonaceous nanoparticles significantly influence toxicity. The use of metallic catalysts to produce CNTs and graphene nanoparticles have shown to be highly toxic when these particles are exposed to cells (Pumera, 2011; Liu et al., 2012). However, surface functionalization and the use of carbonaceous nanoparticles at low concentration in a polymeric matrix is shown to reduce agglomeration and the subsequent slow release of the low concentration of the nanoparticles significantly reduces cytotoxicity (Khabashesku et al., 2005; Gutiérrez-Praena et al., 2011; Vardharajula et al., 2012).

Nanofibrous composites prepared with carbonaceous nanofillers of high-surface area help to improve physical, mechanical, and biological properties of the polymer fibers (Qi et al., 2013). The presence of carbonaceous nanoparticles strengthens the fiber matrix providing for calcification for hard tissue engineering. Aside from strengthening the fibers, the particle size, orientation, chemistry, and distribution can significantly enhance biological properties of the composites.

3.3.5.1 CNT-Reinforced Nanofibers for Bone Tissue Engineering

CNTs being cylindrical and porous are believed to be able to mimic collagen fibers and have been shown to enhance cell attachment, growth, and differentiation (X. Zhang et al., 2008; D. Zhang et al., 2010). CNTs have shown to adsorb serum proteins from culture medium, which improves interactions with cells (Li et al., 2009). In addition, functionalization of CNTs with chemical or polymeric moieties was shown to further improve the state of dispersion and biological properties of CNTs (Bianco et al., 2005; Armentano et al., 2008).

Studies have demonstrated that aligned CNTs on a glass substrate significantly enhanced MSC growth and differentiation compared to the nonaligned ones (Namgung et al., 2011). These findings encouraged research studies to use electrospinning method for CNTs alignment in the polymer, which influence cell growth and directional migration (Saeed et al., 2006; Meng et al., 2010). During electrospinning, the elongated polymer jet tends to align CNTs along the fiber axis. Aligned electrospun fibers have shown to disperse nanoparticles more effectively in comparison to random fibers (Baji et al., 2010). Shao et al. showed that the osteoblasts respond differently on aligned and random nanofibers of PLA/CNT composites with more cellular extensions and outgrowth on aligned fibers (Shao et al., 2011). CNTs have the natural ability to influence the formation of HA on the surface when osteoblasts are cultured on the CNT surface (Zanello et al., 2006).

Incorporation of CNTs into soft electrospun nanofibers have shown that it not only strengthens but also improves electrical properties of the polymer nanofiber (Sen et al., 2004). Strong electrically conducting biomaterials can influence mechano-transduction and electrophysiological cell response for bone and neural tissues (Kam et al., 2008). Electrically conductive electrospun fibers having CNTs showed enhanced osteoblasts growth along the direction of the electric current (Shao et al., 2011). Osteoblasts cultured on PLLA/MWNT composites with alternating current stimulus showed enhanced extracellular calcium mineral deposition (Supronowicz et al., 2002). Hybrid composites of CNT and nano-HA in nanofiber of a polymer matrix exhibit synergetic effects accrued from the properties of individual nanoparticles. As a result, multifunctional electrospun nanofiber composites show improved properties of mechanical, electrical, and bioactivity with addition of HA and CNT (Mei et al., 2007; Misra et al., 2007).

3.3.5.2 Graphene-Reinforced Nanofiber for Bone Tissue Engineering

Over the years, graphene has shown to be a promising candidate for variety of applications including electronic, energy, medical imaging, and more recently in gene delivery and tissue engineering applications (Feng et al., 2011). Graphene and graphene-derived nanoparticles such as graphene oxide (GO) and reduced graphene oxide (RGO) are carbonaceous nanoparticles that can be synthesized without the use of a metallic catalyst. These graphene-derived nanoparticles differ mainly in terms of composition, surface chemistry, electrical property, and the number of stacked carbon sheets.

RGO having high electrical, thermal property, and being hydrophobic in nature exhibits weak π–π interactions with biomolecules and drugs (Bagri et al., 2010). High electrical conductivity of graphene particles is potentially useful for preparing biomedical composites. A conducting composite not only directs cell proliferation, but can also electrically stimulate bone cells for faster healing (Spadaro, 1977). Furthermore, good thermal property of

RGO can be used for measuring cell potential and in developing thermoconductive cell substrates (Artiles et al., 2011; Cohen-Karni et al., 2012).

GO has many oxygen-containing functional groups such as hydroxyl, epoxy, and carboxyl moieties. The presence of these hydrophilic groups can facilitate chemical functionalization and interaction with the polymer enhancing interfacial strength between the filler and the matrix resulting in improved mechanical properties of the composite. Apart from strengthening, functional groups of GO have shown high affinity for the adsorption of proteins and growth factors. Stem cells grown on the GO surface in the presence of osteogenic supplements results in increased differentiation toward the bone lineage (Lee et al., 2011). GO also tend to form metal ion complexes owing to polar and negative charge of the graphene basal plane. Hence, GO acts as an amphiphilic molecule showing higher basal reactivity than RGO; as a result GO finds extensive use in biomedical applications (Goenka et al., 2014).

Reinforcement of GO in PVA electrospun fiber enhanced strength and wettability. PVA/GO fiber surface was biocompatible with osteoblasts without affecting cell viability (Qi et al., 2013). Addition of GO in PLGA resulted in improved mechanical and thermal properties. Reinforced GO acted as the heteronucleating agent, increasing the percentage crystallinity, which further improved tensile modulus. GO also showed chemical interaction with PLGA resulting in overall improvement of the physicochemical properties of the PLGA/GO composite (Yoon et al., 2012). In another study, GO showed chemical bonding with natural polymer chitosan. The carboxyl group on the GO surface reacted with amine group of chitosan forming strong amide bonds. It not only enhanced mechanical property but also improved biocompatibility and bioactivity of chitosan scaffolds for osteoblast adhesion and growth (Depan et al., 2011). The presence of negative charge functional groups on the GO surface has proved to be effective for cell–scaffold interactions at the biomaterial interface (Depan et al., 2011). Addition of GO in PCL fiber showed increased bioactivity due to the presence of negatively charged functional groups providing active sites for biomineralization (Wan and Chen, 2011). In fibers of a PVA/chitosan blend, GO reinforcement significantly improved the antibacterial property offering another indicating potential advantage for bone tissue engineering (Liu et al., 2014). In recent work, we have shown that the amine functionalized GO are efficient fillers to enhance mechanical strength of the composites, promote osteogenic differentiation, and impart bactericidal activity (Kumar et al., 2015). Cells on polymer/graphene fiber composites exhibit polygonal shape with extensions in contrast to more rounded cells with fewer extensions on the neat polymer (Liu et al., 2010; Qi et al., 2013), which is suggestive of strong cell attachment to the biomaterial surface. Lee et al. has shown an interesting approach where GO-decorated electrospun hybrid fiber sheets of PLGA and collagen were prepared by dual electrospinning technique (Lee et al., 2014). The presence of GO and collagen improved wettability of the fiber mat influencing cell attachment and enhanced proliferation on the hybrid fibers compared to neat PLGA fiber. A few other reports have demonstrated that spin coating of GO or spraying of GO solution on polymeric electrospun fiber helps in stem cell differentiation. Coating or spraying of GO on fiber mat provides unique topographical and microenvironment regulating intracellular signaling for selective differentiation of stem cells (Shah et al., 2014; Chaudhuri et al., 2015).

Fabrication of hybrid polymer scaffolds incorporating bioactive and strong nanoparticles offers a combination of biological and mechanical properties to yield attractive biomaterials for bone tissue engineering. Hybrid PLA/HA/GO electrospun composites showed significant improvement in both mechanical and biological performance (Ma et al., 2012). Hybrid composites showed mature osteoblast cells with spread and extended morphology on its surface and stimulated cell growth and differentiation (Ma et al., 2012). While

HA imparted bioactivity to PLA, GO reinforcement improved strength and hydrophilicity, and provided topographical features for strong attachment of osteoblasts to synergistically improve mechanical and biological properties of PLA. In another similar study, hybrid composites of nanogold-deposited GO in PVA electrospun fiber showed enhanced conductivity, thermal stability, and mechanical strength with no cytotoxicity on L929 fibroblasts (Ma et al., 2012; Yu et al., 2014). Hybrid graphene particles of metal nanoparticles on graphene sheets can also be added to a polymer matrix to induce osteogenesis for bone regeneration (Kumar and Chatterjee, 2015) as we have demonstrated recently. Thus, by synthesizing hybrid or ternary nanocomposite scaffolds, multifunctional properties can be imparted to the scaffolds.

3.3.5.3 ND-Reinforced Electrospun Fibers for Bone Tissue Engineering

NDs have shown better cytocompatiblity than CNTs and graphene (Zhang et al., 2012). Studies have shown that thin film of crystalline NDs deposited on biomaterial surface promoted proliferation of bone and various cell lines (Amaral et al., 2008; Grausova et al., 2011). In certain other studies researchers have demonstrated that the incorporation of ND in a polymer film significantly enhanced growth and differentiation of osteoblasts (Zhang et al., 2011). Wang et al. reported that NDs mechanically reinforced PVA matrix and also provided additional morphological features to ND/PVA fibers (Wang et al., 2013).

Parizek et al. showed that the addition of NDs in PLGA fibers led to beaded nanoclusters on the fiber surface. These nanoclusters created nanofeatures, which enhanced bioactivity of osteoblasts on the scaffold. Cells on electrospun fiber with additional nanostructure formed well-developed focal adhesion plaques (Parizek et al., 2012). In another report, PLLA/NDs composite fiber did not show a promising response on the proliferation or differentiation of bone-derived cells. One possible explanation for the less favorable cellular response was the release of NDs into culture medium (L. Bacakova et al., 2014). Salaam and coworkers have demonstrated the effect of ND reinforcement in PVA on three different cell lines. Low loading (0.1 wt%) of ND in PVA showed improved cell response over neat PVA fibers. However, further increase in the ND content in the PVA fiber matrix resulted in concentration-dependent cytotoxicity in all the three cell lines (Salaam et al., 2014).

Surface of NDs can be functionalized with different functional groups to further improve bioactivity of these nanoparticles (Krueger, 2008). Although ND shows least toxicity among carbonaceous nanoparticles, functionalization of ND further reduces its toxicity (Schrand et al., 2007). Studies have shown that the functionalized ND promoted cellular attachment and growth (Krueger, 2008; Hopper et al., 2014). Little work has been reported on the use of functionalized NDs as filler particles in polymer fiber matrix for tissue engineering. However, functionalized NDs still holds great potential for bone tissue engineering application. Further research is needed to fully explore the prospective of the use of functionalized NDs as filler particles in polymer fiber matrix for bone tissue regeneration.

3.4 Summary

Although many different approaches for preparing scaffolds for bone tissue engineering are available, electrospun polymeric nanofibrous scaffolds are one of the most promising classes as they closely mimic the native bone architecture. With the development of novel techniques within electrospinning setup as well as in combination, it is now possible to make complex structures with tailored porosity, thickness, and strength useful for bone repair and regeneration. In this chapter, we discussed the progress in improving the equipment design to overcome the limitations of electrospinning to prepare scaffolds that can be used clinically as bone graft substitutes. The wide variety of polymers available to prepare electrospun fibers was also discussed. These polymers can be improved by preparing blends. Further improvement can be achieved by preparing composites that mimic ECM composition and architecture. Many such systems are now being evaluated *in vitro* followed by promising outcomes in preliminary attempts *in vivo*. More long-term animal studies are required to fully understand the performance of the scaffold *in vivo* before clinical use.

Acknowledgments

Kaushik Chatterjee acknowledges the Ramanujan fellowship from the Department of Science and Technology (DST), India. Financial support from Nanomission Program of DST is acknowledged. We acknowledge the work of all the researchers in this field, which helped us compile this chapter and apologize to others whose work was inadvertently omitted.

References

Afanasov, I., Morozov, V., Kepman, A., Ionov, S., Seleznev, A., Van Tendeloo, G., Avdeev, V. 2009. Preparation, electrical and thermal properties of new exfoliated graphite-based composites. *Carbon.* 47: 263–270.

Ali, U., Zhou, Y., Wang, X., Lin, T. 2011. Electrospinning of continuous nanofiber bundles and twisted nanofiber yarns. In *Nanofibers—Production, Properties and Functional Applications,* ed., Lin, T., Croatia: InTech, 154–174.

Ali, U., Zhou, Y., Wang, X., Lin, T. 2012. Direct electrospinning of highly twisted, continuous nanofiber yarns. *J Text I.* 103: 80–88.

Amaral, M., Dias, A., Gomes, P., Lopes, M., Silva, R., Santos, J., Fernandes, M. 2008. Nanocrystalline diamond: *In vitro* biocompatibility assessment by MG63 and human bone marrow cells cultures. *J Biomed Mater Res A.* 87: 91–99.

Amruthwar, S. S., Janorkar, A. V. 2013. *In vitro* evaluation of elastin-like polypeptide–collagen composite scaffold for bone tissue engineering. *Dental Mater.* 29: 211–220.

Arinzeh, T. L., Tran, T., Mcalary, J., Daculsi, G. 2005. A comparative study of biphasic calcium phosphate ceramics for human mesenchymal stem-cell-induced bone formation, *Biomaterials.* 26: 3631–3638.

Armentano, I., Álvarez-Pérez, M. A., Carmona-Rodríguez, B., Gutiérrez-Ospina, I., Kenny, J. M., Arzate, H. 2008. Analysis of the biomineralization process on SWNT-COOH and F-SWNT films. *Mater Sci Eng C.* 28: 1522–1529.

Artiles, M. S., Rout, C. S., Fisher, T. S. 2011. Graphene-based hybrid materials and devices for biosensing. *Adv Drug Deliv Rev.* 63: 1352–1360.

Bacakova, L., Kopova, I., Stankova, L., Liskova, J., Vacik, J., Lavrentiev, V., Kromka, A., Potocky, S., Stranska, D. 2014. Bone cells in cultures on nanocarbon-based materials for potential bone tissue engineering: A review. *Physica Status Solidi (A).* 211: 2688–2702.

Bacakova, M., Lopot, F., Hadraba, D., Varga, M., Zaloudkova, M., Stranska, D., Suchy, T., Bacakova, L. 2014. Effects of fiber density and plasma modification of nanofibrous membranes on the adhesion and growth of HaCaT keratinocytes. *J Biomater Appl.* 29: 837–853.

Badylak, S. F., Freytes, D. O., Gilbert, T. W. 2009. Extracellular matrix as a biological scaffold material: Structure and function. *Acta Biomater.* 5: 1–13.

Bagchi, A., Meka, S. R. K., Rao, B. N., Chatterjee, K. 2014. Perovskite ceramic nanoparticles in polymer composites for augmenting bone tissue regeneration. *Nanotechnology.* 25: 485101.

Bagri, A., Mattevi, C., Acik, M., Chabal, Y. J., Chhowalla, M., Shenoy, V. B. 2010. Structural evolution during the reduction of chemically derived graphene oxide. *Nat Chem.* 2: 581–587.

Baji, A., Mai, Y.-W., Wong, S.-C., Abtahi, M., Chen, P. 2010. Electrospinning of polymer nanofibers: Effects on oriented morphology, structures and tensile properties. *Compos Sci Technol.* 70: 703–718.

Bandyopadhyay-Ghosh, S. 2008. Bone as a collagen-hydroxyapatite composite and its repair. *Trends Biomater Artif Organs.* 22: 116–124.

Beachley, V., Hepfer, R. G., Katsanevakis, E., Zhang, N., Wen, X. 2014. Precisely assembled nanofiber arrays as a platform to engineer aligned cell sheets for biofabrication. *Bioengineering.* 1: 114–133.

Bhattarai, S. R., Bhattarai, N., Yi, H. K., Hwang, P. H., Cha, D. I., Kim, H. Y. 2004. Novel biodegradable electrospun membrane: Scaffold for tissue engineering. *Biomaterials.* 25: 2595–2602.

Bianco, A., Kostarelos, K., Partidos, C. D., Prato, M. 2005. Biomedical applications of functionalised carbon nanotubes. *Chem Comm.* 571–577.

Bishop, A., Balazsi, C., Yang, J. H., Gouma, P. I. 2006. Biopolymer-hydroxyapatite composite coatings prepared by electrospinning. *Polym Adv Technol.* 17: 902–906.

Blair, T. (eds.) 2015. *Biomedical Textiles for Orthopaedic and Surgical Applications: Fundamentals, Applications and Tissue Engineering.* Cambridge, UK: Elsevier Woodhead Publishing, 1–65.

Blanchard, C. R., Timmons, S. F., Smith, R. A. 1999. Keratin-based hydrogel for biomedical applications and method of production. Google Patents. (US5932552).

Boccafoschi, F., Habermehl, J., Vesentini, S., Mantovani, D. 2005. Biological performances of collagen-based scaffolds for vascular tissue engineering. *Biomaterials.* 26: 7410–7417.

Boland, E. D., Coleman, B. D., Barnes, C. P., Simpson, D. G., Wnek, G. E., Bowlin, G. L. 2005. Electrospinning polydioxanone for biomedical applications. *Acta Biomater.* 1: 115–123.

Boland, E. D., Matthews, J. A., Pawlowski, K. J., Simpson, D. G., Wnek, G. E., Bowlin, G. L. 2004. Electrospinning collagen and elastin: Preliminary vascular tissue engineering. *Front Biosci.* 9: C1432.

Borchard, G. 2001. Chitosans for gene delivery. *Adv Drug Deliver Rev.* 52: 145–150.

Buchko, C. J., Kozloff, K. M., Martin, D. C. 2001. Surface characterization of porous, biocompatible protein polymer thin films. *Biomaterials.* 22: 1289–1300.

Burg, K. J., Porter, S., Kellam, J. F. 2000. Biomaterial developments for bone tissue engineering. *Biomaterials.* 21: 2347–2359.

Cai, Y. Z., Zhang, G. R., Wang, L. L., Jiang, Y. Z., Ouyang, H. W., Zou, X. H. 2012. Novel biodegradable three-dimensional macroporous scaffold using aligned electrospun nanofibrous yarns for bone tissue engineering. *J Biomed Mater Res A.* 100: 1187–1194.

Cao, D., Fu, Z., Li, C. 2011. Heat and compression molded electrospun poly(l-lactide) membranes: Preparation and characterization. *Mater Sci Eng B.* 176: 900–905.

Casper, C. L., Stephens, J. S., Tassi, N. G., Chase, D. B., Rabolt, J. F. 2004. Controlling surface morphology of electrospun polystyrene fibers: Effect of humidity and molecular weight in the electrospinning process. *Macromolecules.* 37: 573–578.

Casper, C. L., Yamaguchi, N., Kiick, K. L., Rabolt, J. F. 2005. Functionalizing electrospun fibers with biologically relevant macromolecules. *Biomacromolecules.* 6: 1998–2007.

Chaudhuri, B., Bhadra, D., Moroni, L., Pramanik, K. 2015. Myoblast differentiation of human mesenchymal stem cells on graphene oxide and electrospun graphene oxide–polymer composite fibrous meshes: Importance of graphene oxide conductivity and dielectric constant on their biocompatibility. *Biofabrication.* 7: 015009.

Chen, J.-P., Su, C. H. 2011. Surface modification of electrospun PLLA nanofibers by plasma treatment and cationized gelatin immobilization for cartilage tissue engineering. *Acta Biomater.* 7: 234–243.

Chen, Z., Wang, P., Wei, B., Mo, X., Cui, F. 2010. Electrospun collagen–chitosan nanofiber: A biomimetic extracellular matrix for endothelial cell and smooth muscle cell. *Acta Biomater.* 6: 372–382.

Cheng, H., Jiang, W., Phillips, F. M., Haydon, R. C., Peng, Y., Zhou, L., Luu, H. H., An, N., Breyer, B., Vanichakarn, P. 2003. Osteogenic activity of the fourteen types of human bone morphogenetic proteins (BMPs). *J Bone Joint Surg.* 85: 1544–1552.

Chevallay, B., Herbage, D. 2000. Collagen-based biomaterials as 3D scaffold for cell cultures: Applications for tissue engineering and gene therapy. *Med Biol Eng Comput.* 38: 211–218.

Cohen-Karni, T., Langer, R., Kohane, D. S. 2012. The smartest materials: The future of nanoelectronics in medicine. *ACS Nano.* 6: 6541–6545.

Crapo, P. M., Medberry, C. J., Reing, J. E., Tottey, S., van der Merwe, Y., Jones, K. E., Badylak, S. F. 2012. Biologic scaffolds composed of central nervous system extracellular matrix. *Biomaterials.* 33: 3539–3547.

Cui, W., Li, X., Xie, C., Zhuang, H., Zhou, S., Weng, J. 2010a. Hydroxyapatite nucleation and growth mechanism on electrospun fibers functionalized with different chemical groups and their combinations. *Biomaterials.* 31: 4620–4629.

Cui, W., Zhou, Y., Chang, J. 2010b. Electrospun nanofibrous materials for tissue engineering and drug delivery. *Sci Technol Adv Mater.* 11: 014108.

Daamen, W. F., Veerkamp, J., Van Hest, J., Van Kuppevelt, T. 2007. Elastin as a biomaterial for tissue engineering. *Biomaterials.* 28: 4378–4398.

Deitzel, J., Kleinmeyer, J., Harris, D., Tan, N. B. 2001. The effect of processing variables on the morphology of electrospun nanofibers and textiles. *Polymer.* 42: 261–272.

Depan, D., Girase, B., Shah, J., Misra, R. 2011. Structure–process–property relationship of the polar graphene oxide-mediated cellular response and stimulated growth of osteoblasts on hybrid chitosan network structure nanocomposite scaffolds. *Acta Biomater.* 7: 3432–3445.

Dong, S., Sun, J., Li, Y., Li, J., Cui, W., Li, B. 2014. Electrospun nanofibrous scaffolds of poly(L-lactic acid)-dicalcium silicate composite via ultrasonic-aging technique for bone regeneration. *Mater Sci Eng C.* 35: 426–433.

Duca, L., Floquet, N., Alix, A. J., Haye, B., Debelle, L. 2004. Elastin as a matrikine. *Crit Rev Oncol/ Hematol.* 49: 235–244.

Edwards, A., Jarvis, D., Hopkins, T., Pixley, S., Bhattarai, N. 2015. Poly(ϵ-caprolactone)/keratin-based composite nanofibers for biomedical applications. *J Biomed Mater Res B.* 103: 21–30.

Erisken, C., Kalyon, D. M., Wang, H. 2008. Functionally graded electrospun polycaprolactone and β-tricalcium phosphate nanocomposites for tissue engineering applications. *Biomaterials.* 29: 4065–4073.

Feng, L., Zhang, S., Liu, Z. 2011. Graphene based gene transfection. *Nanoscale.* 3: 1252–1257.

Fiore, G. L., Jing, F., Young, Jr V. G., Cramer, C. J., Hillmyer, M. A. 2010. High T g aliphatic polyesters by the polymerization of spirolactide derivatives. *Polym Chem.* 1: 870–877.

Francis, L., Venugopal, J., Prabhakaran, M. P., Thavasi, V., Marsano, E., Ramakrishna, S. 2010. Simultaneous electrospin–electrosprayed biocomposite nanofibrous scaffolds for bone tissue regeneration. *Acta Biomater.* 6: 4100–4109.

Freitag, R. (eds.) 2003. *Synthetic Polymers for Biotechnology and Medicine.* Georgetown, TX: Eurekah. com/Landes Bioscience, 19–37.

Gibson, M., Beachley, V., Coburn, J., Bandinelli, P. A., Mao, H. Q., Elisseeff, J. 2014. Tissue extracellular matrix nanoparticle presentation in electrospun nanofibers. *Biomed Res Int.* 2014: 469120.

Giusti, P., Lazzeri, L., De Petris, S., Palla, M., Cascone, M. 1994. Collagen-based new bioartificial polymeric materials. *Biomaterials.* 15: 1229–1233.

Goenka, S., Sant, V., Sant, S. 2014. Graphene-based nanomaterials for drug delivery and tissue engineering. *J Control Release.* 173: 75–88.

Grausova, L., Kromka, A., Burdikova, Z., Eckhardt, A., Rezek, B., Vacik, J., Haenen, K., Lisa, V., Bacakova, L. 2011. Enhanced growth and osteogenic differentiation of human osteoblast-like cells on boron-doped nanocrystalline diamond thin films. *PloS One.* 6: e20943.

Gutiérrez-Praena, D., Pichardo, S., Sánchez, E., Grilo, A., Cameán, A. M., Jos, A. 2011. Influence of carboxylic acid functionalization on the cytotoxic effects induced by single wall carbon nanotubes on human endothelial cells (HUVEC). *Toxicol In Vitro.* 25: 1883–1888.

Ha, Y. M., Amna, T., Kim, M. H., Kim, H. C., Hassan, M. S., Khil, M. S. 2013. Novel silicificated PVAc/POSS composite nanofibrous mat via facile electrospinning technique: Potential scaffold for hard tissue engineering. *Colloids Surfaces B.* 102: 795–802.

Harris, S., Bonewald, L., Harris, M., Sabatini, M., Dallas, S., Feng, J., Ghosh-Choudhury, N., Wozney, J., Mundy, G. 1994. Effects of transforming growth factor β on bone nodule formation and expression of bone morphogenetic protein 2, osteocalcin, osteopontin, alkaline phosphatase, and type I collagen mRNA in long-term cultures of fetal rat calvarial osteoblasts. *J Bone Miner Res.* 9: 855–863.

Hassan, C. M., Peppas, N. A. 2000. Structure and applications of poly(vinyl alcohol) hydrogels produced by conventional crosslinking or by freezing/thawing methods. In *Biopolymers·PVA Hydrogels, Anionic Polymerisation Nanocomposites.* Vol. 153. Berlin, Heidelberg: Springer, 37–65.

He, C., Jin, X., Ma, P. X. 2014. Calcium phosphate deposition rate, structure and osteoconductivity on electrospun poly(L-lactic acid) matrix using electrodeposition or simulated body fluid incubation. *Acta Biomater.* 10: 419–427.

He, J. X., Qi, K., Zhou, Y. M., Cui, S. Z. 2014. Fabrication of continuous nanofiber yarn using novel multi-nozzle bubble electrospinning. *Polym Int.* 63: 1288–1294.

Hong, S., Kim, G. 2011. Fabrication of size-controlled three-dimensional structures consisting of electrohydrodynamically produced polycaprolactone micro/nanofibers. *Appl Phys A: Mater.* 103: 1009–1014.

Hopley, E. L., Salmasi, S., Kalaskar, D. M., Seifalian, A. M. 2014. Carbon nanotubes leading the way forward in new generation 3D tissue engineering. *Biotechnol Adv.* 32: 1000–1014.

Hopper, A. P., Dugan, J. M., Gill, A. A., Fox, O. J. L., May, P. W., Haycock, J., Claeyssens, F. 2014. Amine functionalized nanodiamond promotes cellular adhesion, proliferation and neurite outgrowth. *Biomed Mater.* 9: 045009.

Huang, C., Chen, S., Lai, C. et al. 2006. Electrospun polymer nanofibres with small diameters. *Nanotechnology.* 17: 1558.

Jagur-Grodzinski, J. 2006. Polymers for tissue engineering, medical devices, and regenerative medicine. Concise general review of recent studies. *Polym Advan Technol.* 17: 395–418.

Jin, H. J., Chen, J., Karageorgiou, V., Altman, G. H., Kaplan, D. L. 2004. Human bone marrow stromal cell responses on electrospun silk fibroin mats. *Biomaterials.* 25: 1039–1047.

Joseph, J., Nair, S. V., Menon, D. 2015. Integrating substrate-less electrospinning with textile technology for creating biodegradable 3D structures. *Nano Lett.* 15: 5420–5426.

Kam, N. W. S., Jan, E., Kotov, N. A. 2008. Electrical stimulation of neural stem cells mediated by humanized carbon nanotube composite made with extracellular matrix protein. *Nano Lett.* 9: 273–278.

Kang, M. S., Kim, J. H., Singh, R. K., Jang, J. H., Kim, H. W. 2015. Therapeutic-designed electrospun bone scaffolds: Mesoporous bioactive nanocarriers in hollow fiber composites to sequentially deliver dual growth factors. *Acta Biomater.* 16: 103–116.

Khabashesku, V., Margrave, J., Barrera, E. 2005. Functionalized carbon nanotubes and nanodiamonds for engineering and biomedical applications. *Diam Relat Mater.* 14: 859–866.

Ki, C. S., Kim, J. W., Hyun, J. H. et al. 2007. Electrospun three-dimensional silk fibroin nanofibrous scaffold. *J Appl Polym Sci.* 106: 3922–3928.

Kidoaki, S., Kwon, I. K., Matsuda, T. 2005. Mesoscopic spatial designs of nano-and microfiber meshes for tissue-engineering matrix and scaffold based on newly devised multilayering and mixing electrospinning techniques. *Biomaterials.* 26: 37–46.

Kim, H.-W., Lee, H.-H., Knowles, J. C. 2008a. Nanofibrous glass tailored with apatite-fibronectin interface for bone cell stimulation. *J Nanosci Nanotechnol.* 8: 3013–3019.

Kim, H.-W., Yu, H. S., Lee, H. H. 2008b. Nanofibrous matrices of poly(lactic acid) and gelatin polymeric blends for the improvement of cellular responses. *J Biomed Mater Res A.* 87: 25–32.

Kim, I. Y., Seo, S. J., Moon, H. S., Yoo, M. K., Park, I. Y., Kim, B. C., Cho, C. S. 2008. Chitosan and its derivatives for tissue engineering applications. *Biotechnol Adv.* 26: 1–21.

Kim, J. E., Noh, K. T., Yu, H. S., Lee, H. Y., Jang, J. H., Kim, H. W. 2010. A fibronectin peptide-coupled biopolymer nanofibrous matrix to speed up initial cellular events. *Adv Eng Mater.* 12: B94–B100.

Kim, K. H., Jeong, L., Park, H. N., Shin, S. Y., Park, W. H., Lee, S. C., Kim, T. I., Park, Y. J., Seol, Y. J., Lee, Y. M. 2005. Biological efficacy of silk fibroin nanofiber membranes for guided bone regeneration. *J Biotechnol.* 120: 327–339.

Kim, S. E., Heo, D. N., Lee, J. B., Kim, J. R., Park, S. H., Jeon, S. H., Kwon, I. K. 2009. Electrospun gelatin/polyurethane blended nanofibers for wound healing. *Biomed Mater.* 4: 044106.

Kim, T. G., Park, T. G. 2006. Biomimicking extracellular matrix: Cell adhesive RGD peptide modified electrospun poly(D,L-lactic-co-glycolic acid) nanofiber mesh. *Tissue Eng.* 12: 221–233.

Klein, B., Schiffer, R., Hafemann, B., Klosterhalfen, B., Zwadlo-Klarwasser, G. 2001. Inflammatory response to a porcine membrane composed of fibrous collagen and elastin as dermal substitute. *J Mater Sci Mater M.* 12: 419–424.

Klokkevold, P. R., Vandemark, L., Kenney, E. B., Bernard, G. W. 1996. Osteogenesis enhanced by chitosan (poly-N-acetyl glucosaminoglycan) *in vitro*. *J Periodontol.* 67: 1170–1175.

Kolambkar, Y. M., Bajin, M., Wojtowicz, A., Hutmacher, D. W., García, A. J., Guldberg, R. E. 2013. Nanofiber orientation and surface functionalization modulate human mesenchymal stem cell behavior *in vitro*. *Tissue Eng A.* 20: 398–409.

Koski, A., Yim, K., Shivkumar, S. 2004. Effect of molecular weight on fibrous PVA produced by electrospinning. *Mater Lett.* 58: 493–497.

Kreppel, F., Kochanek, S. 2008. Modification of adenovirus gene transfer vectors with synthetic polymers: A scientific review and technical guide. *Mol Ther.* 16: 16–29.

Kretlow, J. D., Mikos, A. G. 2007. Review: Mineralization of synthetic polymer scaffolds for bone tissue engineering. *Tissue Eng.* 13: 927–938.

Krueger, A. 2008. New carbon materials: Biological applications of functionalized nanodiamond materials. *Chem Eur J.* 14: 1382–1390.

Kumar, G., Tison, C. K., Chatterjee, K. et al. 2011. The determination of stem cell fate by 3D scaffold structures through the control of cell shape. *Biomaterials.* 32: 9188–9196.

Kumar, S., Chatterjee, K. 2015. Strontium eluting graphene hybrid nanoparticles augment osteogenesis in a 3D tissue scaffold. *Nanoscale.* 7: 2023–2033.

Kumar, S., Raj, S., Kolanthai, E., Sood, A. K., Sampath, S., Chatterjee, K. 2015. Chemical functionalization of graphene to augment stem cell osteogenesis and inhibit biofilm formation on polymer composites for orthopedic applications. *ACS Appl Mater Inter.* 7: 3237–3252.

Lee, C. H., Singla, A., Lee, Y. 2001. Biomedical applications of collagen. *Int J Pharmaceut.* 221: 1–22.

Lee, E. J., Lee, J. H., Shin, Y. C., Hwang, D.-G., Kim, J. S., Jin, O. S., Jin, L., Hong, S. W., Han, D.-W. 2014. Graphene oxide-decorated PLGA/collagen hybrid fiber sheets for application to tissue engineering scaffolds. *Biomater Res.* 18: 18–24.

Lee, J. H, Lee, Y. J., Cho, H. J., Shin, H. 2013. Guidance of *in vitro* migration of human mesenchymal stem cells and *in vivo* guided bone regeneration using aligned electrospun fibers. *Tissue Eng A.* 20: 2031–2042.

Lee, K.-W., Wang, S., Fox, B. C., Ritman, E. L., Yaszemski, M. J., Lu, L. 2007. Poly(propylene fumarate) bone tissue engineering scaffold fabrication using stereolithography: Effects of resin formulations and laser parameters. *Biomacromolecules.* 8: 1077–1084.

Lee, K.-W., Wang, S., Lu, L., Jabbari, E., Currier, B. L., Yaszemski, M. J. 2006. Fabrication and characterization of poly(propylene fumarate) scaffolds with controlled pore structures using 3-dimensional printing and injection molding. *Tissue Eng.* 12: 2801–2811.

Lee, W. C., Lim, C. H. Y., Shi, H., Tang, L. A., Wang, Y., Lim, C. T., Loh, K. P. 2011. Origin of enhanced stem cell growth and differentiation on graphene and graphene oxide. *ACS Nano.* 5: 7334–7341.

Leung, L. H., Fan, S., Naguib, H. E. 2012. Fabrication of 3D electrospun structures from poly(lactide-co-glycolide acid)–nano-hydroxyapatite composites. *J Polym Sci B: Polym Phys.* 50: 242–249.

Lewandrowski, K.-U., Gresser, J. D., Wise, D. L., White, R. L., Trantolo, D. J. 2000. Osteoconductivity of an injectable and bioresorbable poly (propylene glycol-co-fumaric acid) bone cement. *Biomaterials*. 21: 293–298.

Li, C., Vepari, C., Jin, H. J., Kim, H. J., Kaplan, D. L. 2006. Electrospun silk-BMP-2 scaffolds for bone tissue engineering. *Biomaterials*. 27: 3115–3124.

Li, D., Wang, Y., Xia, Y. 2004. Electrospinning nanofibers as uniaxially aligned arrays and layer-by-layer stacked films. *Adv Mater*. 16: 361–366.

Li, F., Song, Y., Zhao, Y. 2010. Core–shell nanofibers: Nano channel and capsule by coaxial electrospinning. In *Nanofibers*, ed., Kumar A., Croatia: INTECH Open Access Publisher, 420–438.

Li, M., He, Y., Xin, C., Wei, X., Li, Q., Lu, C., Juang, Y. 2008. Dual electrode mode electrospinning of biodegradable polymers. *Appl Phys Lett*. 92: 213114.

Li, M., Mondrinos, M. J., Gandhi, M. R., Ko, F. K., Weiss, A. S., Lelkes, P. I. 2005. Electrospun protein fibers as matrices for tissue engineering. *Biomaterials*. 26: 5999–6008.

Li, M., Mondrinos, M. J., Chen, X., Gandhi, M. R., Ko, F. K., Lelkes, P. I. 2006. Co-electrospun poly (lactide-co-glycolide), gelatin, and elastin blends for tissue engineering scaffolds. *J Biomed Mater Res A*. 79: 963–973.

Li, Q., Wei ,Q., Wu, N., Cai, Y., Gao, W. 2008. Structural characterization and dynamic water adsorption of electrospun polyamide6/montmorillonite nanofibers. *J Appl Polym Sci*. 107: 3535–3540.

Li, X., Gao, H., Uo, M., Sato, Y., Akasaka, T., Feng, Q., Cui, F., Liu, X., Watari, F. 2009. Effect of carbon nanotubes on cellular functions *in vitro*. *J Biomed Mater Res A*. 91: 132–139.

Li, Z., Zhang, M. 2005. Chitosan–alginate as scaffolding material for cartilage tissue engineering. *J Biomed Mater Res A*. 75: 485–493.

Liao, G. Y., Jiang, S., Xia, H., Jiang, K. 2012. Preparation and characterization of aligned PLLA/PCL/HA composite fibrous membranes. *J Macromol Sci A*. 49: 946–951.

Liu, W., Wei, Y., Zhang, X., Xu, M., Yang, X., Deng, X. 2013. Lower extent but similar rhythm of osteogenic behavior in hBMSCs cultured on nanofibrous scaffolds versus induced with osteogenic supplement. *ACS Nano*. 7: 6928–6938.

Liu, Y., Park, M., Shin, H. K., Pant, B., Choi, J., Park, Y. W., Lee, J. Y., Park, S.-J., Kim, H.-Y. 2014. Facile preparation and characterization of poly (vinyl alcohol)/chitosan/graphene oxide biocomposite nanofibers. *J Ind Eng Chem*. 20: 4415–4420.

Liu, Y., Yu, D., Zeng, C., Miao, Z., Dai, L. 2010. Biocompatible graphene oxide-based glucose biosensors. *Langmuir*. 26: 6158–6160.

Liu, Y., Zhao, Y., Sun, B., Chen, C. 2012. Understanding the toxicity of carbon nanotubes. *Acc Chem Res*. 46: 702–713.

Lu, H. H., El-Amin, S. F., Scott, K. D., Laurencin, C. T. 2003. Three-dimensional, bioactive, biodegradable, polymer–bioactive glass composite scaffolds with improved mechanical properties support collagen synthesis and mineralization of human osteoblast-like cells *in vitro*. *J Biomed Mater Res A*. 64: 465–474.

Lu, Q., Ganesan, K., Simionescu, D. T., Vyavahare, N. R. 2004. Novel porous aortic elastin and collagen scaffolds for tissue engineering. *Biomaterials*. 25: 5227–5237.

Luu, Y., Kim, K., Hsiao, B., Chu, B., Hadjiargyrou, M. 2003. Development of a nanostructured DNA delivery scaffold via electrospinning of PLGA and PLA–PEG block copolymers. *J Control Release*. 89: 341–353.

Ma, H., Su, W., Tai, Z., Sun, D., Yan, X., Liu, B., Xue, Q. 2012. Preparation and cytocompatibility of polylactic acid/hydroxyapatite/graphene oxide nanocomposite fibrous membrane. *Chin Sci Bull*. 57: 3051–3058.

Madurantakam, P. A., Rodriguez, I. A., Garg, K., McCool, J. M., Moon, P. C., Bowlin, G. L. 2013. Compression of multilayered composite electrospun scaffolds: A novel strategy to rapidly enhance mechanical properties and three dimensionality of bone scaffolds. *Adv Mater Sci Eng*. 2013: 1–9.

Mallick, K. 2014. *Bone Substitute Biomaterials*. Cambridge, UK: Elsevier Woodhead Publishing, 352.

Mano, J., Silva, G., Azevedo, H. S., Malafaya, P., Sousa, R., Silva, S., Boesel, L., Oliveira, J. M., Santos, T., Marques, A. 2007. Natural origin biodegradable systems in tissue engineering and regenerative medicine: Present status and some moving trends. *J R Soc Interface.* 4: 999–1030.

Mansouri, S., Lavigne, P., Corsi, K., Benderdour, M., Beaumont, E., Fernandes, J. C. 2004. Chitosan-DNA nanoparticles as non-viral vectors in gene therapy: Strategies to improve transfection efficacy. *Eur J Pharm Biopharm.* 57: 1–8.

Martins, A., Chung, S., Pedro, A. J. et al. 2009. Hierarchical starch-based fibrous scaffold for bone tissue engineering applications. *J Tissue Eng Regen Med.* 3: 37–42.

Matthews, J. A., Wnek, G. E., Simpson, D. G., Bowlin, G. L. 2002. Electrospinning of collagen nanofibers. *Biomacromolecules.* 3: 232–238.

Mei, F., Zhong, J., Yang, X., Ouyang, X., Zhang, S., Hu, X., Ma, Q., Lu, J., Ryu, S., Deng, X. 2007. Improved biological characteristics of poly (L-lactic acid) electrospun membrane by incorporation of multiwalled carbon nanotubes/hydroxyapatite nanoparticles, *Biomacromolecules.* 8: 3729–3735.

Meinel, L., Karageorgiou, V., Hofmann, S. et al. 2004. Engineering bone-like tissue *in vitro* using human bone marrow stem cells and silk scaffolds. *J Biomed Mater Res A.* 71: 25–34.

Meng, J., Han, Z., Kong, H., Qi, X., Wang, C., Xie, S., Xu, H. 2010. Electrospun aligned nanofibrous composite of MWCNT/polyurethane to enhance vascular endothelium cells proliferation and function. *J Biomed Mater Res A.* 95: 312–320.

Meng, W., Kim, S.-Y., Yuan, J., Kim, J. C., Kwon, O. H., Kawazoe, N., Chen, G., Ito, Y., Kang, I.-K. 2007. Electrospun PHBV/collagen composite nanofibrous scaffolds for tissue engineering. *J Biomater Sci.* 18: 81–94.

Meng, Z., Li, H., Sun, Z., Zheng, W., Zheng, Y. 2013. Fabrication of mineralized electrospun PLGA and PLGA/gelatin nanofibers and their potential in bone tissue engineering, *Mater Sci Eng C: Mater Biol Appl.* 33: 699–706.

Meng, Z., Wang, Y., Ma, C., Zheng, W., Li, L., Zheng, Y. 2010. Electrospinning of PLGA/gelatin randomly-oriented and aligned nanofibers as potential scaffold in tissue engineering. *Mater Sci Eng C.* 30: 1204–1210.

Meng, Z., Zeng, Q., Sun, Z., Xu, X., Wang, Y., Zheng, W., Zheng, Y. 2012. Immobilizing natural macromolecule on PLGA electrospun nanofiber with surface entrapment and entrapment-graft techniques. *Colloids Surf B: Biointerfaces.* 94: 44–50.

Mickova, A., Buzgo, M., Benada, O., Rampichova, M., Fisar, Z., Filova, E., Tesarova, M., Lukas, D., Amler, E. 2012. Core/shell nanofibers with embedded liposomes as a drug delivery system. *Biomacromolecules.* 13: 952–962.

Middleton, J. C., Tipton, A. J. 2000. Synthetic biodegradable polymers as orthopedic devices. *Biomaterials.* 21: 2335–2346.

Misra, S. K., Watts, P., Valappil, S. P., Silva, S., Roy, I., Boccaccini, A. 2007. Poly (3-hydroxybutyrate)/bioglass® composite films containing carbon nanotubes. *Nanotechnology.* 18: 075701.

Mit-uppatham, C., Nithitanakul, M., Supaphol, P. 2004. Ultrafine electrospun polyamide-6 fibers: Effect of solution conditions on morphology and average fiber diameter. *Macromol Chem Phys.* 205: 2327–2338.

Mochalin, V. N., Shenderova, O., Ho, D., Gogotsi, Y. 2012. The properties and applications of nanodiamonds. *Nat Nanotechnol.* 7: 11–23.

Nam, J., Huang, Y., Agarwal, S., Lannutti, J. 2007. Improved cellular infiltration in electrospun fiber via engineered porosity. *Tissue Eng.* 13: 2249–2257.

Namgung, S., Baik, K. Y., Park, J., Hong, S. 2011. Controlling the growth and differentiation of human mesenchymal stem cells by the arrangement of individual carbon nanotubes. *ACS Nano.* 5: 7383–7390.

Nardecchia, S., Carriazo, D., Ferrer, M. L., Gutiérrez, M. C., del Monte, F. 2013. Three dimensional macroporous architectures and aerogels built of carbon nanotubes and/or graphene: Synthesis and applications. *Chem Soc Rev.* 42: 794–830.

Nazre, A. T., Lin, S. 1994. Theoretical strength comparison of bioabsorbable (PLLA) plates and conventional stainless steel and titanium plates used in internal fracture fixation. In *Clinical and Laboratory Performance of Bone Plates*, ed., Harvey, J. P., Games, R. F., ASTM Special Technical Publication. 1217: 53–53.

Ng, A. M., Tan, K. K., Phang, M. Y., Aziyati, O., Tan, G., Isa, M., Aminuddin, B., Naseem, M., Fauziah, O., Ruszymah, B. 2008. Differential osteogenic activity of osteoprogenitor cells on HA and TCP/HA scaffold of tissue engineered bone. *J Biomed Mater Res A.* 85: 301–312.

Nivison-Smith, L., Rnjak, J., Weiss, A. S. 2010. Synthetic human elastin microfibers: Stable cross-linked tropoelastin and cell interactive constructs for tissue engineering applications. *Acta Biomater.* 6: 354–359.

Okamoto, M., John, B. 2013. Synthetic biopolymer nanocomposites for tissue engineering scaffolds. *Prog Polym Sci.* 38: 1487–1503.

Panzavolta, S., Gioffrè, M., Focarete, M. L., Gualandi, C., Foroni, L., Bigi, A. 2011. Electrospun gelatin nanofibers: Optimization of genipin cross-linking to preserve fiber morphology after exposure to water. *Acta Biomater.* 7: 1702–1709.

Parizek, M., Douglas, T. E., Novotna, K., Kromka, A., Brady, M. A., Renzing, A., Voss, E., Jarosova, M., Palatinus, L., Tesarek, P. 2012. Nanofibrous poly(lactide-co-glycolide) membranes loaded with diamond nanoparticles as promising substrates for bone tissue engineering. *Int J Nanomed.* 7: 1931.

Park, J., Kelly, B., Kenner, G., von Recum, A., Grether, M., Coffeen, W. 1981. Piezoelectric ceramic implants: *In vivo* results. *J Biomed Mater Res A.* 15: 103–110.

Park, S. H., Kim, T. G., Kim, H. C., Yang, D. Y., Park, T. G. 2008. Development of dual scale scaffolds via direct polymer melt deposition and electrospinning for applications in tissue regeneration. *Acta Biomater.* 4: 1198–1207.

Patlolla, A., Collins, G., Arinzeh, T. L. 2010. Solvent-dependent properties of electrospun fibrous composites for bone tissue regeneration. *Acta Biomater.* 6: 90–101.

Paule, W., Bernick, S., Strates, B., Nimmi, M. 1992. Calcification of implanted vascular tissues associated with elastin in an experimental animal model. *J Biomed Mater Res A.* 26: 1169–1177.

Peng, F., Yu, X., Wei, M. 2011. *In vitro* cell performance on hydroxyapatite particles/poly(L-lactic acid) nanofibrous scaffolds with an excellent particle along nanofiber orientation. *Acta Biomater.* 7: 2585–2592.

Petreaca, M., Martins-Green, M. 2013. The dynamics of cell-ECM interactions, with implications for tissue engineering. In *Principles of Tissue Engineering*, ed., Lanza, R., Langer, R., Vacanti, J. P., Burlington, MA: Academic Press.

Pham, Q. P., Sharma, U., Mikos, A. G. 2006. Electrospun poly (ε-caprolactone) microfiber and multilayer nanofiber/microfiber scaffolds: Characterization of scaffolds and measurement of cellular infiltration. *Biomacromolecules.*7: 2796–2805.

Phipps, M. C., Clem, W. C., Grunda, J. M., Clines, G. A., Bellis, S. L. 2012. Increasing the pore sizes of bone-mimetic electrospun scaffolds comprised of polycaprolactone, collagen I and hydroxyapatite to enhance cell infiltration. *Biomaterials.* 33: 524–534.

Pumera, M. 2011. Nanotoxicology: The molecular science point of view. *Chem Asian J.* 6: 340–348.

Qi, Y., Tai, Z., Sun, D., Chen, J., Ma, H., Yan, X., Liu, B., Xue, Q. 2013. Fabrication and characterization of poly(vinyl alcohol)/graphene oxide nanofibrous biocomposite scaffolds. *J Appl Polym Sci.* 127: 1885–1894.

Ramalingam, M., Young, M. F., Thomas, V., Sun, L., Chow, L. C., Tison, C. K., Chatterjee, K., Miles, W. C., Simon, C. G. 2013. Nanofiber scaffold gradients for interfacial tissue engineering. *J Biomater Appl.* 27: 695–705.

Rao, C., Sood, A., Voggu, R., Subrahmanyam, K. 2010. Some novel attributes of graphene. *J Phys Chem Lett.* 1: 572–580.

Ravichandran, R., Venugopal, J. R., Sundarrajan, S., Mukherjee, S., Ramakrishna, S. 2012. Precipitation of nanohydroxyapatite on PLLA/PBLG/collagen nanofibrous structures for the differentiation of adipose derived stem cells to osteogenic lineage. *Biomaterials.* 33: 846–855.

Rodgers, U. R., Weiss, A. S. 2005. Cellular interactions with elastin. *Pathol-Biol.* 53: 390–398.

Roozbahani, F., Sultana, N., Ismail, A. F., Nouparvar, H. 2013. Effects of chitosan alkali pretreatment on the preparation of electrospun PCL/chitosan blend nanofibrous scaffolds for tissue engineering application. *J Nanomater* 2013: 1–6.

Saeed, K., Park, S.-Y., Lee, H.-J., Baek, J.-B., Huh, W.-S. 2006. Preparation of electrospun nanofibers of carbon nanotube/polycaprolactone nanocomposite. *Polymer.* 47: 8019–8025.

Saito, R., Dresselhaus, G., Dresselhaus, M. S. 1998. *Physical Properties of Carbon Nanotubes.* Vol. 35, London, UK: Imperial College Press.

Salaam, A. D., Mishra, M., Nyairo, E., Dean, D. 2014. Electrospun polyvinyl alcohol/nanodiamond composite scaffolds: Morphological, structural, and biological analysis. *J Biomater Tissue Eng.* 4: 173–180.

Schneider, O. D., Weber, F., Brunner, T. J., Loher, S., Ehrbar, M., Schmidlin, P. R., Stark, W. J. 2009. *In vivo* and *in vitro* evaluation of flexible, cottonwool-like nanocomposites as bone substitute material for complex defects. *Acta Biomater.* 5: 1775–1784.

Schrand, A. M., Huang, H., Carlson, C., Schlager, J. J., Osawa, E., Hussain, S. M., Daim, L. 2007. Are diamond nanoparticles cytotoxic? *J Phys Chem B.* 111: 2–7.

Seal, B., Otero, T., Panitch, A. 2001. Polymeric biomaterials for tissue and organ regeneration. *Mat Sci Eng R.* 34: 147–230.

Sell, S. A., Wolfe, P. S., Garg, K., McCool, J. M., Rodriguez, I. A., Bowlin, G. L. 2010. The use of natural polymers in tissue engineering: A focus on electrospun extracellular matrix analogues. *Polymers.* 2: 522–553.

Sellaro, T. L., Ravindra, A. K., Stolz, D. B., Badylak, S. F. 2007. Maintenance of hepatic sinusoidal endothelial cell phenotype *in vitro* using organ-specific extracellular matrix scaffolds. *Tissue Eng.* 13: 2301–2310.

Sen, R., Zhao, B., Perea, D., Itkis, M. E., Hu, H., Love, J., Bekyarova, E., Haddon, R. C. 2004. Preparation of single-walled carbon nanotube reinforced polystyrene and polyurethane nanofibers and membranes by electrospinning. *Nano Lett.* 4: 459–464.

Shah, S., Yin, P. T., Uehara, T. M., Chueng, S. T. D., Yang, L., Lee, K. B. 2014. Guiding stem cell differentiation into oligodendrocytes using graphene-nanofiber hybrid scaffolds. *Adv Mater* 26: 3673–3680.

Shalumon, K., Binulal, N., Selvamurugan, N., Nair, S., Menon, D., Furuike, T., Tamura, H., Jayakumar, R. 2009. Electrospinning of carboxymethyl chitin/poly(vinyl alcohol) nanofibrous scaffolds for tissue engineering applications. *Carbohyd Polym.* 77: 863–869.

Shao, S., Zhou, S., Li, L., Li, J., Luo, C., Wang, J., Li, X., Weng, J. 2011. Osteoblast function on electrically conductive electrospun PLA/MWCNTs nanofibers. *Biomaterials.* 32: 2821–2833.

Shim, I. K., Jung, M. R., Kim, K. H., Seol, Y. J., Park, Y. J., Park, W. H., Lee, S. J. 2010. Novel three-dimensional scaffolds of poly(L-lactic acid) microfibers using electrospinning and mechanical expansion: Fabrication and bone regeneration. *J Biomed Mater Res B: Appl Biomater.* 95: 150–160.

Shim, I. K., Suh, W. H., Lee, S. Y., Lee, S. H., Heo, S. J., Lee, M. C., Lee, S. J. 2009. Chitosan nano-/microfibrous double-layered membrane with rolled-up three-dimensional structures for chondrocyte cultivation. *J Biomed Mater Res A.* 90: 595–602.

Sill, T. J., von Recum, H. A. 2008. Electrospinning: Applications in drug delivery and tissue engineering. *Biomaterials.* 29: 1989–2006.

Singh, R. K., Jin, G. Z., Mahapatra, C., Patel, K. D., Chrzanowski, W., Kim, H.-W. 2015. Mesoporous silica-layered biopolymer hybrid nanofibrous scaffold: A novel nanobiomatrix platform for therapeutics delivery and bone regeneration. *ACS Appl Mater Interface.* 7: 8088–8098.

Singh, R. K., Patel, K. D., Lee, J. H., Lee, E.-J., Kim, J.-H., Kim, T.-H., Kim, H.-W. 2014. Potential of magnetic nanofiber scaffolds with mechanical and biological properties applicable for bone regeneration. *PloS One.* 9: e91584.

Sionkowska, A. 2011. Current research on the blends of natural and synthetic polymers as new biomaterials: Review. *Prog Polym Sci.* 36: 1254–1276.

Sisson, K., Zhang, C., Farach-Carson, M. C., Chase, D. B., Rabolt, J. F. 2010. Fiber diameters control osteoblastic cell migration and differentiation in electrospun gelatin. *J Biomed Mater Res A.* 94: 1312–1320.

Smit, E., Büttner, U., Sanderson, R. D. 2005. Continuous yarns from electrospun fibers. *Polymer.* 46: 2419–2423.

Soliman, S., Pagliari, S., Rinaldi, A. et al. 2010. Multiscale three-dimensional scaffolds for soft tissue engineering via multimodal electrospinning. *Acta Biomater.* 6: 1227–1237.

Spadaro, J. A. 1977. Electrically stimulated bone growth in animals and man: Review of the literature. *Clin Orthop Relat R.* 122: 325–332.

Srouji, S., Ben-David, D., Lotan, R., Livne, E., Avrahami, R., Zussman, E. 2010. Slow-release human recombinant bone morphogenetic protein-2 embedded within electrospun scaffolds for regeneration of bone defect: *In vitro* and *in vivo* evaluation. *Tissue Eng A.* 17: 269–277.

Su, Y., Su, Q., Liu, W., Lim, M., Venugopal, J. R., Mo, X., Ramakrishna, S., Al-Deyab, S. S., El-Newehy, M. 2012. Controlled release of bone morphogenetic protein 2 and dexamethasone loaded in core–shell PLLACL–collagen fibers for use in bone tissue engineering. *Acta Biomater.* 8: 763–771.

Supronowicz, P., Ajayan, P., Ullmann, K., Arulanandam, B., Metzger, D., Bizios, R. 2002. Novel current-conducting composite substrates for exposing osteoblasts to alternating current stimulation. *J Biomed Mater Res A.* 59: 499–506.

Teo, W., Liao, S., Chan, C., Ramakrishna, S. 2008. Remodeling of three-dimensional hierarchically organized nanofibrous assemblies. *Curr Nanosci.* 4: 361–369.

Teo, W. E., Gopal, R., Ramaseshan, R., Fujihara, K., Ramakrishna, S. 2007. A dynamic liquid support system for continuous electrospun yarn fabrication. *Polymer.* 48: 3400–3405.

Thomas, V., Dean, D. R., Jose, M. V., Mathew, B., Chowdhury, S., Vohra, Y. K. 2007. Nanostructured biocomposite scaffolds based on collagen coelectrospun with nanohydroxyapatite. *Biomacromolecules.* 8: 631–637.

Thompson, C., Chase, G., Yarin, A., Reneker, D. 2007. Effects of parameters on nanofiber diameter determined from electrospinning model. *Polymer.* 48: 6913–6922.

Tian, L., Zhao, C., Li, J., Pan, Z. 2014. Multi-needle, electrospun, nanofiber filaments: Effects of the needle arrangement on the nanofiber alignment degree and electrostatic field distribution. *Text Res J.* 8: 621–631.

Tuzlakoglu, K., Bolgen, N., Salgado, A., Gomes, M. E., Piskin, E., Reis, R. 2005. Nano-and micro-fiber combined scaffolds: A new architecture for bone tissue engineering. *J Mater Sci Mater M.* 16: 1099–1104.

Van Dyke, M. E. 2012a. Wound healing compositions containing keratin biomaterials. Google Patents. (US20080274165).

Van Dyke, M. E. 2012b. Clotting and healing compositions containing keratin biomaterials. Google Patents. (US 8299013 B2).

Van Dyke, M. E. 2014. Keratin bioceramic compositions. Google Patents. (WO 2007050387 A3).

Vaquette, C., Cooper-White, J. J. 2011. Increasing electrospun scaffold pore size with tailored collectors for improved cell penetration. *Acta Biomater.* 7: 2544–2557.

Vardharajula, S., Ali, S. Z., Tiwari, P. M., Eroğlu, E., Vig, K., Dennis, V. A., Singh, S. R. 2012. Functionalized carbon nanotubes: Biomedical applications. *Int J Nanomed.* 7: 5361.

Verreck, G., Chun, I., Peeters, J., Rosenblatt, J., Brewster, M. E. 2003. Preparation and characterization of nanofibers containing amorphous drug dispersions generated by electrostatic spinning. *Pharm Res.* 20: 810–817.

Wan, C., Chen, B. 2011. Poly(ε-caprolactone)/graphene oxide biocomposites: Mechanical properties and bioactivity. *Biomed Mater.* 6: 055010.

Wang, J., Yu, X. 2010. Preparation, characterization and *in vitro* analysis of novel structured nanofibrous scaffolds for bone tissue engineering. *Acta Biomater.* 6: 3004–3012.

Wang, M. 2003. Developing bioactive composite materials for tissue replacement. *Biomaterials.* 24: 2133–2151.

Wang, W., Itoh, S., Matsuda, A., Ichinose, S., Shinomiya, K., Hata, Y., Tanaka, J. 2008. Influences of mechanical properties and permeability on chitosan nano/microfiber mesh tubes as a scaffold for nerve regeneration. *J Biomed Mater Res B: Appl Biomater.* 84: 557–566.

Wang, Y., Wang, G., Chen, L. et al. 2009. Electrospun nanofiber meshes with tailored architectures and patterns as potential tissue-engineering scaffolds. *Biofabrication.* 1: 015001.

Wang, Z., Cai, N., Zhao, D., Xu, J., Dai, Q., Xue, Y., Luo, X., Yang, Y., Yu, F. 2013. Mechanical reinforcement of electrospun water-soluble polymer nanofibers using nanodiamonds. *Polym Composites.* 34: 1735–1744.

Weadock, K. S., Miller, E. J., Bellincampi, L. D., Zawadsky, J. P., Dunn, M. G. 1995. Physical crosslinking of collagen fibers: Comparison of ultraviolet irradiation and dehydrothermal treatment. *J Biomed Mater Res A.* 29: 1373–1379.

Wei, Y., Zhang, X., Song, Y., Han, B., Hu, X., Wang, X., Lin, Y., Deng, X. 2011. Magnetic biodegradable Fe3O4/CS/PVA nanofibrous membranes for bone regeneration. *Biomed Mater.* 6: 055008.

Whited, B. M., Whitney, J. R., Hofmann, M. C., Xu, Y., Rylander, M. N. 2011. Pre-osteoblast infiltration and differentiation in highly porous apatite-coated PLLA electrospun scaffolds. *Biomaterials.* 32: 2294–2304.

Woodruff, M. A., Hutmacher, D. W. 2010. The return of a forgotten polymer—Polycaprolactone in the 21st century. *Prog Polym Sci.* 35: 1217–1256.

Wu, Y., Jiang, W., Wen, X., He, B., Zeng, X., Wang, G., Gu, Z. 2010. A novel calcium phosphate ceramic–magnetic nanoparticle composite as a potential bone substitute. *Biomed Mater.* 5: 015001.

Wutticharoenmongkol, P., Sanchavanakit, N., Pavasant, P., Supaphol, P. 2006. Preparation and characterization of novel bone scaffolds based on electrospun polycaprolactone fibers filled with nanoparticles. *Macromol Biosci.* 6: 70–77.

Yang, Q., Li, Z., Hong, Y. et al. 2004. Influence of solvents on the formation of ultrathin uniform poly (vinyl pyrrolidone) nanofibers with electrospinning. *J Polym Sci B: Polym Phys.* 42: 3721–3726.

Yoo, C. R., Yeo, I.-S., Park, K. E., Park, J. H., Lee, S. J., Park, W. H., Min, B.-M. 2008. Effect of chitin/silk fibroin nanofibrous bicomponent structures on interaction with human epidermal keratinocytes. *Int J Biol Macromol.* 42: 324–334.

Yoon, O. J., Sohn, I. Y., Kim, D. J., Lee, N.-E. 2012. Enhancement of thermomechanical properties of poly(D,L-lactic-co-glycolic acid) and graphene oxide composite films for scaffolds. *Macromol Res.* 20: 789–794.

Yoshimoto, H., Shin, Y., Terai, H., Vacanti, J. 2003. A biodegradable nanofiber scaffold by electrospinning and its potential for bone tissue engineering. *Biomaterials.* 24: 2077–2082.

Yousefzadeh, M., Latifi, M., Amani-Tehran, M., Teo, W. E., Ramakrishna, S. 2012. A note on the 3D structural design of electrospun nanofibers. *J Eng Fibr Fabr.* 7: 7–23.

Yu, D. G., Li, X., Wang, X., Yang, J., Bligh, S. A., Williams, G. R. 2015. Nanofibers fabricated using triaxial electrospinning as zero order drug delivery systems. *ACS Appl Mater Interfaces.* 7: 18891–18897.

Yu, Y.-H., Chan, C.-C., Lai, Y.-C., Lin, Y.-Y., Huang, Y.-C., Chi, W.-F., Kuo, C. W., Lin, H. M., Chen, P.-C. 2014. Biocompatible electrospinning poly(vinyl alcohol) nanofibres embedded with graphene-based derivatives with enhanced conductivity, mechanical strength and thermal stability. *RSC Adv.* 4: 56373–56384.

Zanello, L. P., Zhao, B., Hu, H., Haddon, R. C. 2006. Bone cell proliferation on carbon nanotubes. *Nano Lett.* 6: 562–567.

Zhang, D., Chang, J. 2008. Electrospinning of three-dimensional nanofibrous tubes with controllable architectures. *Nano Lett.* 8: 3283–3287.

Zhang, D., Yi, C., Qi, S., Yao, X., Yang, M. 2010. Effects of carbon nanotubes on the proliferation and differentiation of primary osteoblasts. In *Carbon Nanotubes*, eds. Balasubramanian, K. and Burghard, M. NY, USA: Humana Press, 41–53.

Zhang, Q., Mochalin, V. N., Neitzel, I., Knoke, I. Y., Han, J., Klug, C. A., Zhou, J. G., Lelkes, P. I., Gogotsi, Y. 2011. Fluorescent PLLA-nanodiamond composites for bone tissue engineering. *Biomaterials.* 32: 87–94.

Zhang, S., Huang, Y., Yang, X., Mei, F., Ma, Q., Chen, G., Ryu, S., Deng, X. 2009. Gelatin nanofibrous membrane fabricated by electrospinning of aqueous gelatin solution for guided tissue regeneration. *J Biomed Mater Res A.* 90: 671–679.

Zhang, X., Hu, W., Li, J., Tao, L., Wei, Y. 2012. A comparative study of cellular uptake and cytotoxicity of multi-walled carbon nanotubes, graphene oxide, and nanodiamond. *Toxicol Res.* 1: 62–68.

Zhang, X., Wang, X., Lu, Q., Fu, C. 2008. Influence of carbon nanotube scaffolds on human cervical carcinoma HeLa cell viability and focal adhesion kinase expression. *Carbon.* 46: 453–460.

Zhang, Y., Ali, S. F., Dervishi, E., Xu, Y., Li, Z., Casciano, D., Biris, A. S. 2010. Cytotoxicity effects of graphene and single-wall carbon nanotubes in neural phaeochromocytoma-derived PC12 cells. *ACS Nano.* 4: 3181–3186.

Zhang, Y., Ouyang, H., Lim, C. T., Ramakrishna, S., Huang, Z. M. 2005. Electrospinning of gelatin fibers and gelatin/PCL composite fibrous scaffolds. *J Biomed Mater Res B.* 72: 156–165.

Zhang, Y., Venugopal, J., Huang, Z.-M., Lim, C., Ramakrishna, S. 2006. Crosslinking of the electrospun gelatin nanofibers. *Polymer.* 47: 2911–2917.

Zhang, Y., Venugopal, J. R., El-Turki, A., Ramakrishna, S., Su, B., Lim, C. T. 2008. Electrospun biomimetic nanocomposite nanofibers of hydroxyapatite/chitosan for bone tissue engineering. *Biomaterials.* 29: 4314–4322.

Zhong, S., Teo, W. E., Zhu, X., Beuerman, R., Ramakrishna, S., Yung, L. Y. L. 2005. Formation of collagen-glycosaminoglycan blended nanofibrous scaffolds and their biological properties. *Biomacromolecules.* 6: 2998–3004.

Zhou, F. L., Gong, R. H. 2008. Manufacturing technologies of polymeric nanofibres and nanofibre yarns. *Polym Int.* 57: 837–845.

Zuo, W., Zhu, M., Yang, W., Yu, H. 2005. Experimental study on relationship between jet instability and formation of beaded fibers during electrospinning. *Polym Eng Sci.* 45: 704.

Zvibel, I., Wagner, A., Pasmanik-Chor, M., Varol, C., Oron-Karni, V., Santo, E. M., Halpern, Z., Kariv, R. 2013. Transcriptional profiling identifies genes induced by hepatocyte-derived extracellular matrix in metastatic human colorectal cancer cell lines. *Clin Exp Metastas.* 30: 189–200.

4

Strategies for Bone Grafting and Bone Tissue Engineering

Brittany L. Taylor and Joseph W. Freeman

CONTENTS

4.1 Introduction

Bone-related disorders associated with cancer, injury, abnormal development, and degenerative conditions dramatically diminish the health and quality of life of millions of people. These disorders can cause significant disability through loss of bone or its functionality, creating a need for bone replacements or effective regenerative strategies. Bone loss and skeletal deficiencies arising from traumatic injury, abnormal development, cancer, and degenerative bone diseases significantly impact the health and mobility of millions of Americans and frequently require surgical intervention. Degenerative bone disorders such as osteoporosis (which affects ~75 million people in Europe, the United States, and Japan) weaken bones, to the extent that even mild stresses like bending over, lifting a vacuum cleaner, or coughing can cause a fracture (Consensus Development Statement, 1997). This leads to dramatic changes in quality of life due to severe pain, loss of mobility, and diminished function. Nearly 30%–50% of women and 15%–30% of men will suffer a fracture related to osteoporosis in their lifetime (Kanis et al., 2000; Melton et al., 1992, 1998; Randell et al., 1995). Over three million orthopedic procedures are performed annually in the United States. Approximately 500,000 of these are bone grafting procedures with an estimated cost of $2.5 billion annually making bone second to blood as the most frequently transplanted material (Consensus Development Statement, 1997; Randell et al., 1995). The bone grafting market in the United States has an estimated value at over $1 billion; this number is expected to increase due to a projected annual increase of 2%–3% in the population over age 65 (Consensus Development Statement, 1997; Kanis et al., 2000; Melton et al., 1992, 1998; Perry, 1999; Shin et al., 2008). The loss of bone due to traumatic injury or disease is a huge problem. In 2005, the American Cancer Society estimated that 2570 people would be diagnosed with bone cancer that year, with osteosarcoma and chondrosarcoma being the two most common primary bone cancers (Schoenstadt, 2013); severe forms can lead to amputation. Every year over 600,000 people in the United States undergo hip- or knee-replacement surgery (Hitti, 2006). In 1999, 500,000–600,000 bone grafting procedures were performed (Khan et al., 2004). Approximately 10% of these procedures included the use of synthetic bone graft substitutes (Khan et al., 2004) and the remaining being autografts and allografts.

4.2 Bone Composition and Structure

Bone is a complex hard tissue with a heterogeneous composition and structure. The main purpose of bone is to protect the body's vital organs by providing structural support and serve as a blood cell reservoir (Hing, 2004). The main components of bone are an organic matrix, collagen, inorganic mineral crystals, calcium phosphate, and water (Hing, 2004; Rho et al., 1998; Wang et al., 2007). Each component plays a role in bone's overall mechanical properties. The organic matrix, mainly type I collagen, contributes to the toughness of bone. The hydrated inorganic mineral phase composed of hydroxyapatite (HAp) and water are responsible for the stiffness and viscoelastic behaviors of bone, respectively. The cells active in bone development and maintenance are osteoblasts, osteocytes, and osteoclasts (Hing, 2004). Osteoblasts, bone making cells, function in groups of connected cells to form the organic matrix of bone. Osteoclasts, bone resorption cells, are the main cell type involved in bone remodeling and repair. Osteocytes, inert cells derived from osteoblasts, are most commonly found in mature bone and responsible for bone molecular synthesis and modification. The interaction between osteoblasts, osteoclasts, and osteocytes is essential for bone homeostasis. Structurally, bone is organized into two distinct types based on its density and location: cortical bone and trabecular bone (Hing, 2004; Rho et al., 1998; Wang and Puram, 2004). Cortical bone or compact bone has a highly organized dense structure composed of tightly packed osteons and is usually found in the outside of bone. The compact architecture of cortical bone, with a porosity ranging between 5% and 30%, contribute to the structural integrity of bone (Yuehuei and Draughn, 1999). The Haversian canals are located in the center of the osteonic subunits and house the blood microvasculature, nerve cells, and osteocytes. Volkmann's canals run perpendicular to the Haversian canals and are responsible for creating structures for vessel sprouting. Blood and nutrient transport are essential for bone remodeling. The highly porous bone structure, trabecular bone, is located inside cortical bone. Trabecular bone or spongy bone, is 90% porous with low strength (Wang and Puram, 2004; Yuehuei and Draughn, 1999). The mechanical properties of cortical bone, trabecular bone, and whole bone are outlined

TABLE 4.1

Mechanical Properties of Trabecular, Cortical, and Whole Bone

	Tensile Strength (MPa)	Young's Modulus (GPa)
Trabecular bone	3–9	0.01–0.9
Cortical bone	167–215	10–20
Whole bone	70	1

Source: Reprinted with permission from Chen, G. et al. 3D scaffolds with different stiffness but the same microstructure for bone tissue engineering. *ACS Appl Mater Interfaces.* 7: 15790–802. Copyright 2015 American Chemical Society.

in Table 4.1 (Wheeler and Enneking, 2005). The difference in the mechanical properties is due to the structure, porosity, and composition of the two bone types.

4.3 Current Treatments for Damaged Bone

Naturally, bone regenerates on its own without scar tissue formation (Frohlich et al., 2008). In the case of bone disease due to abnormal bone development and physiology or significant skeletal bone loss, the natural healing process is compromised. Surgical intervention is required to replace the damaged bone and provide structural support while the bone regeneration process takes place. In the United States, there are approximately 500,000 bone grafting treatment performed annually resulting in $2.5 billion expenditure (Perry, 1999). Bone is the second most transplanted tissue next to blood making the bone grafting industry a $1 billion market. These values are expected to increase as people are living past the average life expectancy age of 65 at a 2%–3% increasing rate per year (Greenwald et al., 2001; Hing, 2004). The gold standard orthopedic procedure to replace damaged bone is autografting. Autografting utilizes an autologous bone tissue source usually harvested from the iliac crest. Autografts provide good mechanical strength upon implantation, disadvantages include limited supply, donor site morbidity, and increased pain, hospital and recovery time, and costs due to two surgeries (harvest and implantation surgery). The second most commonly used biological graft is allografts. Allografting procedures use donated bone tissue from a cadaveric source. There is an abundant supply of allografts, but there is a risk of disease transmission associated with the allogenic source and there is a 30%–60% risk of failure over 10 years due to the decrease of mechanical properties *in vivo* (Wheeler and Enneking, 2005). Xenografts, bone taken from animals, also have risk of disease transmission, difficulty of processing, and uncertain immune response. Alternatives such as metallic implants (used in joint replacement) lack the ability to bond with surrounding bone, whereas bone cements cannot be used exclusively to repair load-bearing bones. Given the drawbacks associated with the use of biological grafts, metallic implants, and cements, there is a need for a tissue-engineered (TE) bone graft.

4.4 TE Graft as a Promising Alternative

The field of tissue engineering is a rising and promising field that combines the use of cells, bioactive molecules, and engineered scaffolds to improve tissue regeneration. The idea behind tissue engineering is the use of a biodegradable scaffold to provide initial structure and support for matrix deposition and tissue formation. Cells are harvested from the patients and cultured and expanded in monolayer. The cells are then seeded in a three-dimensional (3D) scaffold with the addition of growth factors, nanoparticles, or secondary cell type to enhance the culturing process and natural cellular activity. With additional culture time, the TE scaffold with cells develops into organized tissue, which is then implanted back into the patient (Dvir et al., 2001). TE grafts have advantageous features such as abundant supply and a low risk of adverse effects. Ideally, the scaffold used in the TE approach should have the ability to promote cellular attachment, proliferation, infiltration, and bone matrix deposition by mimicking the extracellular matrix. In order to meet these requirements, the scaffold must be biocompatible, osteoconductive (allows bone to grow on the surface), osteoinductive (able to differentiate osteoprogenitor cells into osteoblasts and begin bone formation), and osteogenic (promotes osteoblasts to lay down new bone material). In addition, the TE scaffold must be porous with favorable degradation rates and mechanical properties comparable to native bone. The desired pores range for a TE scaffold designed to promoted bone growth is 5–200 μm. This pore range allows for the infiltration of osteoblastic cells, nutrients, and connective soft tissue. The scaffold serves as a temporary matrix for tissue formation, therefore the degradation rate should be proportional to bone renewal and growth rate. To reduce the risk of mechanical failure *in vivo*, the scaffold should process mechanical properties that match the surrounding tissue's mechanical properties. Although TE bone replacements have enormous potential, aspects such as cellular infiltration, vascularization, comparable mechanical strength and osteoblastic differentiation limit development of truly viable and functional bone. Many researchers have develop scaffold, which mimic only the porous trabecular structure, leading to a TE graft that has lower end mechanical properties for nonload-bearing applications. The calcium phosphate and ceramic-based bioactive TE grafts have enhanced mechanical strength, but lack osseointegration (ability of an implant to integrate with the surrounding tissue). Furthermore, very few effective strategies exist for stimulating osteoblastic and vascular differentiation simultaneously. The presence of newly forming osteoblastic tissue and vasculature is crucial for long-term mechanics and graft viability. Growth factors such as bone morphogenetic proteins (BMP), to induce osteoblastic differentiation can have adverse effects such as an overexpression of bone development leading to atopic bone formation. Future directions to enhance vascularization in bone regeneration are largely aimed at enhancing early vascular support using prevascularization of tissue-engineered constructs (Krishnan et al., 2014; Novosel et al., 2011). The following two sections will focus on recent research and insights in the area of bone grafting and bone tissue engineering and patented devices in bone grafting and tissue engineering. This will give the readers both a view of some of the cutting edge research in this area and also allow them to see what ideas have been able to reach a point where they are patented and in some cases ready for commercialization.

4.5 Novel Research in Bone Grafts and Bone Tissue Engineering Scaffolds

Recent advances in bone tissue engineering focus on addressing three main issues: developing a biomimetic porous scaffold to allow for the migration of cells and nutrient transport, increasing the scaffold's robustness and mechanical stability for load-bearing applications, and promoting early vascularization to enhance the scaffold's integration *in vivo*. In addition, the scaffold must be 3D, biocompatible, and exhibit osteoinductive behaviors. In this section, we will discusses three recent technologies that attempt to address one of the main issue discussed above. More detailed work is outlined in the cited research articles.

4.5.1 Varying Scaffold Stiffness for Cellular Response

Chen et al. developed a novel 3D scaffold with varying degrees of stiffness while maintaining the microstructure of native bone (Chen et al., 2015). They achieved this by using decellularized trabecular bone as the scaffold base with a collagen/hydroxyapatite (HAp) mixture. They aimed to alter the scaffold's stiffness by varying the collagen to HAp proportions and modulating stem cell adhesion, proliferation, migration, differentiation, and signaling. They hypothesized that the collagen/HAp coating incorporated into decellularized trabecular bone would promote the surrounding biological environment to facilitate osseointegration and mitigate possible adverse tissue responses. Pure collagen type I sponge from a bovine tendon and HAp powder fabricated from calcium nitrate tetrahydrate $(Ca(NO_3)_2 \cdot 4H_2O)$ and sodium phosphate tribasic $(Na_3PO_4 \cdot 12H_2O)$ were magnetically stirred to prepare mixtures of HAp in collagen solutions. Decellularized porcine trabecular bone was then dipped in mixtures of different collagen/HAp concentration ratios. Scanning electron microscopy (SEM) images of the coated scaffold showed the maintained porous interconnected architecture with a mean pore diameter of 398.3 ± 134.9 μm and 74% porosity was confirmed by micro computed tomography, μ-CT, analysis (Figure 4.1).

There was a direct correlation between the concentration of collagen in the collagen/HAp coating mixture and the scaffold's overall compressive elastic modulus with the greatest average moduli being 23.61 ± 8.06 kPa. Rat mesenchymal stem cells (MSCs) seeded on the collagen/HAp composites expressed osteopontin (OPN) and osteocalcin (OC); two specific protein markers involved in osteogenic differentiation. Immunohistochemistry staining on histological sections showed an increase in OPN and OC expressional over a

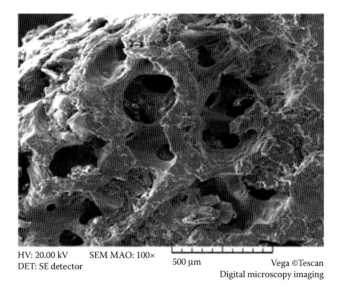

HV: 20.00 kV   SEM MAO: 100×
DET: SE detector   500 μm   Vega ©Tescan
                                        Digital microscopy imaging

FIGURE 4.1
SEM micrographs of decellularized cancellous bone. The SEM image shows the porous structure of decellularized cancellous bone. The scale bar indicates 500 μm. (From Chen, G. et al. 2015. *ACS Appl Mater Interfaces.* 7: 15790–802. With permission.)

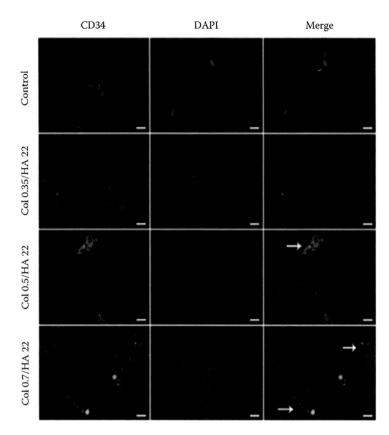

FIGURE 4.2

Immunofluorescent detection of CD34+ cells in scaffold with varying stiffness after 6 months of subcutaneous implantation (the arrow indicates blood vessel). Scale bar = 100 μm. (Reprinted with permission from Chen, G. et al. 3D scaffolds with different stiffness but the same microstructure for bone tissue engineering. *ACS Appl Mater Interfaces.* 7: 15790–802. Copyright 2015 American Chemical Society.)

3-week time period. In addition, the scaffolds with the higher stiffness exhibited significantly higher expressions of OPN and OC, suggesting that the 3D scaffold's microenvironment significantly affects the differentiation behaviors of MSCs. *In vivo* subcutaneous cell-free scaffold implantation in a Sprague–Dawley rat model demonstrated the scaffold's biocompatibility. The histological results indicate the cells infiltrated into the scaffolds and secreted their own extracellular matrix (ECM) with gradual expression of OPN and OC over time and recruited MSCs from the subcutaneous tissue. The immunofluorescence detection of CD34+ cells, a primary vascular endothelial marker, was confirmed after 1 month implantation and appeared to form a blood vessel in two-dimension (Figure 4.2). The information from this study proved cell-free scaffolds to be promising for bone tissue engineering and future clinical applications. The data highlight the ability of the scaffold to provide a favorable environment for enhanced endothelial cells attachment and proliferation with the addition of angiogenin (ANG) to promote neovascularization *in vivo*.

4.5.2 Addressing Angiogenesis with Growth Factors

A technology developed by Kim et al. (2015) utilizes an ANG-loaded scaffold to stimulate angiogenesis *in vivo*. ANG is a potent growth factor that has been found to stimulate blood vessel formation. The scaffolds were developed by rapid blending of calcium phosphate-coated bovine bone powder, fibrin glue, recombinant human ANG, and thrombin. The polymerized mixture was then freeze-dried to obtain a fibrin/bone (FB) powder scaffold. Scaffold surface characterization of the fabricated scaffolds by SEM images and mercury liquid extrusion porosimetry yielded an average porosity of $61.94 \pm 0.52\%$ with numerous micro-pores throughout the scaffold formed by the fibrin network. This porous network is necessary for angiogenesis, nutrient transport, and cell migration. Furthermore, the compressive strength of the FB/ANG scaffold was 0.95 ± 0.04 MPa. *In vitro* biocompatibility was evaluated with human umbilical vein endothelial cells (HUVECs). Live dead stain and metabolic assay analysis concluded increased cellular proliferation and viability as the concentration of added ANG was increased; indicating the angiogenic benefits of the growth factor to scaffolds. This was confirmed in SEM images, which showed that more HUVECs attached to the FB/ANG scaffold can control FB scaffold. The scaffolds were then implanted into a critical-size calvarial defect in New Zealand rabbits to determine the effects of ANG containing FB scaffolds on bone regeneration *in vivo*. At 2 weeks postimplantation, more blood vessel formation was observed in the FB/ANG scaffold than the control FB scaffold and the number of blood vessels increased with increasing concentrations of ANG in the scaffold (Figure 4.3). In addition, mature bone was observed at 8-week postimplantation of the FB/ANG scaffold, whereas fibrous tissue was observed in the groups with untreated defects. Quantifying images of bone regeneration were

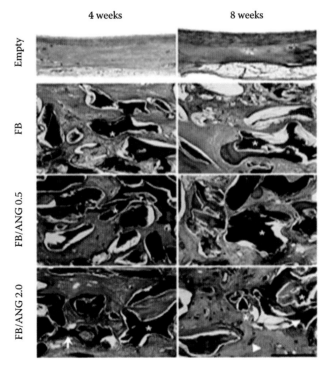

FIGURE 4.3
Masson trichrome staining of regenerated bone in the calvarial defect at 4 weeks after scaffold implantation. Mature bone (arrow) and blood vessels (arrow head) observed treatment groups containing angiogennin. Scale bar = 250 μm. (Reprinted with permission from Chen, G. et al. 3D scaffolds with different stiffness but the same microstructure for bone tissue engineering. *ACS Appl Mater Interfaces*. 7: 15790–802. Copyright 2015 American Chemical Society.)

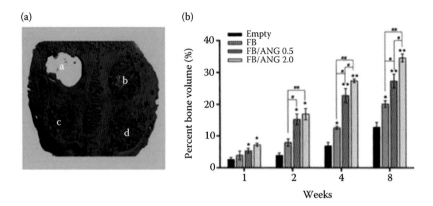

FIGURE 4.4
(a) 3D images of calvarial defects 8 weeks after implantation (a) empty, (b) FB, (c) FB/ANG 0.5, and (d) FB/ANG 2.0. (b) The percentage of bone volume generated in the bone defects. The amount of new bone significantly increased in the FB/ANG-implanted groups. Each column value represents the mean ± SD. * and # indicates significant difference when compared with empty and FB scaffold groups, respectively ($n = 4$, *, #$P < 0.05$ and **, ##$P < 0.01$). (Adapted from Kim, B.S. et al. 2015. *Biomater Res.* 19: 18.)

consistent with the histological analysis (Figure 4.4). Micro-CT revealed significant differences in bone formation between the untreated defects and defects. This group was successful in creating a scaffold for bone tissue regeneration with favorable microenvironment for enhanced endothelial cell proliferation and adhesion using an angiogenic growth factor, ANG. This study highlights the future of combing recombinant growth factors with a biological scaffold for bone tissue engineering applications.

4.5.3 Enhancing Mechanical Strength while Maintaining Biological Functionality

Porous 3D β-tricalcium phosphate (TCP) scaffolds are popular in the field of bone tissue regeneration due to their good biocompatibility and osteoconductivity, but scaffolds of this composition tend to lack structural stability and mechanical robustness due to their brittle nature. Recent research by Yang et al. (2015) focuses on combining high elastic polymers, such as poly(glycerol sebacate) (PGS), with -TCP to create a scaffold with elastic properties similar to native tissue. The advantage of using PGS is the ability to prepare the prepolymer by polycondensation that can then be crosslinked by heat treatment. This allows for homogenous coating of PGS onto B-TCP scaffolds to improve the robustness of the β-TCP scaffold without interfering with the β-TCP-induced osteoactivity. Figure 4.5 depicts the process by which the PGS coated β-TCP scaffolds (β-TCP/PGS) are fabricated yield. SEM images confirm the porous architecture of the β-TCP scaffold and uniform coating of the PGS (Figure 4.6).

The enhanced elastic behavior of the scaffold with the addition of PGS is seen with a simple compression test as demonstrated in Figure 4.7. The ability for the scaffold to recover to its original shape upon release of the load and exhibit shape memory characteristics is desirable in filling bone defects. Furthermore, to confirm the addition of the PGS would not have a cytotoxic response *in vivo*, *in vitro* biocompatibility testing with rat bone marrow stromal cells (rBMSc) and HUVECs was performed. The results concluded the rBMSCs and HUVECS attached and proliferated on the scaffold. This recent technology is one of few that addresses biological, mechanical, and structural issue commonly seen with bone tissue engineering technologies by increasing the elastic properties of β-TCP scaffolds without altering the biological response.

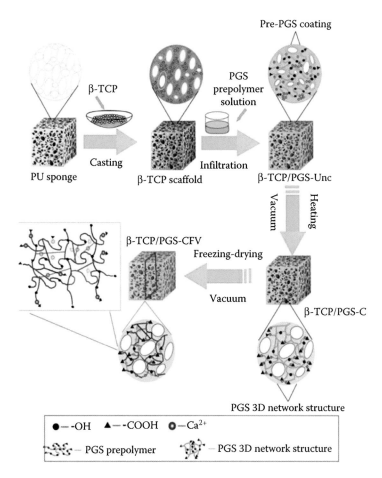

FIGURE 4.5
Illustration of preparation of porous β-TCP/PGS scaffold. In the acronym "CFV" the "C" stands for heat treatment under vacuum and "FV" means freeze dry under vacuum. (Adapted from Kim, B.S. et al. 2015. *Biomater Res.* 19: 18.)

4.5.4 Biomimetic Mechanically Enhanced Scaffold

Research in the Freeman group address the issue of lack of mechanical strength and graft integration by developing an innovative mechanically enhanced composite polymeric-based structurally biomimetic TE graft. Recent published research focuses on the development of the biomimetic trabecular and cortical scaffolds (Andric et al., 2011; Taylor and Freeman, 2015; Wright et al., 2010). They hypothesize that the joining of a porous trabecular scaffold with the addition of HAp, prevascularized cortical bone scaffold, and HAp columns will promote differentiation of human mesenchymal stromal cells (hMSCs) into osteoblasts and vascular endothelial cells in appropriate areas in the scaffolds *in vitro* and *in vivo* and provide long-term graft viability and mechanics. The composite scaffold is composed of electrospun Food and Drug Administration (FDA) approved polymers poly-L-lactide (PLLA) and poly-D-lactide, 10% bovine gelatin, and inorganic HAp to promote the osteogenic differentiation. The trabecular scaffold was fabricated by electrospinning onto a rotating mandrel with salt crystals acting as porogens. The biomimetic cortical scaffold is fabricated by electrospinning PLLA/gel onto a rotating water soluble polymer polyethylene oxide and PLLA twist. All scaffolds were crosslinked previous to leaching with a FDA-approved enzymatic

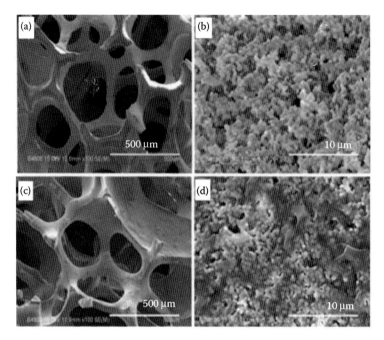

FIGURE 4.6
SEM images of (a and b) porous scaffolds of B-TCP and (c and d) B-TCP/PGS. (Reprinted from *Mater Sci Eng C: Mater Biol Appl.*, 56, Yang, K. et al., Beta-tricalcium phosphate/poly(glycerol sebacate) scaffolds with robust mechanical property for bone tissue engineering, 37–47, Copyright 2015, with permission from Elsevier.)

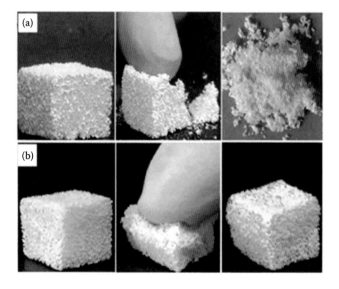

FIGURE 4.7
Optical images of (a) β-TCP and (b) β-TCP/15P-CFV scaffolds upon compressive loading and unloading switch. (Reprinted from *Mater Sci Eng C: Mater Biol Appl.*, 56, Yang, K. et al., Beta-tricalcium phosphate/poly(glycerol sebacate) scaffolds with robust mechanical property for bone tissue engineering, 37–47, Copyright 2015, with permission from Elsevier.)

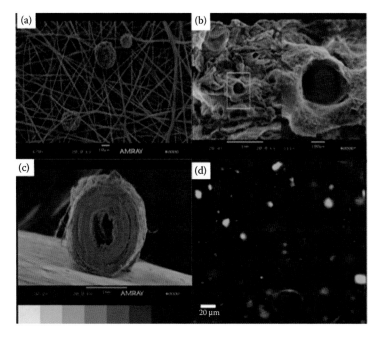

FIGURE 4.8
SEM images of (a) HAp nanopowder in scaffold; scale bar = 10 μm, (b) porous trabecular scaffold; scale bar = 1 mm, (c) cortical scaffold; scale bar = 1 mm, and (d) fluorescent immunostained hMSCs (blue = nuclei) and VEGF (green) on decellularized scaffolds; scale bar = 20 μm. (Reprinted from *Mater Sci Eng C: Mater Biol Appl.*, 56, Yang, K. et al., Beta-tricalcium phosphate/poly(glycerol sebacate) scaffolds with robust mechanical property for bone tissue engineering, 37–47, Copyright 2015, with permission from Elsevier.)

crosslinking agent transglutaminase (mTG) to increase strength and prevent gelatin leaching and mineralized in simulate body fluid. Material characterization confirmed the presence of HAp crystals embedded in the trabecular scaffold (Figure 4.8a). Liquid extrusion porosimetry analysis yielded pore ranges within the 5–10 and 100–300 μm (Figure 4.8b). These pore ranges are desirable and necessary for neovascularization and osteoblast infiltration. *In vitro* analysis concluded that the presence of HAp statistically increases the amount of hMSCs calcium deposition in comparison to the control scaffolds. SEM images of the fabricated osteon yielded an average inner diameter of 0.495 ± 44 μm, similar to a native osteon (Figure 4.8c). Confocal images of the cortical scaffold prove that the osteonic structure promotes endothelial development circumferentially when seeded with HUVECs. The decellularized scaffolds exhibited an 86% decrease in cellular viability with a 94% maintained collageneous matrix. In addition, hMSCs seeded on the decellularized scaffold expressed vascular endothelial growth factor (VEGF), an early angiogenesis marker and cellular morphology indicative of endothelial lumen development (Figure 4.8d). Studies discussed demonstrate the scaffold's biomimetic trabecular and cortical structure and the ability to promote osteogenic and angiogenic stem cell differentiation. Ongoing subcutaneous *in vivo* murine studies are being performed to further validate the TE graft's biocompatibility and differentiation potential. This technology is transformative because it will be the first synthetic bone graft to contain both trabecular and cortical bone structures, designed for vascularized bone growth and load-bearing applications. The recent findings discussed in this section highlight the advancements in the field of bone tissue regeneration research. An optimal scaffold for bone tissue engineering should process the biological and material characteristics necessary to allow for long-term graft viability and mechanics by providing structural support while promoting tissue development. The future of composite scaffolds and stem cells for bone tissue engineering is promising as researchers are getting closer and closer to developing scaffolds that "look" and "act" like native bone.

4.6 Patented Novel Grafting and Tissue Engineering Options

As there are limitations with autografts (limited supply, donor site pain, and donor site morbidity) and allografts (resorption, mechanical properties, and potential for disease transfer), researchers have been actively searching for the right blend of materials, architecture, and factors for the construction of synthetic bone grafts. In this search, researchers have focused primarily on three major areas in the improvement of graft performance: porosity, mechanical strength, and biocompatibility/osteocompatibility. The porosity of a bone graft is extremely important as it directly affects cell and nutrient infiltration (which will enhance compatibility). Many researchers are looking to further enhance compatibility through the addition of various calcium phosphates and biomacromolecules such as collagen or fibrinogen. In order to enhance the mechanical properties, calcium phosphate and bioactive glasses (which may also contain calcium phosphate) have been added to grafting materials. The devices in this section are all recently patented and have used the previously described strategies to improve their performance.

4.6.1 Porous Composite Bone Grafts

A disadvantage of current commercially available bone grafts is their poor mechanical properties, which limits their use to nonload-bearing applications. Some researchers have chosen to overcome this limitation by producing materials which enhanced the mechanical properties by incorporating porous ceramics with degradable polymers. These composites have enhanced strength without the risk of articulating debris. Smith et al. (2011) (US 7,875,342 B2, 2011) have developed a porous ceramic composite that incorporates biodegradable polymers (polycaprolactone) into the matrix. The biodegradable polymer improves mechanical properties of the implant (decreasing brittleness) and allows for the delivery of a variety of agents throughout the porous ceramic matrix. It is designed for use as a bone substitute or TE scaffold in the fields of orthopedics and dentistry. This bone graft is a porous substitute that can limit fragmentation and migration of debris during standard orthopedic fixation. The graft is composed of a porous osteoinductive ceramic matrix and a biodegradable polymer. The composite possesses optimum pore size, pore size distribution, porosity, and pore connectivity that promotes rapid bone tissue ingrowth. In comparison to prior ceramic bone grafts, this graft has advantageous mechanical properties as a result of repeatedly coating the organic substrate with a mixture of thickening agents (slurries) varying in solid loading. The coated structure is heated to burn away the flexible organic foam and then sintered, creating a fused, ceramic foam with interconnected voids.

4.6.2 Improving Biocompatibility

Erbe et al. have developed a resorbable, composite bone graft with polymeric and inorganic material that exhibit macro-, meso-, and microporosites (US 7,189,263 B2, 2007) (Erbe et al., 2007). The graft incorporates the benefits of inorganic-shaped bodies with a macro, meso, and microporosity and polymers such as collagen (a natural polymer). Different stoichiometric compositions of calcium phosphate such as hydroxyapatite (HAp), TCP, tretacalcium phosphate, and other calcium phosphate salts and minerals, have all been used to match the biocompatibility, structure, and strength of natural bone. The pore size and porosity are critical as they aid in promoting revascularization, healing, and remodeling of bone. The porosity of this graft is enhanced by the oxidation–reduction product of at least one metal cation, oxidizing agent, and oxidization precursor anion. The reaction products may be inorganic, calcium phosphate compositions such as biphasic calcium phosphate or beta tricalcium phosphate (β-TCP). The oxidation–reduction product gives the graft the macro, meso, and microporosity, which grant the graft extraordinary absorption properties. The inclusion of a polymer, such as the structural protein collagen, decreases graft brittleness and increases flexibility. The granulated form gives the final material a great deal of porosity and large pore distribution (1–1000 μm), which increases the ability of the graft to imbibe fluids such as bone marrow aspirate, blood, or saline and cell loaded solutions (e.g., fibroblasts, mesenchymal, stromal, marrow, and stem cells) for use *in vivo*. This porosity also allows the material to incorporate growth factors such as BMP into the graft to enhance healing. The granulated form allows the clinician the flexibility to produce grafts of various shapes, including cylinder, blocks, strips, sheets, and wedges. This graft may also serve as a coating on any orthopedic implant. Further, unlike traditional bone graft substitutes, this granulated material is highly compressible and therefore can be packed into a gap to insure maximum contact with adjacent bone for beneficial healing of a bony defect.

4.6.3 Bioactive Bone Graft Substitute

Among those grafts designed to improve biocompatibility/osteocompatibility is a device by Clineff et al. (2008) (US 2010/0215718 A1) composed of resorbable calcium phosphate, collagen, and bioactive glass. This composite is a biocompatible, resorbable, homogeneous blend of materials with a calcium phosphate phase that has macro-, meso-, and microporosity. The graft replicates the natural osteoactivity of native bone through the addition of a bioactive glass. Bioactive glasses that have been utilized by Clineff et al. (2008) include glass–ceramics, crystalline phase materials, and a combination of acrylic polymerizable species. The bioactive glass reacts as it comes in contact with physiologic fluids, such as blood and serum, leading to the formation of an apatite layer on the graft surface. The bioactive glass phase has a glass–ceramic composition with heterogeneous particles of irregular morphologies and regions of crystallinity.

The bioactive glass and calcium phosphate are combined with collagen by blending to form a homogeneous mixture that leads to a composite matrix. The collagen not only increases graft bioactivity, but also aids in material handling and flexibility. The inclusion of the collagenous phase allows the graft to be more easily shaped or cut by scalpels and scissors. The graft has been formed into basic shapes such as a disk, semi-sphere, semi-tube, or torus. Once implanted, the material may act as a barrier to prevent the migration of other implants or graft materials and serve as a resorbable, osteoconductive bone graft capable of promoting bone formation. The bone graft is designed to reabsorb over time following delivery to the surgical site.

4.6.4 Two-Phase Polymeric Bone Defect Filler

Another material proposed as a bone defect filler by Deslauriers et al. (2011) (US 2011/0201711 A1) consists of a particulate polymer distributed within a polymeric binder.

The particulate polymer is made up of particles with a wide range of sizes and may be the same material (a polyurethane) as the polymeric binder. The particles within the particulate polymer may have a variety of shapes and/or sizes in order to enhance pore interconnectivity and create space for material expansion within the bone defect filler. The combination of polymer particulate and binder gives this bone defect filler sufficient mechanical strength and handling characteristics for bone repair applications. The degradability is one characteristic that makes this polymeric bone defect filler advantageous to current synthetic bone defect fillers. Current commercially available devices or materials are not degradable and maintain their chemical and mechanical properties, such as titanium or poly methylmethacrylate (PMMA). The synthetic bone fillers may have poor tensile and shear properties, as well as poor adhesion properties. This combination can cause the materials to be washed out of the defect area before new bone ingrowth occurs. Conventional bone grafting technologies, such as the use of PMMA, are problematic because as permanent bone filler they are not resorbable and/or cannot be molded and shaped for *in situ* curing. This combination of particulate and filler material is also an improvement over a similar bone technology, the use of particulate polymer mixed with biological fluids. Unlike the particulate-filler combination, the particulate polymer and fluid mixtures tend to adhere poorly to the surround bone and exhibit low initial mechanical properties (tensile, compressive, and shear) after implantation (Weibrich et al., 2000). Creating the particulate and binder phases from the same biocompatible polyurethane allows the material in both phases to have similar mechanical properties. By having similar responses to stress and strain in the two phases, there is a reduction in stress concentrations where the phases meet in the cured bone defect filler, which can increase product life. The mechanical properties of the graft can be altered to match the native bone surrounding the defect area, by varying porosity and particulate concentration. Increased porosity and/or increased interconnectivity also improves bone ingrowth, but will lead to a decrease in strength with the addition of more void spaces. Therefore, the size of the pores may be varied for the intended application, nonloading bearing bone versus load-bearing bone. In addition, this graft can be molded or shaped *in situ* to fill the bone defect with varying mechanical properties.

4.6.5 Bone Graft with Growth Factor Encapsulation System

A grafting technology developed by Lu et al. (2006) (US 2006/0159663) enhances bone formation through the release of various growth factors and/or platelet-rich plasma (PRP) from a solid material. PRP is known to contain a number of autologous thrombocytic growth factors that may aid in the acceleration of bone regeneration (Weibrich et al., 2000). These growth factors include platelet-derived growth factor (PDGF) and transforming growth factors β1 (TGF-β1); these factors are produced by platelets and released during granulation. TGF-β1 stimulates proliferation and collagen synthesis by osteoblasts and osteoblast precursors and PDGF stimulates mitogenesis of osteoblastic recursors. PRP gel has also been used as an adhesive with cancellous bone particles in oral and maxillofacial surgery bone grafting procedures. This graft comprises a capsule of protein-permeable material, releasable porous calcium alginate beads with encapsulated growth factors, a PRP gel, and a bone regeneration facilitating material. The bone regeneration facilitating material is a solid scaffold that supports bone-forming cells. Bone regeneration facilitating materials include collagen, BioOss (calcium phosphate-based bone graft substitute), Pepgen P-15 (synthetic P-15 peptide bound to natural form of hydroxylapatite), and AlloGraft (demineralized bone matrix (DBM), allograft-based bone graft substitute).

The alginate porous beads contain autologous PRP. This allows the contained growth factors to be released from the PRP and then from the bead to the surrounding area, the defect location. The controlled release of factors from this graft is crucial to the enhancement of bone regeneration because the growth factors can be released at varying stages throughout the natural healing process. Chitosan beads have been investigated as a possible vehicle for the growth factors/PRP. This novel hydrogel delivery system permits prolonged and modulated release of growth factors relevant to bone regeneration.

4.6.6 Natural Bone Graft Materials

Conner et al. have developed hydrated mixtures of fragments of acellular tissue matrix (ATM) and fragments of DBM that can be dried and blended and hydrated to form an osteoinductive bone graft composition that can retain its osteoinductivity upon long-term storage (US 2007/0248575 A1) (Connor et al., 2007). The ATM and DBM mixture is a semisolid putty that can be shaped prior to drying. The advantage of this invention is that the ATM and DBM mixture retains most of the biological functions of its constitutive materials, native collagen, and other extracellular matrix proteins, calcium phosphate, etc., even during long-term storage. The acellular tissue mixture can be made from human tissue, genetically engineered nonhuman mammalian tissue lacking expression of α-1,3-galactosyl residues or any other collagen-containing tissues. The α-1,3-galactosyl gene found in nonmammalian tissue has been shown to cause rejection from xenograft procedures. The tissue obtained from the ATM does not need to be structurally identical to the surrounding host tissue because it can be remodeled by infiltrating cells of the relevant host tissue, stem cell, or progenitor cells. Optionally, the ATM can be made up from the recipient's own tissue (collagen based) without altering it biochemically or structurally. The DBM is from long bone, calvaria, or any other type of bone. The bone has been treated to remove nearly all of the inorganic, mineral components. The DBM possesses most of the biological properties of native bone that are important for successful bone grafting. The bone morphogenic proteins still present in the DBM signal stem cells to differentiate into osteoprogenitor cells to produce new bone, making the DBM osteoinductive. The DBM also supports neovascularization and osteoblast infiltration. The DBM can be made from the same species as the recipients or from a different species, with similar genetic alterations as the ATM. The ATM and DBM can be made into multiple forms such as threads, fibers, and particles. The final bone graft can be composed of any combinations of forms of ATM and any form of DBM (e.g., fibers of ATM and particles of DBM) and then freeze-dried for prolonged storage. This bone graft can be held in place by sutures, wrapped around a damaged or defective bone, placed on top of an area of bone that is damaged or defective, or placed at a nonbony site to induce bone formation.

4.6.7 BMP Releasing Bone Graft Materials

Just as in other areas of the body, the gold standard for bone grafting in spinal fusion is autograft from the iliac crest. However, this method presents the same challenges as autograft from other sites (described earlier), including pseudarthrosis and a fracture nonunion due to the slow rate of fusion. As a result, there is a large effort to develop bone technologies that cannot only reduce or replace the need for harvest of autogenous bone but also accelerate the rate of fusion (arthodesis) for spinal applications. For decades, researchers have investigated the benefits of growth factors in regenerative medicine. In particular, members of the bone morphogenic protein (BMP) family have shown clinical benefit in treatment of bone defects, injuries, disorders, or diseases. In particular, BMP-2 and BMP-7 have shown benefits in the treatment of bone fractures and spine fusions. Among the synthetic grafts to harvest the power of BMP is a device by Melican et al. (2011) (US 2011/0117165 A1) for spinal fusion. The device is an implantable bone graft comprising a resorbable ceramic phase and a resorbable polymer phase. A growth factor binding peptide is covalently attached to the polymer phase, allowing BMP to be presented to seeded cells. Osteoconductivity of novel bone grafting technology for spinal fusion is enhanced by the use of a porous ceramic such as beta-TCP (β-TCP), which has a total porosity of 50% greater and a particle size ranging from 100 to about 300 μm. TCP-based bone graft substitutes often contain collagen and are commonly used in lumbar spinal fusion because TCP is resorbed over months as the native bone heals. In addition, BMP is covalently bonded to the polymeric phase of the graft to promote bone growth facilitated by a "spacer"; A "spacer" is the compound moiety inserted between the BMP-binding peptide and polymer and to enhance the stability of the BMP. Spacers can increase flexibility and accessibility of the BMP-binding peptide and the BMP-binding peptide density on the polymer surface. The attachment of the correct concentration of BMP onto a resorbable polymer–βTCP composite is presented as a safe, cost-effective osteoinductive injectable bone technology to promote spinal fusion.

4.6.8 Granulated Bone Grafting Material

One solution to bone grafting nonuniform shapes is a powder made from actual bone (DBM), Long et al. (2004) (US 2004/0019132 A1). Clinicians often perform bone grafting procedures to fill a bone void created by loss of bone or compaction of cancellous bone. In many instances, the clinician also may rely on the bone graft material to provide some measure of mechanical support. In these instances, the clinicians pack grafting material into the defect, creating a stable base to support the surrounding tissue and hardware. Past solutions to this problem have included gel, putty, paste, formable strips, and tablets. Irregularly shaped bone chips alone are not optimal for these applications because they lack an interlocking shape and do no compact sufficiently. Therefore, the bone graft material created by Long et al. is a granule product for use in powder compaction to provide a scaffold structure for ingrowth from the host bone and for the purpose of easy delivery. The granulated material is formed by pulverizing bone and then subjecting it to a powder compaction. The pulverized material is a composition comprising particles of various sizes (grains, granules, and powder). The material can be molded and shaped using a moveable die with a moveable upper and lower punch. The first punch creates a relief profile onto the surface of the granulated bone material. The second punch creates a second contact surface; the moveable die has a cavity into which the material is introduced. The upper and lower punches create the shaped bone graft substitute necessary to fit the desired bone void. Its granular nature allows this bone graft substitute to absorb factors or agents that can enhance or augment bone growth. Fibrinogen, for example, has been added; fibrin (which is obtained after cleavage by thrombin) enhances the structural integrity of the bone graft, can cause angiogenesis (growth of blood vessels), and acts as an instigator for bone growth.

References

Andric, T., Sampson, A.C., Freeman, J.W. 2011. Fabrication and characterization of electrospun osteon mimicking scaffolds for bone tissue engineering. *Mater Sci Eng C.* 31: 2–8.

Chen, G., Dong, C., Yang, L., Lv, Y. 2015. 3D scaffolds with different stiffness but the same microstructure for bone tissue engineering. *ACS Appl Mater Interfaces*. 7: 15790–802.

Clineff, T.D., Koblish, A., Bagga, C.S., Erbe, E.M., Nagvajara, G.M., Darmoc, M.M., inventors; Orthovita, Inc., assignee. 2008. Bioactive Bone Graft Substitute (US 2008/0187571 A1).

Connor, J., Qui, Q.Q., inventors; Connor, J., Qui, Q.Q., assignee. 2007. Bone Graft Composition (US 2007/0248575 A1).

Consensus Development Statement. 1997. Who are candidates for prevention and treatment for osteoporosis? *Osteoporos Int*. 7: 1–6.

Deslauriers, R., Kolb, E., Boxberger, J., inventors; Doctors Research Group, Inc., assignee. 2011. Polymeric Bone Defect Filler (US 2011/0201711 A1).

Dvir, T., Timko, B.P., Kohane, D.S., Langer, R. 2001. Nanotechnological strategies for engineering complex tissues. *Nat Nanotechnol*. 6: 13–22.

Erbe, E.M., Clineff, T.D., Bagga, C.S., Nagvajara G.M., Koblish, A., inventors; Vita Special Purpose Corporation, assignee. 2007. Biocompatible Bone Graft Material (US 7,189,263 B2).

Frohlich, M., Grayson, W.L., Wan, L.Q., Marolt, D., Drobnic, M., Vunjak-Novakovic, G. 2008. Tissue engineered bone grafts: Biological requirements, tissue culture and clinical relevance. *Curr Stem Cell Res Ther*. 3: 254–64.

Greenwald, S., Boden, S.D., Goldber, V.M., Khan, T., Laurensin, C., Rosier, R.N. 2001. Bone-graft substitutes: Facts, fictions, and applications. *J Bone Joint Surg Am*. 83A: 98–103.

Hing, K.A. 2004. Bone repair in the twenty-first century: Biology, chemistry or engineering? *Philos Trans A: Math Phys Eng Sci*. 362: 2821–50.

Hitti, M. 2006. Patients Rate Knee, Hip Replacement: WebMD (updated May 5, 2006; cited July 17, 2008). http://www.webmd.com/news/20060505/patients-rate-knee-hip-replacement.

Kanis, J.A., Johnell, O., Oden, A. et al., 2000. Long-term risk of osteoporotic fracture in Malmo. *Osteoporos Int*. 11: 669–74.

Khan, Y.M., Katti, D.S., Laurencin, C.T. 2004. Novel polymer-synthesized ceramic composite-based system for bone repair: An *in vitro* evaluation. *J Biomed Mater Res A*. 69: 728–37.

Kim, B.S., Kim, J.S., Yang, S.S., Kim, H.W., Lim, H.J., Lee, J. 2015. Angiogenin-loaded fibrin/bone powder composite scaffold for vascularized bone regeneration. *Biomater Res*. 19: 18.

Krishnan, L., Willett, N.J., Guldberg, R.E. 2014. Vascularization strategies for bone regeneration. *Ann Biomed Eng*. 42: 432–44.

Long, M., Cooper, M.B., Kinnane, K.M., Allen, T., Schryver, J.E., inventors; Marc Long, Michael B. Cooper, Keith M. Kinnane, Trevor Allen, Jeffrey E. Schryver assignee. 2004. Bone Graft Substitutes (US 2004/0019132 A1).

Lu, H., Landesberg, R., Vo, J.M., Tsay, R., Peng, H., inventors; Lu, H., Landesberg, R., Vo, J.M., Tsay, R., Peng, H., assignee. 2006. Growth Factor Encapsulation System for Enhancing Bone Formation (US20060159663 A1).

Melican, M.C., Hamilton, P.T., Hodges, J.A., Nair, S.A., Chen, Y., inventors; Affinergy, Inc., assignee. 2011. Implantable Bone Graft Materials (US 2011/0117165 A1).

Melton, L.J., Atkinson, E.J, O'Connor, M.K., O'Fallon, W.M., Riggs, B.L. 1998. Bone density and fractures risk in men. *J Bone Miner Res*. 13: 1915–23.

Melton, L.J. 3rd, Chrischilles, E.A., Cooper, C., Lane, A.W., Riggs, B.L. 1992. Perspective: How many women have osteoporosis? *J Bone Miner Res*. 7: 10005–1010.

Novosel, E.C., Kleinhans, C., Kluger, P.J. 2011. Vascularization is the key challenge in tissue engineering. *Adv Drug Deliv Rev*. 63: 300–11.

Perry, C.R. 1999. Bone repair techniques, bone graft, and bone graft substitutes. *Clin Orthop Relat Res*. 360: 71–86.

Randell, A., Sambrook, P.N., Nguyen, T.V., Lapsley, H., Jones, G., Kelly, P.J., Eisman, J.A. 1995. Direct clinical and welfare costs of osteoporotic fractures in elderly men and women. *Osteoporos Int*. 5: 427–32.

Rho, J.Y., Kuhn-Spearing, L., Zioupos, P. 1998. Mechanical properties and the hierarchical structure of bone. *Med Eng Phys*. 20: 92–102.

Schoenstadt, A., 2013. Bone Cancer Statistics: Clinaero, Inc., (updated July 14, 2013). http://bone-cancer.emedtv.com/bone-cancer/bone-cancer-statistics.html (accessed August, 2015).

Shin, M., Abukawa, H., Troulis, M.J., Vacanti, J.P. 2008. Development of a biodegradable scaffold with interconnected pores by heat fusion and its application to bone tissue engineering. *J Biomed Mater Res A*. 84: 702–9.

Smith, T.J., Jason, H., Sydney, M.P., Reginald, S., inventors; Warsaw Orthopedic, Inc., assignee. 2011. Porous Ceramic Composite Bone Grafts (US7875342 B2).

Taylor, B., Freeman, J. 2015. Evaluation of a pre-vascularized osteoinductive polymeric scaffold for bone tissue regeneration. *Presented at the Society for Biomaterials Annual Meeting*, Charlotte, North Carolina.

Wang, H., Li, Y., Zuo, Y., Li, J., Ma, S., Cheng L. 2007. Biocompatibility and osteogenesis of biomimetic nanohydroxyapatite/polyamide composite scaffolds for bone tissue engineering. *Biomaterials*. 28: 3338–48.

Wang, X., Puram, S. 2004. The toughness of cortical bone and its relationship with age. *Ann Biomed Eng*. 32: 123–35.

Weibrich, G., Kleis, W., Hafner, G., Hitzler, W. 2000. Growth factor levels in platelet-rich plasma and correlations with donor age, sex, and platelet count. *J Craniomaxillofac Surg*. 30: 97–102.

Wheeler, D.L., Enneking, W.F. 2005. Allograft bone decreases in strength *in vivo* over time. *Clin Orthop Relat Res*. 435: 36–42.

Wright, L.D., Young, R.T., Andric, T., Freeman J.W. 2010. Fabrication and mechanical characterization of 3D electrospun scaffolds for tissue engineering. *Biomed Mater*. 5: 055006.

Yang, K., Zhang, J., Ma, X., Ma, Y., Kan, C., Ma, H., Li, Y., Yuan, Y., Liu, C. 2015. Beta-tricalcium phosphate/poly(glycerol sebacate) scaffolds with robust mechanical property for bone tissue engineering. *Mater Sci Eng C: Mater Biol Appl*. 56: 37–47.

Yuehuei, H.A., Draughn, R.A. 1999. *Mechanical Testing of Bone and the Bone-Implant Interface*. Boca Raton, Florida: CRC Press.

5

Biomaterials and Designs Supporting Cartilage Regeneration

Rahul V. G. and Prabha D. Nair

CONTENTS

5.1 Introduction

More than 15 million people each year suffer from diseases such as osteoarthritis and chondrosarcoma, which damage cartilage and severely affect the quality of their daily life (Martin and Bucklwater, 2002). Cartilage is an avascular, alymphatic, aneural connective tissue present in different parts of the body. Depending on the location, its function and composition varies. Mechanically, cartilage is stiff but not hard as bone. The cartilage lines the bone surface at the joints, protecting the bone from wear and tear. Hence, cartilage should have enough mechanical strength to resist the compression and tear. The extracellular matrix (ECM) components of the cartilage are responsible for imparting its functional properties. The collagen fibers impart tensile strength and the glycosaminoglycan is responsible for the resilience to resist the compression. In native cartilage, the chondrocytes are dispersed in a very specialized ECM made of dense fibrillary network of collagen type-II and negatively charged glycosaminoglycan. The cells are responsible for the maintenance of the ECM by secreting the ECM components in response to the signals stored in the matrix.

There are three different types of cartilage seen in our body:

1. *Hyaline cartilage.* Hyaline cartilage appears bluish white in color and is seen in joints, sternum, ribs, etc.

2. *Fibro cartilage.* It appears glistening white and is seen in symphysis pubis, intervertebral discs, menisci, etc. It is the only cartilage containing collagen type-I.

3. *Elastic cartilage.* This type of cartilage has yellowish appearance. It is present in ear pinna, epiglottis, nose, etc. It contains a network of elastin fibers, which is responsible for its flexibility.

Articular cartilage is a hyaline cartilage that cushions the bones at the joints preventing its wear and tear and allows painless movement, but with limited intrinsic regeneration and self-healing capacity through the natural healing processes in the body, due to its innate avascular nature. Loss of cartilage results in pain and immobility. Most of the diseases such as osteoarthritis affecting cartilage cause deterioration of cartilage, and presently there are not many effective methods to cure this condition. The available treatment involves pain killers and anti-inflammatory drugs. Cartilage transplantation strategies have not been considered safe due to the scarcity and morbidity of donor site. This lack of effective treatment methods indicates that cartilage replacement with artificial cartilage would be a better and effective strategy for treating such conditions.

Two-dimensional cultures fail to recreate the native cell–cell and cell–ECM interaction and hence affect the cellular response. In a three-dimensional (3D) culture system, the scaffold serves as a "Support" for the cells to proliferate and grow better. The main motto behind tissue engineering is to recreate the mechanical features and the microenvironment of the native tissue so that the cells respond in the same way as that of the native tissue. Most of the tissue engineering strategies involve three components: (1) scaffolds, (2) cells, and (3) bioactive molecules. Even though cells give better response in the natural scaffolds, synthetic polymeric scaffolds are widely used because of its varied desirable properties like tailorable and reproducible synthesis, range of mechanical strength and biodegradation, and easy to functionalize or modify. Another goal of tissue engineering is the use of stem cells and differentiating them into the desired cell. There are many studies showing scaffolds incorporated with chondrogenic factors formed cartilage-like tissue when seeded with adipose-derived mesenchymal stem cells. The field of tissue engineering is progressing toward a promising method of tissue replacement that eliminates the need of donors and provides autologous replacements.

5.2 History of Biological Scaffolds

In 1985, Paul S. Russel suggested primary cells isolated from a tissue can be transplanted (Chaignaud et al., 1997). Even though the isolated cells can form tissue structures, the approach had limitations as the cells lack matrix for attachment. John F. Burke and Ioannis Yannas were the first to make artificial skin using collagen matrix. They found collagen matrix implanted on a wound enhances skin regeneration (Yannas and Burke, 1980; Yannas et al., 1982). Combining both these principles, Vacanti first developed the idea of creating artificial organs using a 3D system, in 1988. They used a biodegradable polymer scaffold for growing parenchymal cells (Vacanti et al., 1988). Although they did not succeed in making a fully functional artificial organ, their work consequently served to understand the different properties required of a scaffold for making an artificial organ or tissue and led to the development of a new field called "Tissue engineering."

5.3 Characteristics of a Scaffold

The first tissue-engineered cartilage was reported by Vacanti et al. in 1991. They seeded chondrocytes on a biodegradable polymer scaffold and on implanting the construct sub-cutaneously in nude mice, succeeded in generating a cartilage of 100 mg weight (Vacanti et al., 1991). The work of Vacanti and other studies that followed, serve to understand the different characteristics required for a scaffold, to create an artificial tissue-engineered cartilage.

5.3.1 3D Porous Structure with Interconnected Pores

In native cartilage, the chondrocytes reside in interconnected porous structures called lacunae. Although porosity does not affect the proliferation of chondrocytes, a scaffold with a pore size of 150–250 µm is considered ideal for cartilage tissue engineering. It has been shown that highly porous scaffolds enhance the expression of aggrecan and collagen-II and produce a cartilage of better mechanical strength (Zhang et al., 2014). This porous architecture also helps in migration of bone marrow stem cells (BMSCs) for cartilage repair (Ikeda et al., 2009) and in diffusion of nutrients and waste products.

5.3.2 Mechanical Properties Similar to Native Cartilage

The compressive stress at the hip joint is about 20 MPa. It is the multiphasic nature of cartilage that imparts the cushioning effect and the resilience to withstand this high amount of stress (Chang and Wang, 2011). The nature of cartilage components is responsible for the multiphasic nature of cartilage. For example, the negative charge and inherent hydrophilicity of the proteoglycans and aggrecans is responsible for attracting water molecules (which makes 70% of total weight). When the cartilage is compressed, the water molecules diffuse and on relaxation of load, the water is absorbed back (Kiani et al., 2002). This is known as the "cushioning" effect of the cartilage.

In cartilage, the collagen fibers are arranged parallel to each other. This anisotropic arrangement is responsible for the compressive, shear, and tensile strength of the cartilage. Even though it is extremely difficult to recreate the native zonal cartilage, through multiphasic scaffolds, some properties like resilience and tensile strength can be reproduced by choosing the appropriate polymer. And most importantly, the scaffold is expected to support the neocartilage formation, which can give similar mechanical strength as that of the native cartilage.

5.3.3 Biocompatible, Bioresorbable, and Biodegradable

A particular material can be considered biocompatible if it is not harmful or toxic to the organism or tissue and integrates well with the surrounding tissue without adverse host-material responses.

The term biodegradable became relevant when the concept of scaffold that slowly degrades away and is replaced by the tissue became popular. In case of bioresorbable materials, the degraded products are metabolized by the body itself. The scaffold is expected to have a controlled degradation rate that match with the tissue growth. The incorporation of organic fillers like hydroxyapatite, starch, etc. can help to tailor the degradation rate of the scaffold. Other factors that could influence the degradation are copolymerization, modification of bulk physical properties, processing techniques, etc. Bulk release of acidic degradation products has been shown to cause inflammatory response, hence these types of composite or modified scaffolds help to avoid inflammatory responses.

5.3.4 Surface Properties of the Scaffold

There are reports (Xu and Siedlecki, 2007; Ranella et al., 2010) that both hydrophobicity and hydrophilicity of scaffolds favor cell attachment. In case of hydrophobic scaffolds, the cells attach to the serum proteins that are adhered on the scaffold surface. Hydrophilicity helps to hold more nutrients and water molecules, although cells have shown good cell spreading, proliferation and attachment on hydrophilic surfaces, too much hydrophilicity (contact angle <65) limits the cell attachment (Vogler, 1999). Our study (Mohan and Nair, 2008) concluded that the surface of the scaffold should not be either too hydrophobic or hydrophilic but maintain a balance of hydrophobic–hydrophilic ratio.

The surface charge of the scaffold is also known to influence the behavior of the cell. The negatively charged surfaces have been shown to have better expression of collagen-II and glycosaminoglycan in chondrocytes when compared to neutral or positive-charged surfaces (Vacanti et al., 1988; Dadsetan et al., 2011).

The scaffold roughness has a direct influence on the proliferation, differentiation, and matrix production. Chondrocytes cultured on microrough surfaces have been shown to have enhanced proliferation, differentiation, and matrix production compared to that cultured on smooth surfaces (Boyan et al., 1999).

5.4 Polymeric Scaffolds for Cartilage Tissue Engineering

Many biomaterials have been exploited as scaffolds for cartilage tissue engineering. Ceramics are not found as suitable candidate materials for cartilage tissue engineering as they induce mineralization of cartilage and their mechanically brittle nature makes them unsuitable for load-bearing applications. However, bioceramics have been used as inserts in osteochondral interfaces of articular cartilage (Bernstein et al., 2013).

Polymers are much preferred in tissue engineering of cartilage because of its mechanical properties and flexibility to fabricate using different methods. A suitable polymer is selected depending on its mechanical properties, cell-matrix response, biocompatibility, porosity, surface properties, method of fabrication, etc. Yet, in most of the cases, a single biomaterial does not comply all these required properties. Copolymers, blends, or composite polymers are used in such situations. Following are some of the commonly used natural and synthetic, biocompatible polymers for cartilage tissue engineering.

5.4.1 Natural Polymers as Scaffolds

Natural polymers usually have excellent biocompatibility, but their common drawbacks, such as weak mechanical properties, lack of reproducibility, unstable degradation rate, and possibility of antigenic reactions, limit its application in tissue engineering. Following are some of the natural materials commonly used for cartilage tissue engineering.

5.4.1.1 Collagen

Collagen is a naturally occurring protein with excellent tissue compatibility, nontoxic, and facile biodegradation; moreover, its degradation products are absorbed mostly without inflammation. Since collagen is a key component of the ECM, collagen-based scaffolds show very good cell attachment and response. There are 28 different types of collagen that have been identified so far, of which collagen-I and II play a major role in bone and cartilage ECM. Collagen-II is favorable for sustenance of cartilage phenotype, while collagen-I causes dedifferentiation of chondrocytes (Sell et al., 2010). Porous scaffolds are made from collagen using different methods like electrospinning, freeze drying, etc. followed by crosslinking. These scaffolds are less immunogenic and give better cell response. Mueller-Rath et al. (2010) attempted a stabilized collagen-I gel seeded with human articular chondrocytes, while Jancár et al. (2007) tested the mechanical properties of collagen and combinations of collagen and hydroxyapatite scaffolds. All of them, however, were limited in usage due to their inferior mechanical properties.

5.4.1.2 Chitosan

Chitosan is a natural biopolymer made of repeating polysaccharide units of β(1–4) 2-amino-2-deoxy-D-glucose. It is prepared by the deacetylation of chitin and hence can be an unlimited natural resource. Chitosan has excellent biocompatibility and can be easily fabricated into porous scaffolds by methods like freeze-drying electrospinning, etc. Chitosan is chemically similar to glycosaminoglycans and hyaluronic acid, which makes them a favorite material for cartilage tissue engineering (Tan et al., 2009). However, chitosan as such is reported to be not a good option for injectable cartilage, because of its slow gelling time and possibility of forming cartilage-like tissue ectopically on account of its flowing out of the joints (Hao et al., 2010). Chitosan solution (Hoemann et al., 2005), chitosan–pluronic injectable gel (Park et al., 2009), and chitosan/polycaprolactone (PCL) blends (Neves et al., 2011) have been used for cartilage repair with chondrocytes with favorable results *in vivo* in rabbit models. While mechanical properties of the chitosan-blended systems are promising, the possibility of some allergic reactions with chitosan as well as its hemostatic potential can limit its widespread use.

5.4.1.3 Fibrin

Fibrin is a fibrous protein responsible for clotting of blood. Fibrin hydrogels are made by crosslinking of fibrinogen from blood. It is widely used for applications such as bioadhesive, sealant, etc. Even though it shows minimal inflammatory responses, it can be isolated from the individual's own blood and can be used as an autologous transplant.

In cartilage tissue engineering, fibrin has been used as an injectable gel. When fibrin gel mixed with chondrocytes was injected into forehead defect of New Zealand white rabbits, it produced neocartilage in 8 weeks (Cakmak et al., 2013). Fibrin gels are Food and Drug Administration (FDA) approved and were extensively studied for cartilage tissue engineering applications (Silverman et al., 1999; Fussengger et al., 2003). Chondrocytes cultured in fibrin hydrogels showed accumulation of glycosaminoglycans (GAGs) and other ECM components. Peretti et al. (2006) demonstrated how autologous chondrocytes suspended in fibrin glue mixed with devitalized cartilage chips resulted in the formation of cartilage-like tissue. However, other studies (Haleem et al., 2010; Rampichová et al., 2010; Scotti et al., 2010) with mesenchymal stem cells or autologous chondrocytes with fibrin gel did not claim full success. Though good matrix turnover is reported, the studies also indicated incomplete closure of defects or inferior mechanical properties and unstable degradation rate, limiting its application in cartilage tissue engineering.

5.4.1.4 Agarose

Agarose is another polysaccharide polymer extracted from seaweed. It is a disaccharide made of D-galactose and 3,6-anhydro-L-galactopyranose. Agarose is widely used for cartilage tissue engineering as it is reported to maintain the chondrogenic phenotype (Darling and Athanasiou, 2005; Mouw et al., 2005). Mouw et al. (2005) demonstrated that chondrocytes cultured in agarose scaffold had highest GAG-to-DNA ratio compared to other scaffolds, and showed a disaccharide ratio similar to native cartilage. In another study, Tan et al. (2010) demonstrated the reparative ability of chondroces encapsulated in agarose hydrogel in *in vitro* conditions. However, chondrocytes show limited interaction and adherence in the agarose gel.

5.4.1.5 Alginate

Alginates are naturally derived polysaccharide extracted from brown algae. They are block copolymers composed of β-D-mannuronic acid (M-blocks) and α-L-guluronic acid (G-blocks), covalently linked in different sequences. In aqueous solution, alginate can form reversible gel on interaction with cations such as Ca^{2+}, Ba^{2+}, and Sr^{2+} (Rowley et al., 1999). Alginate gels are widely used for cartilage tissue engineering applications (Grandolfo et al., 1993; Guo et al., 1989; Paige et al., 1995; Aydelotte et al., 1998). The chondrocytes cultured in alginate gel shows differentiated phenotype and synthesized cartilage-specific markers (Benya and Shaffer, 1982; Glowacki et al., 1983; Aydelotte and Kuettner, 1988). However, in another study, cells cultured in alginate gel *in vitro* (Wong et al., 2001) for over several week, failed to regenerate native-like ECM, limiting its use for clinical application.

5.4.1.6 Hyaluronan

Hyaluronan is a glycosaminoglycan having alternative units of D-glucuronic acid and D-N-acetylglucosamine. It is an essential component of native cartilage, which supports cell proliferation, differentiation, and cell migration. Because of its easy processibility and bioactivity, hyaluronan is highly preferred for cartilage tissue engineering. Hyaff-11 is benzylic ester of hyaluronan, which is a commercially available hyaluronan-based biodegradable scaffold. It has been widely used for cell delivery, cartilage repair, and other cell-based therapeutic strategies (Aigner et al., 1998; Solchaga et al., 1999; Radice et al., 2000). Lisignoli et al. (2005) reported Hyaff-11 supports differentiation of human mesenchymal stem cells (hMSCs) into chondrocytes. In this study, TGFβ-1 was used to differentiate hMSC seeded on Hyaff-11 into chondrocytes. Interestingly, without TGFβ-1, the cells did not survive. In another study, chondrocytes seeded in hydrogels made of methacrylated hyaluronan showed matrix deposition, but failed to show good mechanical strength (Nettles et al., 2004).

5.4.2 Synthetic Polymers as Scaffolds for Cartilage Tissue Engineering

Unlike natural polymers, synthetic polymers are inexpensive and easily available. They can be easily molded and their mechanical properties, degradation rate, etc. can be desirably tailored. Typical synthetic biodegradable polymers that have been used for cartilage tissue engineering are PCL, polyglycolic acid (PGA), or poly(lactic-co-glycolic acid) (PLGA) copolymers. Other polymer blends and composites have also found use as scaffold material.

5.4.2.1 Polycaprolactone

PCL is a synthetic biodegradable polyester. It was less preferred during the early days due to its slow biodegradation rate (3–4 years). Since studies showing tailoring of PCL degradation rate started appearing, it has resurged again into the arena of tissue engineering. PCL is much preferred now because of its mechanical strength and low Tg value (60°C). PCL is FDA approved biocompatible polymer. PCL can maintain phenotype and promote chondrocyte proliferation. The most significant advantages of PCL are slow degradation rate and high drug permeability. But it also has drawbacks such as poor hydrophilicity and acidic degradation products which may cause inflammation (Baker et al., 2012). There are many *in vivo* studies showing chondrocyte seeded PCL scaffolds when implanted into the articular defect of rabbit, integrated well with the surrounding tissue and also showed accumulation of collagen-II and glycosaminoglyacan. The defect also showed an elastic modulus very similar to the native cartilage (Martinez-Diaz et al., 2010).

5.4.2.2 PLGA

PLGA has been widely used for tissue engineering (Stoop, 2008). PLGA is a copolymer of lactic acid and glycolic acid and reported to have good biocompatible property. However, as synthetic materials, they are expensive and have weak cell adhesive ability. PLGA degrades by hydrolysis to form the biological metabolites lactic acid and glycolic acid. PLGA is easy to process and has good mechanical strength. Unlike other synthetic polymers, it is easy to make a highly porous scaffold with interconnected pores using PLGA, a characteristic which is very important for a cartilage scaffold. People have used various methods like electrospinning and freeze drying, to fabricate PLGA-based scaffolds. Jing et al. made highly porous PLGA scaffolds of different shapes using compression molding and particulate leaching method. PLGA has excellent processibility, which makes them highly preferred for making scaffolds of desired properties. However, when it comes to cartilage tissue engineering, culturing chondrocytes for long term has been shown to decrease the expression of collagen-II and aggrecan genes (Jeon et al., 2007). It, however, acts as a good temporary matrix for cartilage tissue engineering.

5.4.2.3 Polyglycolic Acid

PGA, a polymer of glycolic acid, has been widely used for suture and other tissue engineering application for decades. It is biocompatible and bioresorbable, degraded in body by hydrolysis, and also absorbed. These properties and its tensile strength makes PGA popular among tissue engineers, though it is expensive and lack in cell adhesive motifs. Freed et al. reconstructed a 3 mm articular cartilage defect in rabbits by implanting PGA scaffold seeded with chondrocytes. After 6 months, the defect was accumulated with collagen-II and glycosaminoglycan and the surface appeared smooth as the native cartilage (Freed et al., 1994). The study showed that both the scaffold without cells and with cells helped in the healing of the defect, but scaffold with cells showed better reconstruction compared to the control.

5.4.2.4 Polyvinyl Alcohol

Polyvinyl alcohol (PVA) is a synthetic polymer having great potential for engineering articular cartilage, because of its hydrophilicity and adhesive properties (Oka et al., 2000). In a new strategy, Holloway et al. (2010) used polyethylene to reinforce PVA hydrogel, which improved its mechanical strength by 1000 times compared to the control. The reinforced PVA hydrogel showed a tensile strength of 258.1 ± 40.1 MPa. However, the potential PVA for tissue engineering application is limited due to its nondegradability. Mohan and Nair (2008) have reported a PVA–PCL interpenetrating network (IPN) with an optimum hydrophobic–hydrophilic balance that has good potential for cartilage tissue engineering and which proved better than natural scaffolds for cartilage regeneration.

5.5 Biomimetic Scaffolds for Cartilage Tissue Engineering

Biomimetic is a term introduced by Otto Schmitt in the 1950s, which means providing all the biological, chemical, physical cues responsible for tissue growth just like in the native tissue. Merely seeding of cells on scaffolds does not form a complete milieu for tissue growth. During the early days, people have been trying to improve the cell attachment by coating the scaffold surface with several factors like RGD peptides. Recent research is focused on making nanosized, isotropic, fibrous scaffolds with growth factors incorporated to it so that cells will attach and behave exactly in the way they do in the native cartilage. With recent advancements in the basic knowledge about the ECM, people are trying to mimic the physical, chemical, and biological characteristics of ECM.

5.5.1 Physical Modifications

The size of native collagen is 50–500 nm in diameter. Culturing chondrocytes on fibrous scaffold with fiber diameter less than 1 μm has shown increased expression of chondrogenic markers and proliferation. The expression of ligament specific marker is also influenced by fiber diameter, wherein fiber with least diameter showed maximum expression. When the fibrous scaffold having nanometer diameter was compared to a porous sponge-like scaffold, two-fold increase in gene expression was observed (Noriega et al., 2012). Depending on the method of fabrication, the scaffolds can be made as aligned fibers or randomly oriented fibers. The orientation of fibers significantly affects the tensile and compressive strength of the scaffold. Apart from increasing the resistance to shear and tear, the cells seeded on the aligned fibers are expected to align in the direction of the fibers and secrete ECM proteins in its direction. Studies have also shown that cells seeded on randomly oriented fibers appear flattened and that on the aligned fibers appears spindle-shaped (Schneider et al., 2012).

5.5.2 Chemical Modifications

Addition of functional groups like –CH3, –OH, –COOH, and –NH2 on scaffold surface has been shown to increase integrin binding. These functional groups also have a direct effect on gene expression (Keselowsky et al., 2003). Hydrophilicity and hydrophobicity of the scaffold has a direct effect on cell attachment. The addition of such functional groups on to the surface of the scaffolds is done by techniques like plasma treatment and corona treatment. In a study by Cheon et al. (2010), oxygen functional groups were introduced on to silk fibroin scaffold by Argon plasma treatment. This improved the hydrophilicity without affecting its bulk characteristics, and further cell studies on this scaffold showed enhanced cell attachment and proliferation. The modification also showed enhanced expression of chondrogenic markers (Cheon et al., 2010).

5.5.3 Biological Modifications

The cell behavior is greatly influenced by soluble and insoluble factors present in the ECM. The different classes of cell receptors present on the chondrocytes, like integrins, leptins, etc. bind to the ECM proteins like collagen and fibronectin and regulate the differentiation, proliferation and matrix remodeling. Apart from these insoluble proteins, there are different soluble factors like TGFβ, bone morphogenetic protein (BMP), Wnt, etc., released by the cells itself, which are responsible for regulating cell differentiation, proliferation, and secretion of ECM.

Recent years have witnessed many studies showing the importance of bioactive molecules in scaffold; such bioactive scaffolds provide a suitable microenvironment for the cells.

When an artificial ECM is made, the presence of these signaling molecules has a key role in regulating the cell behavior. Many studies have shown that controlled release of growth factors have resulted in improved cell response. TGFβ and chondroitin sulfate (CS) incorporated freeze-dried collagen/chitosan scaffold has shown enhanced cartilage formation and cell proliferation (Lee et al., 2004). Remya and Nair (2013) have shown that a biomimetic chitosan–hyaluronic acid diacetate (HDA) hydrogel can support chondrogenesis. Previous studies have shown chondrocytes seeded on chitosan scaffold maintain their round morphology and release ECM components collagen-II and glycosaminoglycans. Cell adhesion can be enhanced by adding ECM components; (Pro-Hyp-Gly)7 is chemically synthesized collagen mimetic peptides, which forms triplex structure (Wang et al., 2005; Mo et al., 2006). Lee et al. (2008) have shown that a CMP/PEODA collagen peptide biomimetic hydrogel provides suitable microenvironment for the differentiation of mesenchymal stem cells into chondrocytes.

Incorporating CMPs into polyethyleneglycol (PEG) hydrogels have been shown to enhance the accumulation of collagen-II and aggrecan (Liu et al., 2010). CMP serves as a promising candidate for making biomimetic scaffolds. Apart from scaffolds and cell sources, growth factors are also an important component for engineering articular cartilage. In native cartilage, TGFβ and BMP-2 are known to induce chondrogenesis. Mohan et al. (2010) used TGFβ-1, TGFβ-3, and BMP-2 in different combinations to differentiate mesenchymal stem cells seeded on PVA–poly(caprolactone). The authors reported ideal combination of TGFβ-3 and BMP-2 that differentiated stem cells into chondrocytes in a synthetic scaffold.

In a clinical study by Kon et al. (2011), young and active patients showed a faster recovery when they were implanted with a biomimetic collagen type 1—hydroxyapatite gradient scaffold. These results encourage further biomimetic cartilage replacements.

In a recent attempt to make hydrogels more biomimetic, Kim et al. (2015) copolymerized methacrylated ECM molecules—hyaluronic acid, CS, and integrin-binding peptides (RGD peptides) were copolymerized with PEG. Their results demonstrated the presence of ECM component and integrin-binding moieties to have a direct effect on cellular morphology and response. The chondrocytes encapsulated on CS-based hydrogel with RGD peptide showed enhanced lubricin, GAG, and collagen expression compared to other hydrogels.

Due to its similarity with the native ECM, fibrous scaffolds are ideal for cartilage tissue engineering. However, these studies often omit the importance of zone-specific organization seen in native cartilage. In a recent attempt to mimic the osteochondral interface with the gradient of biological cues, Mohan et al. (2015) incorporated gradients of CS and sol–gel-derived bioactive glass (BG) into an electrospun fiber assembled hydrogel. Gradient of chondroitin sulfate and BG were incorporated in a fibrous scaffold so that it generates opposing gradients of chondrogenic and mineralization signals as the CS and BG signals diffuse from the fibers. In response to the chondrogenic–osteogenic signals, chondrocytes seeded on CS region secreted cartilage markers—glycosaminoglycans, collagen-II, and aggrecan, and chondrocytes on BG region secreted bone marker proteins—collagen type X and osteocalcin. This construct is expected to integrate well with the surrounding tissue accelerating the osteochondral regeneration *in vivo*.

5.6 Recent Advancements

Cartilage tissue engineering is greatly enhanced through the use of scaffolds and hydrogel matrices. Researchers are attempting various studies trying to combine different concepts, as outlined in the previous sections, to regenerate functional cartilage with greater success. In an effort to mimic the mechanical properties of native cartilage, multiphasic woven fibrous scaffold was made (Moutos et al., 2007). The woven fibers were reinforced with agarose gel, in this study, the woven fiber mimicked the fibrous ECM and the gel reproduced the aqueous phase and tensile strength of native cartilage. Mechanical tests showed that the scaffold has the same magnitude of tensile, and compressive strength as that of the native cartilage. Another recent trend in tissue engineering is 3D bioprinting of ECM mixed polymer. A disadvantage of using decellularized ECM as a scaffold is the lack of sufficient mechanical strength. Mixing decellularized matrix with synthetic polymers is an innovative way of overcoming this problem. In a study, a porous 3D-printed PCL scaffold was filled with a gel prepared from decellularized cartilage matrix. Mesenchymal stem cells cultured on such scaffold showed greater expression of Sox 9, which is an early marker for chondrogenesis (Pati et al., 2014). The future of cartilage tissue engineering hence lies in the integration of different concepts of basic research of cells and materials and elegant fabrication methods to create a better biocompatible, biomimetic artificial cartilage.

References

Aigner, J., Tegeler, J., Hutzler, P. et al. 1998. Cartilage tissue engineering with novel nonwoven structured biomaterial based on hyaluronic acid benzyl ester. *J Biomed Mater Res.* 42: 172–81.

Aydelotte, M.B., Kuettner, K.E. 1988. Differences between sub-populations of cultured bovine articular chondrocytes. I. Morphology and cartilage matrix production. *Connect Tissue Res.* 18: 205–22.

Aydelotte, M.B., Thonar, E.J., Mollenhauer, J., Flechtenmacher, J. 1998. Culture of chondrocytes in alginate gel: Variations in conditions of gelation influence the structure of the alginate gel, and the arrangement and morphology of proliferating chondrocytes. *In Vitro Cell Dev Biol Anim.* 34: 123–30.

Baker, M.I., Walsh, S.P., Schwartz, Z., Boyan, B.D. 2012. A review of polyvinyl alcohol and its uses in cartilage and orthopaedic applications. *J Biomed Mater Res B: Appl Biomater.* 100: 1451–7.

Benya, P.D., Shaffer, J.D. 1982. Dedifferentiated chondrocytes reexpress the differentiated collagen phenotype when cultured in agarose gels. *Cell.* 30: 215–24.

Bernstein, A., Niemeyer, P., Salzmann, G. et al. 2013. Microporous calcium phosphate ceramics as tissue engineering scaffolds for the repair of osteochondral defects. *Acta Biomater.* 9: 7490–505.

Boyan, B.D., Lincks, J., Lohmann, C.H. et al. 1999. Effect of surface roughness and composition on costochondral chondrocytes is dependent on cell maturation state. *J Orthop Res.* 17: 446–57.

Cakmak, O., Babakurban, S.T., Akkuzu, H.G. et al. 2013. Injectable tissue-engineered cartilage using commercially available fibrin glue. *Laryngoscope.* 123: 2986–92.

Chaignaud, B.E., Langer, R., Vacanti, J.P. 1997. The history of tissue engineering using synthetic biodegradable polymer scaffolds and cells. In *Synthetic Biodegradable Polymer Scaffolds*, A. Atala and D.J. Mooney (eds), 1–14. Birkhäuser, Boston, Massachusetts.

Chang, H., Wang, Y. 2011. Cell responses to surface and architecture of tissue engineering scaffolds. In *Regenerative Medicine and Tissue Engineering—Cells and Biomaterials*, D. Eberli (ed.), 569–88. INTECH Open.

Cheon, Y.W., Lee, W.J., Baek, H.S. et al. 2010. Enhanced chondrogenic responses of human articular chondrocytes onto silk fibroin/wool keratose scaffolds treated with microwave-induced argon plasma. *Artif Organs.* 34: 384–92.

Dadsetan, M., Pumberger, M., Casper, M.E. et al. 2011. The effects of fixed electrical charge on chondrocyte behavior. *Acta Biomater.* 7: 2080–90.

Darling, E.M., Athanasiou, K.A. 2005. Retaining zonal chondrocyte phenotype by means of novel growth environments. *Tissue Eng.* 11: 395–403.

Freed, L.E., Vunjak-Novakovic, G., Biron, R.J. et al. 1994. Biodegradable polymer scaffolds for tissue engineering. *Biotechnology (NY).* 12: 689–93.

Fussengger, M., Meinhart, J., Hobling, W. et al. 2003. Stabilized autologous fibrin-chondrocyte constructs for cartilage repair *in vivo*. *Ann Plast Surg.* 51: 493–8.

Glowacki, J., Trepman, E., Folkman, J. 1983. Cell shape and phenotypic expression in chondrocytes. *Proc Soc Exp Biol Med.* 172: 93–8.

Grandolfo, M., D'Andrea, P., Paoletti, S. et al. 1993. Culture and differentiation of chondrocytes entrapped in alginate gels. *Calcif Tissue Int.* 52: 42–8.

Guo, J.F., Jourdian, G.W., MacCallum, D.K. 1989. Culture and growth characteristics of chondrocytes encapsulated in alginate beads. *Connect Tissue Res.* 19: 277–97.

Haleem, A.M., Singergy, A.A., Sabry, D. et al. 2010. The clinical use of human culture-expanded autologous bone marrow mesenchymal stem cells transplanted on platelet-rich fibrin glue in the treatment of articular cartilage defects: A pilot study and preliminary results. *Cartilage.* 1: 253–61.

Hao, T., Wen, N., Cao, J.K. et al. 2010. The support of matrix accumulation and the promotion of sheep articular cartilage defects repair *in vitro* by chitosan hydrogels. *Osteoarthr. Cartilage.* 18: 257–65.

Hoemann, C.D., Sun, J., Legare, A., McKee, M.D., Buschmann, M.D. 2005. Tissue engineering of cartilage using injectable and adhesive chitosan-based cell-delivery vehicle. *Osteoarthr Cartilage.* 13: 318–29.

Holloway, J.L., Lowman, A.M., Palmese, G.R. 2010. Mechanical evaluation of poly(vinyl alcohol)-based fibrous composites as biomaterials for meniscal tissue replacement. *Acta Biomater.* 6: 4716–24.

Ikeda, R., Fujioka, H., Nagura, I. et al. 2009. The effect of porosity and mechanical property of a synthetic polymer scaffold on repair of osteochondral defects. *Int Orthop.* 33: 821–8.

Jancár, J., Slovíková, A., Amler, E. et al., 2007. Mechanical response of porous scaffolds for cartilage. *Physiol Res.* 56: 17–25.

Jeon, Y.H., Choi, J.H., Sung, J.K. et al. 2007. Different effects of PLGA and chitosan scaffolds on human cartilage tissue engineering. *J Craniofac Surg.* 18: 1249–58.

Keselowsky, B.G., Collard, D.M., García, A.J. 2003. Surface chemistry modulates fibronectin conformation and directs integrin binding and specificity to control cell adhesion. *J Biomed Mater Res A.* 66: 247–59.

Kiani, C., Chen, L., Wu, Y.J., Yee, A.J., Yang, B.B. 2002. Structure and function of aggrecan. *Cell Res.* 12: 19–32.

Kim, H.D., Heo, J., Hwang, Y. et al. 2015. Extracellular-matrix-based and Arg-Gly-Asp-modified photopolymerizing hydrogels for cartilage tissue engineering. *Tissue Eng A.* 21: 757–66.

Kon, E., Delcogliano, M., Filardo, G. et al. 2011. Novel nano-composite multilayered biomaterial for osteochondral regeneration. *Am J Sports Med.* 39: 1180–90.

Lee, H.J., Christopher, Y.U., Thanissara, C.B.S. et al. 2008. Enhanced chondrogenesis of mesenchymal stem cells in collagen mimetic peptide-mediated microenvironment. *Tissue Eng A.* 14: 1843–51.

Lee, J.E., Kim, K.E., Kwon, I.C. et al. 2004. Effects of the controlled-released TGF-beta 1 from chitosan microspheres on chondrocytes cultured in a collagen/chitosan/glycosaminoglycan scaffold. *Biomaterials.* 25(18): 4163–73.

Lisignoli, G., Cristino, S., Piacentini, A. et al. 2005. Cellular and molecular events during chondrogenesis of human mesenchymal stromal cells grown in a three-dimensional hyaluronan based scaffold. *Biomaterials.* 26: 5677–86.

Liu, S.Q., Tian, Q., Hedrick, J.L. et al. 2010. Biomimetic hydrogels for chondrogenic differentiation of human mesenchymal stem cells to neocartilage. *Biomaterials.* 31: 7298–307.

Martin, J.A., Bucklwater, J.A. 2002. Aging, articular cartilage chondrocyte senescence and osteoarthritis. *Biogerontology.* 3: 257–64.

Martinez-Diaz, S., Garcia-Giralt, N., Lebourg, M. et al. 2010. *In vivo* evaluation of 3-dimensional polycaprolactone scaffolds for cartilage repair in rabbits. *Am J Sports Med.* 38: 509–19.

Mo, X., An, Y., Yun, C.S., Yu, S.M. 2006. Nanoparticle-assisted visualization of binding interactions between collagen mimetic peptide and collagen fibers. *Angew Chem Int Ed Engl.* 45: 2267–70.

Mohan, N., Nair, P.D. 2008. Polyvinyl alcohol-polycaprolactone semi IPN scaffold with implication for cartilage tissue engineering. *J Biomed Mat Res B: Appl Biomater.* 84: 584–94.

Mohan, N., Nair, P.D., Tabata, Y. 2010. Growth factor-mediated effects on chondrogenic differentiation of mesenchymal stem cells in 3D semi-IPN poly(vinyl alcohol)-poly(caprolactone) scaffolds. *J Biomed Mater Res A.* 94: 146–59.

Mohan, N., Wilson, J., Joseph, D., Vaikkath, D., Nair, P.D. 2015. Biomimetic fiber assembled gradient hydrogel to engineer glycosaminoglycan enriched and mineralized cartilage: An *in vitro* study. *J Biomed Mater Res A.* 103: 3896–906.

Moutos, F.T., Freed, L.E., Guilak, F. 2007. A biomimetic three-dimensional woven composite scaffold for functional tissue engineering of cartilage. *Nat Mater.* 6: 162–7.

Mouw, J.K., Case, N.D., Guldberg, R.E., Plaas, A.H., Levenston, M.E. 2005. Variations in matrix composition and GAG fine structure among scaffolds for cartilage tissue engineering. *Osteoarthr Cartilage.* 13: 828–36.

Mueller-Rath, R., Gavenis, K., Andereya, S. et al. 2010. Condensed cellular seeded collagen gel as an improved biomaterial for tissue engineering of articular cartilage. *Biomed Mater Eng.* 20: 317–28.

Nettles, D.L., Vail, T.P., Morgan, M.T., Grinstaff, M.W., Setton, L.A. 2004. Photocrosslinkable hyaluronan as a scaffold for articular cartilage repair. *Ann Biomed Eng.* 32: 391–7.

Neves, S.C., Moreira Teixeira, L.S., Moroni, L. et al. 2011. Chitosan/poly(3-caprolactone) blend scaffolds for cartilage repair. *Biomaterials.* 32: 1068–79.

Noriega, S.E., Hasanova, G.I., Schneider, M.J., Larsen, G.F., Subramanian, A. 2012. Effect of fiber diameter on the spreading, proliferation and differentiation of chondrocytes on electrospun chitosan matrices. *Cells Tissues Organs.* 195: 207–21.

Oka, M., Ushio, K., Kumar, P. et al. 2000. Development of artificial articular cartilage. *Proc Inst Mech Eng H.* 214: 59–68.

Paige, K.T., Cima, L.G., Yaremchuk, M.J., Vacanti, J.P., Vacanti, C.A. 1995. Injectable cartilage. *Plast Reconstr Surg.* 96: 1390–8.

Park, K.M., Lee, S.Y., Joung, Y.K., Na, J.S., Lee, M.C., Park, K.D. 2009. Thermosensitive chitosan–pluronic hydrogel as an injectable cell delivery carrier for cartilage regeneration. *Acta Biomater.* 5: 1956–65.

Pati, F., Jang, J., Ha, D.H., Won Kim, S., Rhie, J.W., Shim, J.H., Kim, D.H., Cho, D.W. 2014. Printing three-dimensional tissue analogues with decellularized extracellular matrix bioink. *Nat Commun.* 5: 3935.

Peretti, G.M., Xu, J.W., Bonassar, L.J., Kirchhoff, C.H., Yaremchuk, M.J., Randolph, M.A. 2006. Review of injectable cartilage engineering using fibrin gel in mice and swine models. *Tissue Eng.* 12: 1151–68.

Radice, M., Brun, P., Cortivo, R., Scapinelli, R., Battaliard, C., Abatangelo, G. 2000. Hyaluronan-based biopolymers as delivery vehicles for bone-marrow-derived mesenchymal progenitors. *J Biomed Mater Res.* 50: 101–9.

Rampichová, M., Filová, E., Varga, F. et al. 2010. Fibrin/hyaluronic acid composite hydrogels as appropriate scaffolds for *in vivo* artificial cartilage implantation. *Am Soc Art Int Org.* 56: 563–8.

Ranella, A., Barberoglou, M., Bakogianni, S., Fotakis, C., Stratakis, E. 2010. Tuning cell adhesion by controlling the roughness and wettability of 3D micro/nano silicon structures. *Acta Biomater.* 6: 2711–20.

Remya, N.S., Nair, P.D. 2013. Engineering cartilage tissue interfaces using a natural glycosaminoglycan hydrogel matrix—An *in vitro* study. *Mater Sci Eng C: Mater Biol Appl.* 33: 575–82.

Rowley, J.A., Madlambayan, G., Mooney, D.J. 1999. Alginate hydrogels as synthetic extracellular matrix materials. *Biomaterials.* 20: 45–53.

Schneider, T., Kohl, B., Sauter, T. et al. 2012. Influence of fiber orientation in electrospun polymer scaffolds on viability, adhesion and differentiation of articular chondrocytes. *Clin Hemorheol Microcirc.* 52: 325–36.

Scotti, C., Mangiavini, L., Boschetti, F. et al. 2010. Effect of *in vitro* culture on a chondrocyte-fibrin glue hydrogel for cartilage repair. *Knee Surg Sports Traumatol Arthrosc.* 18: 1400–6.

Sell, S.A., Wolfe, P.S., Koyal, G., McCool, J.M., Rodriguez, I.A., Bowlin, G.L. 2010. The use of natural polymers in tissue engineering: A focus on electrospun extracellular matrix analogues. *Polymers.* 2: 522–53.

Silverman, R.P., Passareti, D., Huang, W., Randolph, M.A., Yaremchuk, M.J. 1999. Injectable tissue-engineered cartilage using a fibrin glue polymer. *Plast Reconstr Surg.* 103: 1809–18.

Solchaga, L.A., Dennis, J.E., Goldberg, V.M., Caplan, A.I. 1999. Hyaluronic acid-based polymers as cell carriers for tissue-engineered repair of bone and cartilage. *J Orthop Res.* 17: 205–13.

Stoop, R. 2008. Smart biomaterials for tissue engineering of cartilage, *Injury.* 39: 77–87.

Tan, A.R., Dong, E.Y., Ateshian, G.A., Hung, C.T. 2010. Response of engineered cartilage to mechanical insult depends on construct maturity. *Osteoarthr Cartilage.* 18: 1577–85.

Tan, H., Chu, C.R., Payne, K., Marra, K.G. 2009. Injectable *in situ* forming biodegradable chitosan–hyaluronic acid based hydrogels for cartilage tissue engineering. *Biomaterials.* 30: 2499–506.

Vacanti, C.A., Langer, R., Schloo, B., Vacanti, J.P. 1991. Synthetic polymers seeded with chondrocytes provide a template for new cartilage formation. *Plast Reconstr Surg.* 88: 753–9.

Vacanti, J.P., Morse, M.A., Saltzman, W.M., Domb, A.J., Perez-Atayde, A., Langer, R. 1998. Selective cell transplantation using bioabsorbable artificial polymers as matrices. *J Pediatr Surg.* 23: 3–9.

Vogler, E.A. 1999. Water and the acute biological response to surfaces. *J Biomater Sci Polym Ed*. 10: 1015–45.

Wang, A.Y., Mo, X., Chen, C.S., Yu, S.M. 2005. Facile modification of collagen directed by collagen mimetic peptides. *J Am Chem Soc*. 127: 4130–1.

Wong, M., Siegrist, M., Wang, X., Hunziker, E. 2001. Development of mechanically stable alginate/ chondrocyte constructs: Effects of guluronic acid content and matrix synthesis. *J Orthop Res*. 19: 493–9.

Xu, L.C., Siedlecki, C.A. 2007. Effects of surface wettability and contact time on protein adhesion to biomaterial surfaces. *Biomaterials*. 28: 3273–83.

Yannas, I.V., Burke, J.F. 1980. Design of an artificial skin. I. Basic design principles. *J Biomed Mater Res*. 14(1): 65–81.

Yannas, I.V., Burke, J.F., Orgill, D.P., Skrabut, E.M. 1982. Wound tissue can utilize a polymeric template to synthesize a functional extension of skin. *Science*. 215: 174–6.

Zhang, Q., Lu, H., Kawazoe, N., Chen, G. 2014. Pore size effect of collagen scaffolds on cartilage regeneration. *Acta Biomater*. 10(5): 2005–13.

Section III

Regeneration of Sensory System

6

Bioengineered Skin: Progress and Prospects

Uma Maheswari Krishnan

CONTENTS

6.1 An Introduction to Tissue Engineering of Skin

Skin is the largest organ in the body and is vital to maintain hydration. It regulates body temperature, facilitates synthesis of vitamin D, aids in the excretion of waste in the form of sweat, and forms a protective barrier against pathogen invasion and chemicals (Metcalfe and Ferguson, 2007a). The skin contains an outer epidermal layer followed by a dermal layer and hypodermis. The epidermis comprises the *stratum corneum, stratum lucidum, stratum granulosum, stratum spinosum,* and *stratum basale* (MacNeil, 2008). In addition to serving as a protective barrier, the epidermal layers are also involved in cell proliferation as well as impart specific coloration to an individual. The innermost basal layer (*stratum basale* or *stratum germinativum*) of the epidermis is involved in producing new cells. It also contains the melanocytes that produce the skin pigment melanin, which offers photoprotection to the deeper tissues. Merkel cells that are of neuronal origin are also found in the basal layer (Eungdamrong et al., 2014). These cells help in distinguishing different types of "touch" sensations. Above the basal layer lies the thickest layer of the epidermis, namely, the *squamous spinosum* that contains the keratinocytes. These cells are produced in the basal layer and are pushed upward. Keratinocytes produce the structural protein keratin that imparts toughness to the cells. These cells are responsible for the barrier function of the cell. The keratinocytes in this layer have spine-like projections on the surface. The Langerhans cells that are part of the immune system also reside in this layer. The keratinocytes are also present in the *stratum granulosum* and *stratum lucidum* layers where their morphology becomes flat. The cells become large, dehydrated, and fuse with each other forming a tough layer containing dead cells. Finally, the dead cells are pushed to the tough layer of *stratum corneum* where the dead cells are constantly shed. Figure 6.1 depicts the various layers present in the skin.

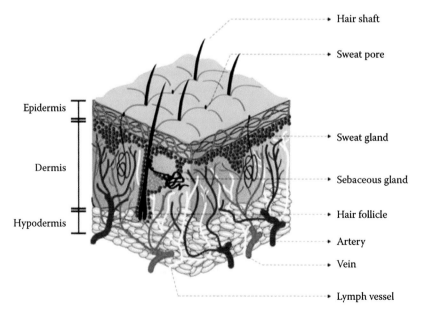

FIGURE 6.1
Various layers and appendages present in skin.

Beneath the epidermal layers lie the dermis that ranges between 1.5 and 4 mm thick. It is the most important layer and is well supplied by blood vessels and lymphatic network. The production of vitamin D occurs in this layer, which is then transported to the other parts of the body by the skin vasculature (Zhang and Michniak-Kohn, 2012). The hair follicles, sweat glands, sebaceous glands, and nerve endings are also found in the dermal layers. The sweat glands regulate body temperature and prevent proliferation of pathogens on the skin. The sebaceous glands are involved in the production of sebum or oil to protect the skin against pathogens as well as maintain the skin texture apart from serving as a waterproof layer. Fibroblasts are the other type of cells found in the dermis. The dermal layer contains rich deposits of elastin and collagen that binds the various layers together and maintains the elastic nature of skin. The hypodermis consists of the subcutaneous layer of fat that serves as a thermal insulator and a shock absorber. The epidermal and dermal layers also contain numerous cytokines and growth factors to regulate cell migration, proliferation, and healing of the tissue after injury.

As skin is constantly in contact with the environment, it is susceptible to damage through mechanical, chemical, and radiation-induced injuries. Restoration of the skin function can be achieved by repair or regeneration. Though in most cases wound healing and skin regeneration are used synonymously, there exists a subtle difference between the two processes. While wound repair represents a process to create continuity in the skin tissue without reconstitution of the tissue, regeneration involves restoration of the function and morphology of the original tissue layers. Wound repair often results in scar formation while regeneration is achieved without scar formation. Natural wound healing process usually results in scarring in most cases, especially if the wound area is large. Modern interventions aim to induce wound healing without scar formation by regenerating the organized layers of the skin.

One of the first reports of scientific interventions leading to skin grafting appeared in *Nonnulla de Regeneratione et Transplantatione* and describes the efforts of the surgeon Johann Friedrich Dieffenbach, considered to be the father of modern plastic and reconstructive surgery, who used pedicled skin grafts in animals and patients to replace damaged skin tissue in the early part of the nineteenth century (Meyer, 2009). Heinrich Christian Bunger is credited with the first clinical autologous skin transplantation while Karl Thiersch employed split thickness skin grafts to replace damaged skin tissue. In the twentieth century, insights on the factors that control cell proliferation and the role of extracellular matrix (ECM) in guiding cell adhesion, growth, and functions led to more successful integration of cells and materials toward the development of skin substitutes. In the early 1970s, Dr. Green sowed the seeds for modern tissue engineering concepts when he predicted that incorporation of viable cells in biocompatible matrices with appropriate geometry and chemical properties can lead to formation of new tissue. This hypothesis was transformed into reality by Yannas and Burke who successfully generated a collagen matrix that supported the adhesion and proliferation of dermal fibroblasts leading to the first tissue-engineered skin substitute (Vacanti, 2006). Later, Dr. Howard Green successfully transplanted a cell sheet of keratinocytes in a burn victim demonstrating the potential of skin tissue engineering in a clinical setup. In 1979, Dr. Bell reported the development of a collagen matrix seeded with fibroblasts as a tissue-engineered dermal substitute (Vacanti, 2006). Since then, many skin substitutes have been introduced in the market for wound healing and replacement of damaged skin tissue (Supp and Boyce, 2005). Table 6.1 summarizes the commercially available skin grafts and their salient characteristics.

Despite the relatively large number of skin substitutes, there are several short comings that limit their use (Nicoletti et al., 2015). Compatibility issues due to allogenic cell sources,

TABLE 6.1

Commercially Available Skin Substitutes

Skin Substitute	Type	Cells Used
Epicel®	Cell-based epidermal substitute	Autologous keratinocytes
CellSpray®	Cell-based epidermal substitute	Autologous keratinocytes
Myskin®	Cell-laden scaffold, epidermal substitute	Autologous keratinocytes
Laserskin®	Cell-laden scaffold, epidermal substitute	Autologous keratinocytes
ReCell®	Cell suspension of autologous epidermal cells, epidermal substitute	Autologous keratinocytes
Integra®	Cell-free dermal substitute	–
Alloderm®	Cell-free dermal substitute	–
Hyalomatrix PA®	Cell-free dermal substitute	–
Dermagraft®	Cell-laden scaffold, dermal substitute	Neonatal allogenic fibroblasts
TransCyte®	Cell-laden scaffold, dermal substitute	Neonatal allogenic fibroblasts
Hyalograft 3D®	Cell-laden scaffold, dermal substitute	Autologous fibroblasts
OrCel®	Cell-laden natural scaffold, dermo-epidermal substitute	Allogenic keratinocytes and fibroblasts
Apligraf®	Cell-laden natural scaffold, dermo-epidermal substitute	Allogenic keratinocytes and fibroblasts
PolyActive®	Cell-laden synthetic scaffold, dermo-epidermal substitute	Autologous keratinocytes and fibroblasts

expensive nature of cell-laden substitutes, lack of skin appendages, and poor vascularization are issues that plague the substitutes. Hence, attempts to develop better substitutes and strategies to regain functional skin postinjury are currently underway.

6.2 Challenges in Skin Tissue Engineering

Most of the skin repair and regeneration attempts have mainly focused on promoting the barrier function of the skin by generating layers of keratinocytes or fibroblasts. However, to maintain a functional live tissue, a well-developed vasculature is essential. In order to ensure good adhesion of the cells on a skin substitute or scaffold, *ex vivo* strategies where the scaffold/substitute is cultured with cells that are then transplanted to the wound site, have been employed. However, if the thickness of this cell-seeded construct is beyond 0.4 mm, vascularization is restricted leading to death of the cells (Eungdamrong et al., 2014). Another concern is the biocompatibility of the constructs employed for reconstruction of the dermal layers. Use of materials from natural sources especially gives rise to safety concerns due to the risk of pathogen transmission and immune rejection. Lack of pigmentation in regenerated skin arising due to depleted numbers of melanocytes is another concern as it involves esthetic issues as well as poor photoprotective functions. As most of the tissue engineering strategies focus on enhancing collagen deposition, this can lead to depletion of the melanocytes at the site of implantation. Moreover, excess collagen deposits can also lead to scar formation instead of a functional elastic skin. Another major limitation in current tissue engineering strategies is skin contraction that is promoted by the large numbers of keratinocytes and fibroblasts found in the skin substitute/scaffold (Eungdamrong et al., 2014). This phenomenon has been attributed to cross-linking of the collagen deposits forming the ECM. The development of an efficient and cost-effective strategy is another challenge for skin tissue engineers. Nevertheless, the promise of rapid repair and regeneration of skin has placed skin tissue engineering at the forefront of strategies to treat chronic injuries.

6.3 Scaffolds for Skin Tissue Engineering

The success of tissue engineering mainly depends upon three main factors commonly referred to as the "tissue engineering triad." These are the scaffold materials, the cells used, and the chemical molecules employed to stimulate growth and proliferation of cells. The general strategy in tissue engineering is to harvest skin cells from a donor, culture them under optimized conditions followed by seeding them on to a substrate with suitable topography and adequate porosity. The cell-seeded scaffold is maintained under regulated conditions to obtain desired proliferation rates. This construct is then implanted in the patient. However, each stage is influenced by numerous factors that need to be optimized to obtain a functional and successful tissue. Figure 6.2 depicts a cartoon that presents an overview of the tissue engineering strategy.

Skin tissue engineering attempts have also focused on identifying the ideal combination of materials, topography, chemical stimulants, and concentrations to be employed to favor the organized arrangement of different cell types. In addition, a fourth major parameter, namely, mechanical stimuli, has been identified to play a crucial role in skin repair and regeneration. The following sections focus on the major parameters that have

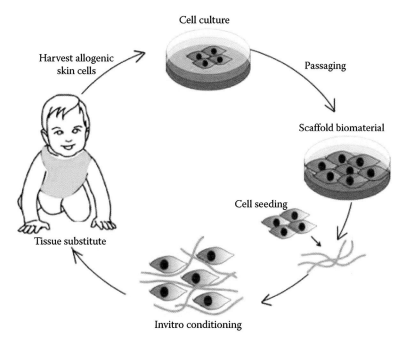

FIGURE 6.2
Tissue engineering strategy.

been investigated for promoting rapid wound healing and regeneration. Several emerging paradigms in the context of developing bioengineered skin constructs have also been discussed.

6.3.1 Scaffold Materials

The chemical nature of the scaffold material influences the nature of cell interactions significantly. Both materials of natural and synthetic origin have been widely explored for skin tissue engineering (MacNeil, 2008). Natural biomaterials have limited availability. Further, several natural polymers have been found to have variable properties owing to the differences in the extraction procedures and sources. Synthetic biomaterials have reproducible properties and are not limited by availability, but tailoring their mechanical properties to match the native skin and avoiding foreign body response in the biological system are major challenges. Regardless of the origin, biomaterials used for skin tissue engineering should possess appropriate water uptake ratio (WUR). This property defines the ability of the material to absorb nutrients and exudates from the wound bed. Full thickness wounds generally contain a large amount of exudates and hence a material with high WUR is preferable. In contrast, partial thickness wounds do not require materials with high WUR and low WUR materials can aid the regeneration process. Another important requisite of biomaterials used for skin regeneration is water vapor permeability (WVP) that depends on the ratio of scaffold area to the water surface area. If a material has very high WVP, it leads to a dry wound bed while materials with very low WVP results in bacterial infection due to accumulation of exudates. It is therefore important to maintain appropriate moisture content in the wound bed for effective skin regeneration and therefore the selection of the scaffold material with adequate WUR and WVP values is critical.

6.3.2 Natural Biomaterials

6.3.2.1 Collagen

As collagen is an important constituent of skin tissue, extensive work has been carried out using collagen-based scaffolds for skin tissue engineering. There are many types of collagen in the biological system. Collagen I is the most abundant form and comprises nearly 90% of the total collagen in the human body. Collagen is mainly produced by the fibroblasts. After their biosynthesis, collagen undergoes posttranslational modification with several proline and lysine residues getting hydroxylated by the respective hydroxylase enzymes. Several lysine residues are also glycosylated. The alpha chains of the collagen self-assemble to form bundles of tropocollagen (Parenteau-Bareil et al., 2010). Once they are released from the excretory vesicles, the collagen undergoes fibrillation to form higher ordered structures known as collagen fibrils with dimensions ranging between 10 and 300 nm. The fibrils undergo aggregation to form large collagen fibers with dimensions ranging from 500 to 3000 nm. Not all types of collagen can form fibrils and fibers. Collagen types I, II, III, V, and XI are fibril-forming collagen and hence can be used for fabricating fibrous scaffolds. Collagen type IX is found to be associated with type II fibrils while collagen type XII associates with type I fibrils. Collagen IV forms a sheet-like network while collagen VII, commonly encountered beneath the stratified squamous epithelial layer, forms a network of anchoring fibrils (Parenteau-Bareil et al., 2010). Collagen is also found widely distributed in other animals. However, their properties are species-specific. Collagen is degraded by the collagenase belonging to the family of matrix metalloproteinases (MMPs).

Collagen I is degraded by MMPs 1, 2, 8, 13, and 14. MMPs initially bind to collagen, unwind the alpha chains of the triple helix, and then cleave the peptide bonds. However, for use in tissue engineering applications, the rate of degradation of collagen needs to be regulated. Hence, cross-linked collagen has been employed to limit the enzyme binding and water permeation.

Physical, chemical, and enzymatic cross-linking strategies have been employed for collagen-based scaffolds (Parenteau-Bareil et al., 2010). Physical cross-linking uses no chemical cross-linkers and hence chemical-associated cytotoxic effects are avoided. Ultraviolet (UV) irradiation of collagen scaffolds has been widely employed for cross-linking through generation of free radical centers. The intensity of the irradiation and duration of exposure determines the extent of cross-linking. Another method that has been employed for cross-linking collagen is dehydrothermal treatment where the scaffold is heated at elevated temperatures for several hours promoting the formation of amide bonds between the amine and carboxylate groups present in the amino acid residues. Typical temperatures range between 105°C and 180°C while the duration could be between 24 and 120 h. About 20%–60% denaturation of collagen occurs due to this method. Also, the long duration required for cross-linking makes it tedious. Though the strength of collagen scaffold increases after cross-linking by both methods, the fragmentation of collagen chains limits their widespread use. Moreover, UV cross-linking is applicable only for thin scaffolds to enable its penetration into the matrix for cross-linking. Chemical cross-linkers have some residual toxicity and in addition, result in alterations in the collagen structure, which may in turn result in modified functions (Parenteau-Bareil et al., 2010). Glutaraldehyde, diisocyanates, carbodiimide, and genipin have been employed for cross-linking collagen.

Blends of collagen with chitosan, glycosaminoglycans, and elastin have been fabricated to bring about cross-linking through electrostatic attractive forces between oppositely charged groups. These blends display enhanced tensile strength and less toxicity owing to the incorporation of biocompatible moieties. However, the incorporation of the second component modifies the cellular response to the scaffold. Enzymatic cross-linking can be brought about using transglutaminase enzymes. This process is highly specific and results in no alterations in the collagen molecular weight and is nontoxic. But the use of enzyme makes the process expensive. One of the drawbacks of using collagen is that conventional sterilization methods modify its structure. Peracetic acid, formic acid, or ethanol treatments are currently employed to sterilize collagen-based scaffolds.

Collagen from a wide range of sources has been fabricated as scaffolds for tissue engineering applications. Exotic sources of collagen such as alligator bones and kangaroo collagen have been investigated for potential tissue engineering applications. However, collagen derived from bovine sources has been used as skin substitutes (Zyderm®) as well as scaffold material for skin regeneration studies due to their similarities with human collagen (Parenteau-Bareil et al., 2010). But, bovine-derived collagen has been found to elicit immune responses and hypersensitivity due to their animal origin. Use of bovine collagen has also been linked with the development of dermatomyositis. Employment of human collagen from cadavers as scaffold materials is limited by their poor availability as well as enhanced risk of disease transmission. Therefore, attempts to derive collagen from other sources have gained momentum.

Collagen from marine organisms represents a source that does not transmit diseases to humans and hence has generated much interest in recent years (Ramanathan et al., 2015). Table 6.2 lists some of the marine sources for collagen and their salient features.

TABLE 6.2

Marine Sources of Collagen

Marine Organism	Biological Name	Source	Salient Features
Jellyfish	*Stomolophus nomurai meleagris*	Whole body	Supported the growth and proliferation of primary fibroblasts and endothelial cells
Red sea cucumber	*Stichopus japonicus*	Body wall	Promoted adhesion and proliferation of human dermal keratinocytes
Marine catfish	*Tachysurus maculatus*	Bladder	Blended with chitosan and PDGF and investigated for dermal regeneration of full thickness wound in female rats
Fish	*Salmo salar*	Skin	Blended with elastin and cross-linked using carbodiimide; supported the proliferation of human dermal fibroblasts and rat fetal fibroblasts *in vitro* and promoted healing of full thickness wound in Wistar rat models
Fish	*Lates calcarifer*	Scales	Promoted the proliferation of human keratinocytes and mouse embryonic fibroblasts *in vitro* when blended with extract of *Macrotyloma uniflorum* plant and cross-linked with glutaraldehyde
Fish	*Oncorhynchus keta*	Skin	Incorporated with DNA and cross-linked using carbodiimide; supported the proliferation of human epidermal keratinocytes and human dermal fibroblasts *in vitro* and promoted healing of full thickness wound in Wistar rats
Fish	*Salmo salar*	Skin	Blended with chitosan and gelatin and cross-linked with genipin; supported the proliferation of fibroblasts *in vitro*
Fish	*Arothron stellatus*	Skin	Promoted the proliferation of fibroblasts and keratinocytes *in vitro*

Generation of human recombinant collagen using bacteria and plants offers a new alternative to the use of bovine collagen. Transgenic tobacco plants were created for the production of human collagen I. The transgenic plants were transformed with two genes encoding for recombinant heterotrimeric collagen type I along with genes for human prolyl-4-hydroxylase and human lysyl hydroxylase-3 enzymes, which are required for the posttranslational modification of collagen. The transgenic plants produced procollagen in the vacuoles that were transformed to collagen using plant ficin protein. The collagen was fibrillated through a series of salt treatment steps. The transgenic human collagen retained the native triple helix structure and conformation of human collagen I. The plant-derived human collagen was less viscous than its bovine counterpart due to the absence of beta and gamma structures. In addition, the plant-derived collagen had slightly higher hydrophilicity and lower mechanical strength and hence scaffolds formed from this plant-derived collagen had smaller pores and lower fiber dimensions (Willard et al., 2013). However, no difference was observed in the adhesion, proliferation, and metabolism of keratinocytes and fibroblasts grown on the plant-derived collagen scaffolds when compared with those grown on bovine collagen scaffolds. The plant-derived collagen scaffolds exhibited superior cell viability owing to better cell–cell communication and cell infiltration. The fibroblasts formed a dense layer on the surface of the scaffold formed from plant-derived collagen that is well suited for rapid epidermal differentiation of the cells. This strategy has the advantage of providing collagen that is less likely to elicit hypersensitive responses *in vivo*.

Despite possessing several advantages, collagen-based scaffolds are not very effective in promoting cell migration. Therefore, recruitment of cells for tissue repair is not adequate. Hence, other scaffold materials have also been investigated.

6.3.2.2 Chitosan

Chitosan is a polysaccharide comprising repeating units of glucosamine and N-acetyl glucosamine. The repeating units are linked through a beta-1,4-glycosidic linkage. It is a partially deacetylated form of the polysaccharide chitin found in the exoskeleton of crabs and mollusks. The free amino groups of chitosan can exist in a protonated form at acidic pH, which enables it to interact with negatively charged moieties including the cell membranes. The hydrophilic nature of chitosan makes it form hydrogels and it swells rapidly in acidic pH. Chitosan also possesses antimicrobial properties due to its affinity for the negatively charged membrane of the pathogens that result in altered permeability and death of the microbe. Further, chitosan has been shown to possess hemostatic properties and hence has been used as wound dressings. It is also been shown to be biocompatible and biodegradable, thereby making it an attractive option for scaffold fabrication and in wound dressing applications (Rodríguez-Vázquez et al., 2015). The amenability of chitosan to be fabricated into a porous scaffold with different kinds of morphology and the ease of surface modification to incorporate biorecognition motifs have resulted in its widespread use as a tissue-engineered scaffold. Chitosan fibers, sponges, gels, and films have been investigated for skin tissue engineering both individually as well as a blend with other polymeric materials. Chitosan-based scaffolds have been demonstrated to support the adhesion, growth, and proliferation of a wide range of cell types including keratinocytes, fibroblasts, and melanocytes. Its hydrogel nature favors cell infiltration. Chitosan scaffolds stimulate the expression of fibroblast growth factors (FGFs), hepatocyte growth factors (HGFs), and mesenchyme-derived growth factors that is responsible for its positive effects on skin regeneration. A photo-cross-linkable chitosan derivative N-methyl acryloyl chitosan containing fibroblasts was fabricated and patterned using lithographic techniques (Li et al., 2015). *In vitro* and *in vivo* studies demonstrated excellent integration with the native tissue and reduced inflammation. Such scaffolds also hold promise for sustained delivery of bioactive molecules and factors to accelerate skin regeneration.

6.3.2.3 Alginate

Alginate is an anionic heteropolysaccharide extracted from the brown seaweed family whose members include *Laminaria japonica*, *Laminaria hyperborea*, *Ascophyllum nodosum*, *Eclonia maxima*, *Lesonia negrescens*, *Macrocystis pyrifera*, and *Sargassum* (Chandika et al., 2015). The repeating units comprise β-D-mannuronic acid and α-L-guluronic acid linked by 1,4-glycosidic bond. Alginates form hydrogels and tend to swell in aqueous medium, especially in alkaline medium, due to the presence of carboxylate groups. The low toxicity and biocompatibility of alginate has been instrumental in its use as a scaffold for tissue engineering both independently as well as in combination with other polymers such as gelatin, chitosan, poly(vinyl alcohol) (PVA), cellulose, etc. As it forms a gel easily, its mechanical properties are not adequate to promote wound healing. Hence, it is cross-linked to improve its stability and mechanical properties. Due to its anionic nature, it is frequently cross-linked using calcium ions or cationic polymers such as chitosan.

When used in combination with gelatin, alginate is oxidized with periodate and cross-linked with gelatin in the presence of borax. Cross-linking with PVA is achieved by means of physical cross-linking using repeated freeze–thaw cycles promoting formation of ester cross-links between the two polymers. The hydrophilic nature of alginate enables maintenance of a moist microenvironment in the scaffold similar to the physiological *milieu*. Alginate scaffolds are also less prone to bacterial infection, which is favorable for wound healing (Chandika et al., 2015). The hydrogel matrix of alginate can serve to accommodate growth factors and pharmacologically active molecules for sustained release over an extended period of time. *In vitro* studies have shown that alginate scaffolds can support the adhesion, growth, and proliferation of fibroblasts and endothelial cells. Alginate matrices have been successfully demonstrated as promising scaffolds for skin regeneration in mice, rats, and rabbits with full thickness wounds. Alginate has also been isolated from several strains of bacteria like *Azotobacter vinelandii* and *Pseudomonas aeruginosa*. The bacterial alginate possess acetylated units of β-1,4-mannuronic acid and α-1,4-guluronic acid, but its potential in wound healing and skin regeneration remains unaltered. It has been accorded Food and Drug administration (FDA) approval for human use and is actively being explored for wound dressing applications.

6.3.2.4 Hyaluronic Acid

Hyaluronan or hyaluronic acid is a glycosaminoglycan that does not possess sulfate functional groups and is an important constituent of extracellular matrices. Chemically it is heteropolysaccharide comprising repeating units of (β-1,4-D-glucuronic acid and β-1,3-N-acetyl-D-glucosamine). Its tendency to form hydrogels enables it to impart compressive resistance properties to the ECM. In addition, it also facilitates diffusion of nutrients that are essential to maintain cell viability (Pardue et al., 2008). Removal of cellular waste is also enabled by hyaluronan. It is abundant in the umbilical cord, the synovial fluid in the articular cartilage, vitreous humor, and both in the epidermis as well as dermis of skin. Hyaluronan facilitates proliferation and migration of fibroblasts and also regulates the inflammatory processes and collagen deposition during wound healing. These properties of hyaluronan have been implicated for its ability to promote scar-less wound healing in fetuses. The glycan structure of hyaluronan makes it amenable for chemical modification as well as cross-linking. Chemical modification with specific recognition motifs can promote adhesion and migration of specific cells at the wound site. For instance, hyaluronan matrix covalently linked with active domains of fibronectin can enhance the spreading of fibroblasts and induce rapid formation of granulation tissue. Cross-linking of hyaluronan imparts superior resistance against enzymatic degradation as well as modulates its stiffness, which can appropriately alter the spreading and production of collagen from fibroblasts. Currently, concerted efforts to isolate hyaluronan from marine organisms are underway to overcome availability issues. Hyaluronic acid has also been isolated from bacteria like *Streptococcus equisimilis* and *Streptococcus zooepidemicus* and has received approval for use in treatment of eye and arthritic complications (Chandika et al., 2015). It had been recognized that the glycosaminoglycan component of the ECM has a major role in regulating the adhesion of cells. The degree of sulfation and the molecular weight of the individual glycosaminoglycan causes differences in the magnitude of cell interactions with the ECM. Sulfated hyaluronic acid was found to enhance the proliferation of dermal fibroblasts and is accompanied by a decrease in the production of ECM components like collagen that augers well for scar-free wound-healing applications. The anionic hyaluronic acid and cationic poly(L-lysine) were deposited in a layer-by-layer manner over a porous hyaluronic acid substrate for coculturing keratinocytes and fibroblasts (Monteiro et al., 2015). It was observed that the keratinocytes preferred to proliferate in the polyelectrolyte layer while the fibroblasts dominated the porous hyaluronic acid layer thereby leading to formation of stratified layers mimicking the epidermal and dermal layers.

6.3.2.5 *Silk Proteins*

Silk, produced by silkworms and certain types of spiders, has been extensively employed as a fabric material. Its impressive mechanical properties, biocompatibility, and amenability for chemical functionalization have resulted in the extension of its applications as a suture material. Silk primarily consists of a protein called fibroin that is coated with a small hydrophilic protein called sericin. The silk fibroin consists of a heavy chain and light chain that are linked together through disulfide bridges formed between cysteine residues. In addition, a 25 kDa protein called P25 also bridges the heavy and light chains through noncovalent interactions (Vepari and Kaplan, 2007). Traditionally, skin proteins, especially sericin, have been used in cosmetics to moisturize and soften the skin due to their hydrophilic nature and high permeability into the skin. In the context of skin tissue engineering, silk fibroin has been extensively used in the form of nanofibers, films, porous sponges, and hydrogels due to their mechanical properties. The orientation of the fibroin proteins in response to tensile and shear stresses during their formation is thought to contribute to their mechanical strength. As a result, nanofibers of silk fibroin also exhibit good mechanical strength. In natural silk fibroin, the oriented segments are crystalline and the other regions are amorphous, which contribute to the elasticity of fibroin. The major amino acid residues found in silk fibroin are glycine, alanine, and serine. The small side groups facilitate formation of beta sheet structures by the protein that are stabilized by intermolecular hydrogen bonding and van der Waals' forces. The beta sheet arrangement augments the stability of fibroin by restricting the access of solvents to the interior. This conformation also renders fibroin more hydrophobic unlike sericin. Silk fibroin is highly stable to hydrolytic degradation and is susceptible to enzymatic degradation by alpha-chymotrypsin, trypsin, and collagenases (Vepari and Kaplan, 2007).

Silk fibroin does not contain the arginyl glycyl aspartic acid RGD motif that aids cell adhesion through binding to integrin receptors on the cell surface. In addition, being a protein, fibroin is highly sensitive to the processing conditions such as pH, temperature, and chemical *milieu* leading to proteins with a wide distribution of properties that is a major drawback in the use of this material. To overcome these drawbacks, chemical functionalization of fibroin or blending with other polymeric systems has been attempted. A commonly adopted strategy is to modify the silk fibroin with RGD motifs to enhance impart biorecognition characteristics. Blending with other polymers such as polyurethane (PU), chitosan, PVA, and polycarbonate urethane or proteins like collagen, fibronectin, elastin, and laminin have also been successfully achieved to promote cell adhesion, proliferation, and infiltration (Vepari and Kaplan, 2007). Fibroblasts have been found to adhere well and proliferate when cultured on fibroin scaffolds, which was comparable to those observed with collagen matrices. They also displayed high levels of collagen deposition indicating the retention of their active functional state on these matrices. Modification of the surface with poly(ethylene oxide) chains has been found to impart hydrophilicity while reducing fibroblast adhesion. Endothelial cells have also been found to proliferate well on silk fibroin nanofibrous scaffolds and form tubes and microvessels suggesting that this scaffold can support neovascularization. *In vivo* studies employing a full thickness wound model in rats were found to heal rapidly within a week when treated with silk fibroin films. The inflammation in the wounded area was also significantly lower when compared with the animals treated with conventional wound dressings. Similarly, sponges composed of a blend of fibroin, chitosan, and PVA were found to effectively regenerate epidermal and dermal layers in a rat model. To overcome its limitation of poor adsorption of growth factors, silk fibroin has been blended with human keratin for dermal regeneration (Bhardwaj et al., 2015). Keratin is a protein found in human hair that possesses the adhesion motifs RGD and LDV (leucine–aspartate–valine) thereby making it a promising substrate for tissue engineering applications. The blend scaffold was found to promote the adhesion, extension, proliferation, and functional expression of fibroblasts.

Silk fibroin is commonly extracted from worms belonging to the order *Lepidoptera* that include butterflies and moths as well as from several species of spiders belonging to the class *Arachnida*. It has now been recognized that there are distinct differences in the silk proteins produced by each species. For example, the silk fibroin extracted from the domesticated silkworm *Bombyx mori* lacks RGD motifs. In contrast, fibroin produced by wild-type silkworms like *Antheraea pernyi* possesses the RGD motif, thereby making them superior substrates for cell adhesion and proliferation (Vepari and Kaplan, 2007). Apart from silkworms, spider silk has also been employed for tissue engineering application. The most extensively investigated spider silk known as "dragline silk" is produced by *Nephilia clavipes*. The spider silk does not contain sericin but is composed of major ampullate spidroins proteins I and II (MaSp-I and MaSp-II) with superior mechanical properties compared to silkworm silk. These proteins are rich in glycine, alanine, glutamate, proline, and arginine residues.

The second major protein from silk worm namely sericin has also been explored for tissue engineering applications due to its biocompatibility and inherent antioxidant, antimicrobial, and antiapoptotic properties (Nayak et al., 2013). Sericin is a highly hydrophilic protein with high amounts of polar amino acid residues such as serine. As it exhibits a tendency to form hydrogels, the mechanical properties of sericin have been improved by cross-linking. Sericin cross-linked with glutaraldehyde had been demonstrated to support the adhesion and proliferation of fibroblasts. Similarly, sericin cross-linked with genipin had been successfully employed to coculture keratinocytes and fibroblasts that displayed increased levels of transforming growth factor (TGF)-beta and FGFs (Nayak et al., 2013). In addition, significant paracrine signaling existed between the keratinocytes and fibroblasts as evidenced from the expression of typical markers such as involucrin, collagen IV, and fibroblast surface proteins. The inflammatory response to these scaffolds was minimal suggesting the potential of these scaffolds for skin regeneration.

6.3.3 Novel Materials of Natural Origin

6.3.3.1 Carrageenan

Carrageenans are marine polysaccharides comprising repeating units of D-galactose that are linked through alternate β-1,4 and α-1,3 glycosidic links (Chandika et al., 2015). They are categorized as kappa, iota, and lambda types based on their degree of sulfation. Kappa carrageenan possesses low viscosity and has a single sulfate group per monomer. It forms brittle gels with monovalent cations like potassium. Iota carrageenan has two sulfate groups per monomer, is a viscous solution, and forms elastic viscous gels with divalent cations like calcium. Lambda carrageenan is a highly sulfated form containing three sulfate groups per monomer. It does not form gels and is highly viscous. Carrageenans are generally isolated from red seaweeds or carrageenophytes like the Irish moss (*Chondrus crispus*), the red algae *Kappaphycus alvarezii* (*cottonii*), *Eucheuma denticulatum* also known as *Euchema spinosum*, *Betaphycus gelatinum*, *Gigartinas kottsbergii*, *Gigartina canaliculata*, *Mastocarpus stellatus*, *Hypnea musciformis*, *Sarcothalia crispate*, and *Mazzaella laminaroides*. Carrageenans possess an inherent antimicrobial and antioxidant activity that can be invaluable for wound-healing applications (Silva and Reis, 2014). Moreover, they also have a tendency to form gels and absorb moisture enabling nutrient and growth factor exchange at the wound site.

6.3.3.2 Ulvan

Ulvan is a sulfated heteropolysaccharide isolated from the green algae (chlorophyta). The repeating units of the linear chains of ulvan comprise glucuronorhamnose-3-sulfate and iduronorhamnose-3-sulfate that closely resemble the glycosaminoglycans present in the ECM. Ulvan possesses intrinsic antioxidant property that can be regulated by altering the degree of sulfation. The similarity in structure of ulvan and other sulfated polysaccharides with heparin imparts anticoagulant property to these molecules. Ulvan can block intrinsic coagulation pathway and formation of fibrin from fibrinogen. Research has also revealed that ulvan possesses anti-hyperlipidemic activity due to its ability to complex bile acids thereby enhancing bile secretion. Immunomodulatory effects have also been identified for ulvan (Chandika et al., 2015). Different morphologies have been fabricated using ulvan. These include nanofibers, particles, hydrogels, and porous three-dimensional (3D) scaffolds. These structures have been explored for drug delivery, bone regeneration, and wound-healing applications. One of the limitations of ulvan is its tendency to form aggregates in aqueous solvents and its insolubility in organic solvents that makes functional modifications challenging.

6.3.3.3 Fucoidan

Fucoidan is a sulfated polysaccharide extracted from brown algae. The composition and structure of fucoidan varies depending on the species from which it is isolated. It consists of fucopyranose units along with mannose, galactose, glucose, xylose, or uronic acids linked via 1,3 and/or 1,4 glycosidic links (Silva and Reis, 2014). The molecular weight of fucoidan also has a wide range depending on the source as well as seasonal variations. It forms viscous solutions and possesses inherent antioxidant, anticoagulant, and anticancer properties that have resulted in its widespread use in the cosmetic industry. The discovery of its ability to activate HGF has spurred research in exploring its potential in healthcare and skin regeneration applications. Due to its inability to form gels, fucoidan has been often blended with other hydrophilic gel forming polymers such as chitosan, alginate, and gelatin. A chitosan–fucoidan hydrogel scaffold has been demonstrated to heal burn injuries indicating its potential in skin regeneration applications (Chandika et al., 2015). Similarly, fucoidan blended with chitosan–alginate hydrogel system has been found to accelerate wound healing in rat models. Yet another linear polysaccharide isolated from brown algae, laminaran, has also been shown to enhance the deposition of collagen and shows promise for dermal reconstruction (Silva and Reis, 2014).

6.3.3.4 Mauran

Mauran is an anionic polysaccharide that is isolated from a halophilic bacteria *Halomonas maura*. The repeating unit of this polysaccharide is highly sulfated and phosphorylated and comprises mannose, glucose, galactose, and glucuronic acid. They exhibit excellent thixotropic properties where the mauran gels undergo shear thinning when subjected to shear forces and regain the original viscosity once the shear stresses are removed. The viscosity of mauran gels remains unaffected by pH, temperature shocks, surfactant, and salt concentrations. Mauran gels display metal adsorbing capabilities that have resulted in their application for remediation applications. Recently, a blend of mauran with PVA cross-linked with glutaraldehyde was electrospun to form defect-free uniform nanofibrous scaffold (Raveendran et al., 2013). This blend scaffold demonstrated excellent adhesion and proliferation of fibroblasts as well as mesenchymal stem cells (MSCs) for over 1 week. The extended morphology of the cells on the blend scaffold was attributed to the presence of a charged surface due to the mauran component that facilitated protein adsorption on the scaffold surface, which augmented cell adhesion and extension. This novel material holds promise for skin tissue engineering applications and needs to be investigated further, especially for its effect on the immune response.

6.3.3.5 Dextran

Dextran is a polymer of glucose that is an exopolysaccharide extracted from bacteria like *Leuconostoc mesenteroides*. It is present in wine and comprises repeating units of glucose linked through α-1,4 and α-1,6 glycosidic links. It represents the first microbial product that has been used for pharmaceutical applications. Conventionally, dextran has been employed for plasma volume expanding applications to control wound shocks. Owing to its hydrophilicity, dextran forms hydrogels that augers well for wound-healing applications.

6.3.3.6 Polyunsaturated Fatty Acids for Skin Regeneration

Lipoic mediators such as alpha lipoic acid regulate many critical stages during the process of wound healing such as chemotaxis, cell adhesion, inflammation, and vascular contraction. These mediators are synthesized from polyunsaturated fatty acids (PUFA) that have a double bond in the third (omega-3 fatty acids) or sixth (omega-6 fatty acids) carbon. These PUFA stimulate epithelial cells and promote rapid wound healing. It has been demonstrated that PUFA enhances the expression of proinflammatory cytokines at the site of skin injury thereby stimulating the healing process. PUFA extracted from various marine sources such as the sea cucumber (*Stichopus chloronotus*), mollusk (*Mytilus galloprovincialis*), and the sea snail (*Tapana venosa*) have been found to aid rapid wound healing (Chandika et al., 2015). PUFA-doped PU hydrogel films have aided accelerated wound healing in full thickness wounds induced in animal models.

6.3.4 Synthetic Scaffold Materials

Although natural materials have been found to possess promising properties for skin repair and regeneration, they are limited by poor availability as well as immunogenicity. In addition, modification of properties to suit diverse applications also is difficult. Hence, synthetic materials mainly comprising polymers and their blends have been extensively investigated for skin tissue engineering applications. Biodegradable polyesters such as poly(L-lactide) (PLLA), poly(lactide-*co*-glycolide) (PLGA), poly(caprolactone) (PCL), and poly(glycolic acid) have been extensively investigated both individually as well as blends for skin regeneration (Metcalfe and Ferguson, 2007b). Poly(3-hydroxy butyrate-*co*-3-hydroxy valerate) is another polyester than has shown much promise as a scaffold material to support the proliferation of keratinocytes and fibroblasts (Kuppan et al., 2011).

The inherent oxygen permeability of this material further aids cell growth and proliferation. The topography of the scaffolds also has an important influence on the successful regeneration of tissues. The nanofibrous morphology mimics the collagen network present in the ECM and hence has been extensively employed. Electrospinning techniques have been used to fabricate nanofibrous scaffolds with either random or aligned morphology to promote the adhesion and expansion of fibroblasts and keratinocytes. Porosity of the scaffolds has also been optimized to ensure adequate permeation of gases and nutrients without compromising the mechanical properties. Other polymers such as PVA. PU, poly acrylates (PAA), and poly(glycerol sebacate) (PGS) have also been investigated for skin tissue engineering. The field still remains wide open, as there are numerous options among synthetic polymers with different mechanical properties and degradation rates. One of the challenges in using synthetic polymeric scaffolds for tissue engineering is the dimensional distortion and shrinkage that occurs when they come in contact with fluids. This phenomenon restricts the adhesion and infiltration of cells. To overcome this limitation, a propylene ring was used to stretch and stabilize nanofibrous mat of PLGA that was found to stimulate proliferation of human skin keratinocytes *in vitro* (Ru et al., 2015). Hybrid scaffolds comprising a natural and synthetic polymer have also been investigated for skin tissue engineering. The synthetic polyester PLLA has been blended with the natural polymer collagen or gelatin to form porous scaffolds that favored the adhesion and proliferation of fibroblasts *in vitro* and promoted rapid healing of full thickness wounds in athymic mice (Lu et al., 2012). The PLLA component provided the mechanical strength to the scaffold while the natural polymer conferred biorecognition and cell adhesion properties. Similarly, a microporous scaffold of PCL–collagen preseeded with fibroblasts for 4 days was found to regenerate the dermal layers with hair follicles in a full thickness wound model in mice (Bonvallet et al., 2014).

In addition to the choice of materials, a large body of the literature exists to incorporate geometrical cues to the cells through patterning of substrates to mimic the topography of the native ECM. The parameters such as mechanical strength, feature sizes, porosity, pore dimensions and cell type, density, and age are factors that influence the adhesion, spreading, proliferation, and functions of the cells on a particular type of scaffold (Oliveira et al., 2015). As geometrical cues alone are insufficient for long-term maintenance of the functional cells, adhesion chemical modifications and stimuli are introduced in the system in an attempt to obtain a functional bioengineered skin.

6.3.5 Chemical Stimuli

Wound healing and skin regeneration involves a complex orchestrated sequence of events that are mediated by cells and growth factors (Yamaguchi et al., 2005). Figure 6.3 summarizes the key events that occur during wound healing and skin repair.

Three major stages are involved in the wound repair process. During the inflammatory phase, the wound area is covered with a blood clot along with increased numbers of activated neutrophils, monocytes, and other leukocytes. This stage is followed by the proliferation phase during which endothelial cells, fibroblasts, and stem cells are recruited to the wound site. Collagen and alpha-actin deposition is stimulated by the proliferating fibroblasts along with development of vascularization. More keratinocytes are pushed in to the wound site in response to the cytokines and growth factors leading to re-epithelialization, revascularization, and formation of a granulation tissue. The final stage is the maturation phase where the epithelial layer and dermal layers undergo remodeling to regain the original elastic nature. However, this phase may last several years (Schreml et al., 2010). The

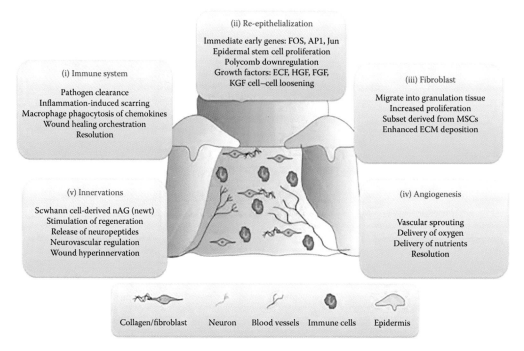

FIGURE 6.3
Various stages that occur during wound healing and skin repair.

various repair and regenerative processes are initiated in response to activation of several genes and production of signaling molecules and growth factors. Investigations using *in vitro* and *in vivo* models have revealed the upregulation of several hundreds of genes that include activator protein (*Ap*)1, *Fos*, *Jun*, and zinc finger transcription factors that stimulate the migration and proliferation of keratinocytes, endothelial cells, and fibroblasts. The migration of cells to the site of repair and regeneration requires extensive modifications of the cell–matrix and cell–cell adhesions and interactions. This involves several matrix remodeling enzymes like the MMPs. A cocktail of growth factors mediate the proliferation and recruitment of specific cell types to the regenerating site (Oliveira et al., 2015).

6.3.5.1 Growth Factors

Growth factors are polypeptides that bind to specific receptors on the cell surface and trigger signaling cascades leading to the proliferation of the specific cell type (Briquez et al., 2015) as depicted in Figure 6.4.

Growth factors also mediate the differentiation, migration, and functions of cells. Table 6.3 summarizes the major growth factors that are involved in skin repair and regeneration (Santoro and Gaudino, 2005).

Exogenous application of the growth factors has been combined with the use of scaffolds to promote regeneration of the skin layers. However, this strategy has been limited by several drawbacks. The highly inflammatory environment in a wound bed characterized by high levels of protease activity limits the influence of growth factors on the healing and regenerative process. Moreover, the large amounts of wound exudates also increase the probability of diffusion and leaching of the growth factors away from the wound site. In

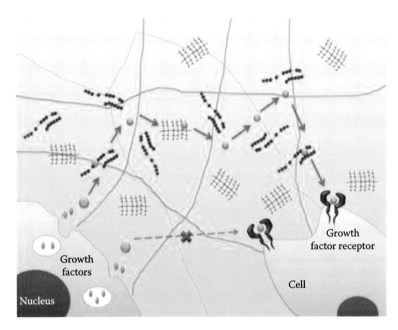

FIGURE 6.4
Stimulation of signaling pathways by growth factors.

addition, the large size of the growth factors limits their permeation into the tissue thereby limiting their availability and efficacy. This necessitates frequent administration of the growth factors, which in turn increases the risk of cancer as well as induces undesirable side effects at the site of administration (Briquez et al., 2015). Hence, there exists the need for a delivery system that will shield the growth factors from the degrading environment, ensure their sustained release and retention at the wound site. Figure 6.5 represents the lytic environment encountered at the site of injury.

6.3.5.2 Drug Delivery Systems for Growth Factor Delivery

A diverse range of delivery systems has been investigated for growth factor delivery in skin tissue engineering (Gainza et al., 2015). The most extensively employed delivery system is based on PLGA, an FDA approved biodegradable polyester. The hydrophobic nature of PLGA restricts its ability to absorb water and therefore ensures enhanced retention of the growth factor at the wound site. Further, PLGA degrades to form lactic acid and ethylene glycol. Lactic acid has been recognized to be proangiogenic. It helps to recruit endothelial progenitor cells (EPCs) to the wound bed and also aids in activation of procollagen factors. Topical application of PLGA spheres of both micron and nanodimensions loaded with recombinant human epidermal growth factor (EGF) was found to enhance fibroblast proliferation when compared with the free growth factor and was characterized with increased levels of proliferation cell nuclear antigen, a proliferation marker, when tested *in vivo*. Localized administration of EGF delivered through PLGA-alginate microspheres was found to be superior to conventional administration of free EGF in bringing about rapid re-epithelialization. Alginate forms hydrogels thereby making encapsulation of growth factors possible under ambient conditions. Moreover, its anionic polysaccharide structure is similar to the glycosaminoglycan content found in the ECM. Hence, several groups have

TABLE 6.3

Growth Factors Involved in Skin Regeneration

Growth Factor	Source	Receptor(s)	Salient Characteristics
EGF	Platelets, macrophages, fibroblasts	EGF receptor	• Stimulates keratinocyte proliferation and migration • Triggers the production of fibronectin and expression of keratin • Enhances fibroblast recruitment
bFGF	Fibroblasts, macrophages, endothelial cells	FGF receptor (interacts with heparin sulfate proteoglycans and heparin)	• Stimulates expression of proinflammatory genes, cytokines, their respective receptors, endothelial cell adhesion molecules, and the prostaglandin pathway • Promotes re-epithelialization, matrix remodeling, and formation of granulation tissue • Pro-angiogenic factor • Stimulates proliferation of fibroblasts and endothelial cells
KGF	Keratinocytes	KGF receptor, FGF receptor	• Promotes migration and proliferation of epithelial cells and keratinocytes
VEGF	Endothelial cells, keratinocytes, platelets, neutrophils, macrophages, smooth muscle cells	VEGF receptors 1 & 2	• Mediates endothelial cell migration and proliferation • Pro-angiogenic factor • Promotes lymphangiogenesis • Involved in formation of granulation tissue
PDGF	Platelets, macrophages, fibroblasts, keratinocytes, endothelium	Alpha and beta PDGF receptors	• Promotes fibroblast proliferation and deposition of ECM proteins • Functions as a chemotactic agent for migration of neutrophils, macrophages, and fibroblasts • Induces secretion of growth factors and TGF-beta by macrophages
IGF	Fibroblasts, hepatocytes, macrophages, neutrophils, skeletal muscle cells	IGF receptors type I and II	• Induces fibroblast proliferation • Promotes re-epithelialization
TGF-beta (TGF-beta)	Fibroblasts, macrophages, platelets, keratinocytes	Heteromeric receptor complexes type I, II, and III	• Promotes granulation tissue formation • Induces proliferation of fibroblasts • Involved in the recruitment of macrophages • Stimulates the expression of integrins and matrix proteins
HGF	Mesenchymal cells	HGF receptor	• Regulates cell growth, motility, and morphogeneis of epithelial and endothelial cells
Macrophage stimulating protein	Hepatocytes	Ron tyrosine kinase receptor	• Activates signaling cascades involved in cell growth, migration, survival, and differentiation • Promotes re-epithelialization

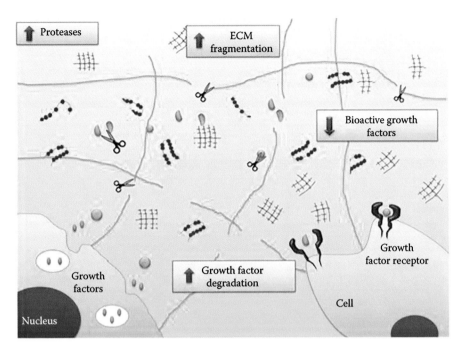

FIGURE 6.5
Degradation of growth factors at the site of injury.

also explored its use for delivering growth factors (Gainza et al., 2015). Alginate microspheres loaded with vascular endothelial growth factor (VEGF) were found to enhance angiogenesis both *in vitro* as well as *in vivo*.

Self-assembled vesicular delivery systems such as liposomes have also been used for growth factor delivery. The ease of formation, biocompatibility, amenability to surface functionalization, and ability to entrap both hydrophilic and hydrophobic entities has made liposomal carriers an attractive choice for growth factor delivery. Insulin-like growth factor (IGF)-1 encapsulated liposomes and EGF-loaded liposomes have been found to enhance the re-epithelialization and formation of strong collagen networks that improved the tensile strength of the newly formed tissue, respectively. However, these systems are severely limited by their poor stability and shelf life. To overcome these limitations of liposomes, other lipid-based carriers such as solid lipid nanoparticles (SLN) and nanostructured lipid carriers (NLC) have been attempted for growth factor delivery (Gainza et al., 2015). These lipid carriers exhibit longer retention time at the wound site and improve the hydration of the skin apart from ensuring sustained release of the growth factors. They also have better shelf life and stability. SLN and NLC encapsulated with recombinant human EGF have been found to accelerate wound healing, improve re-epithelialization, and wound maturity when evaluated using mice models.

Hydrogels are another class of materials that have been extensively explored for skin regeneration applications due to their ability to promote skin hydration and also ensure sustained release of functional growth factors when employed as delivery systems (Gainza et al., 2015). Chitosan hydrogels have been loaded with EGF and have yielded promising results in a burn injury wound model in mice wherein the EGF-encapsulated chitosan resulted in thicker epidermis and faster healing. Similarly, chitosan–collagen system encapsulating platelet-derived growth factor (PDGF) was found to enhance fibroblast proliferation and collagen deposition. A cross-linked chitosan system encapsulating basic FGF (bFGF) was found to effectively contribute to the formation of new blood vessels and accelerated wound closure in diabetic mice (Yang et al., 2012). Fibrin is another naturally occurring hydrogel that can serve as a matrix for skin regeneration as well as contribute to hemostatic effects. bFGF-loaded fibrin gels have been demonstrated to produce neoangiogenesis and faster rates of wound repair in mice. Other hydrogels investigated for growth factor delivery include hyaluronic acid, chondroitin sulfate, heparin, and self-assembling peptides that have been used to deliver EGF, IGF, vitronectin, and bFGF in various wound models and have shown improved performance. Synthetic hydrogels such as the family of poly(ethylene oxide)-*co*-poly(propylene oxide)-*co*-poly(ethylene oxide) surfactants commonly referred to as pluronics and carboxymethyl cellulose have also been investigated for growth factor delivery. The carboxymethyl cellulose-based system for delivery of PDGF was introduced commercially as a topical formulation with the trade name Regranex®, which is, however, not extensively used due to its increased risk of carcinogenesis.

Nanofibrous scaffolds made from biodegradable and biocompatible polymers have been extensively used for skin tissue engineering due to their similarity with the collagen-network topography found in ECM. A blend of gelatin and chondroitin sulfate was fabricated as a nanofibrous scaffold and was found to support the adhesion and proliferation of human dermal fibroblasts (Pezeshki-Modaress et al., 2015). Such nanofibrous scaffolds have also been used to deliver growth factors to provide the appropriate chemical cues to restore the skin layers. Two types of strategies can be adopted for immobilization of the growth factors—entrapment or surface modification of the nanofibers with the growth factor. While in the former case, there is a gradual release of the growth factor with time due to the degradation of the fibers, in the latter case, the growth factors are constantly presented to the environment due to their surface localization. Both strategies have been reported to yield promising results. However, a majority of the work focuses on encapsulated growth factors as their gradual release will present different concentrations of the growth factors in a temporal manner. Silk fibroin nanofibers loaded with EGF have been found to display superior wound healing, re-epithelialization, and collagen deposition in animal models when compared to their blank counterparts. A core–sheath system comprising the biodegradable poly(ethylene glycol)-*co*-poly(lactide) and basic FGF exhibited sustained release of the bFGF over a month and resulted in rapid wound closure, re-epithelialization and regeneration of the dermal layers, collagen network in the ECM, and skin appendages that closely resembled the normal tissue. In an interesting attempt to mimic the different concentration profiles of growth factors available at the wound site, a blend of PCL and poly(ethylene glycol) was fabricated in to coaxial nanofibers for delivery of EGF and bFGF. The EGF was immobilized on the surface while bFGF was encapsulated in the core. This ensured that the EGF was constantly presented to the wound *milieu*, while the bFGF was delivered in a sustained manner after a burst release of 30%. This strategy resulted in improved proliferation of epidermal cells and enhanced keratin and collagen deposition in diabetic mice model when compared to delivery of single growth factors. Another core–shell nanofibrous system made of gelatin–poly(lactide-*co*-caprolactone) blend encapsulating EGF and poly(3-hexylthiophene) was used to promote the differentiation of adipose-derived stem cells (ASCs) in to keratinocytes and enhance wound healing in a stimuli-responsive manner. The incorporation of poly(3-hexylthiophene), which is a conducting polymer, produces a photocurrent in response to optical stimulation that aids the skin regeneration process. Poly(3-hydroxy butyrate-3-valerate) nanofibers coated with R-spondin, a type of thrombospondin that activates the Wnt signaling pathway and promotes angiogenesis was found to enhance rapid wound closure, re-epithelialization along with development of new blood vessel networks in mice with full thickness wounds (Kuppan et al., 2011).

Scaffold-based delivery has been extensively attempted with other morphologies also (Wang et al., 2015). Chitosan films loaded with bFGF have shown improved granulation tissue formation and maintained the functionality of the encapsulated growth factor. Collagen sponges loaded with growth factors such as EGF have been most beneficial in regeneration of epidermal and dermal layers with organized collagen fibers. Chitosan–collagen sponges with FGF have also proved beneficial for accelerated wound healing. Hyaluronan sponges and hyaluronan–collagen sponges loaded with EGF have been shown to promote wound healing by stimulating cytokine production. A comparison of the effect of EGF delivery and bFGF delivery using the same delivery system revealed that while EGF was more beneficial in promoting epidermal cell proliferation, bFGF was superior in stimulating fibroblast proliferation and generation of VEGF and HGF. This clearly indicates that multiple growth factors are more beneficial than single growth factor. An emerging paradigm in the development of bioengineered skin is to embed delivery systems into scaffolds to deliver different growth factors at different rates so that a closer mimic of the native tissue is achieved. Chitosan microspheres loaded with EGF and VEGF were incorporated in a dextran matrix and were found to enhance re-epithelialization and neoangiogenesis in mice models when compared with other treatment modalities. Chitosan–poly(ethylene glycol) nanofibers containing VEGF- and PDGF-loaded PLGA nanoparticles were found to provide an antimicrobial environment due to the chitosan, while the growth factors enhanced angiogenesis and re-epithelialization and remodeling of the ECM (Xie et al., 2013). In another interesting work on multiple growth factor delivery, VEGF and PDGF were encapsulated in gelatin nanoparticles that were embedded in to collagen–hyaluronic acid nanofibers containing EGF and bFGF. This system resulted in an accelerated regeneration of the skin layers due to a phased release of different growth factors. Gelatin microspheres entrapping EGF were embedded in a gelatin sponge over which another layer of a mucoadhesive poly(urethane) was found to effectively contribute to rapid wound closure in rabbit models. These examples indicate that the sustained delivery of growth factors individually or in combination at the wound site augers well for regeneration of the skin layers.

Extracts from natural sources have also been found to display wound healing and regenerative properties. For instance, exogenous application of an ointment containing the powdered shell from the mollusk *Cypraea moneta* was reported to aid skin repair due to its antibacterial property. Similarly, amino acids isolated from two mollusk species namely, *Rapana venosa* and *Myttlys galloprovinsialis* exhibited anti-inflammatory properties, rapid wound coverage, enhanced angiogenesis, collagen deposition, and recruitment of stem cells at the site of burn injury in rats. The seaweed *Eucheuma cottonii* extract had also shown promise for skin repair by promoting re-epithelialization and hair growth in rat models (Chandika et al., 2015). However, integration of these extracts in scaffolds is yet to be realized. Moreover, the natural origin and multi-ingredient nature of these extracts makes it difficult to achieve reproducibility and also possess availability issues. Recently, a human acellular dermis was modified with the thrombin-derived peptides GKY20 and GKY25 (Kasetty et al., 2015). These peptides conferred antimicrobial and endotoxin resistance properties to the graft that may be useful in skin repair and regeneration strategies.

6.3.6 Role of *mi*-RNA in Skin Regeneration

Micro-RNA or *mi*-RNA are short oligonucleotide sequences about 19–22 base pairs long that are noncoding. They are involved in regulating gene expression through formation of a complex with mRNA causing their degradation or deadenylation thereby hastening their degradation. The complexation with *mi*-RNA prevents the translation of the mRNA in to a functional protein. The function of *mi*-RNA is similar to that of small interference RNA (*si*-RNA), the difference being the location of these noncoding segments in RNA. Since the first report of their discovery in 1993, concerted efforts have been made to identify many more *mi*-RNA from plant and mammalian systems. Recently, a strong correlation between skin morphogenesis and development and *mi*-RNA expression levels has been identified. *mi*-RNA levels regulate critical processes like maturation, migration, remodeling ECM, onset of senescence, and epithelial–mesenchymal transition. Currently, attempts to utilize *mi*-RNA as mediators to regulate cell behavior in tissue engineering strategies have gained momentum. Numerous *mi*-RNA have been found to be involved in regulation of the functions of fibroblasts, keratinocytes, melanocytes, follicular cells, and endothelial cells constituting the different skin layers and appendages (Miller et al., 2015).

Pro-proliferative *mi*-RNA regulate the proliferation of cells by transforming quiescent cells to the proliferation stage by inducing their entry into the cell cycle. Some of the *semi*-RNA inhibits interferon activity and several others modulate the anti-proliferative p53 levels. Many of these pro-proliferative *mi*-RNA act on the PI3 K/Akt pathway. While quiescent cells are mitotically inactive cells, another category of cells known as senescent cells are those that are trapped in the G1 phase of the cell cycle and hence are not proliferative. Controlling cellular senescence is a major challenge in skin tissue engineering. High throughput screening has revealed the role of many pro-senescence *mi*-RNA and the search for anti-senescence *mi*-RNA is actively underway. The epithelial–mesenchymal transition has been implicated as one of the causative factors for organ fibrosis and onset of cell senescence. In context to skin regeneration, epithelial–mesenchymal transition appears to favor migration and proliferation of keratinocytes and fibroblasts, and enhances fibroblast responses to TGF-beta. The epithelial–mesenchymal transition is regulated by two proteins, the zinc finger enhancing binding (ZEB) protein and the zinc finger protein SNAIL, that have opposing actions. While ZEB favors epithelial phenotypes, SNAIL expression promotes the mesenchymal phenotypes. Recently, two *mi*-RNA, namely, miR-34 and miR-200, have been discovered, which exhibit similar type of regulatory function on the epithelial–mesenchymal transition (Miller et al., 2015). While miR-200 favors mesenchymal phenotype, miR-34 promotes epithelial phenotypes. Thus, the preferred form of fibroblasts can be promoted during skin regeneration by introducing the appropriate *mi*-RNA.

Another important feature of wound healing is the transdifferentiation of fibroblasts into a more contractile phenotype known as myofibroblasts. This transdifferentiation is mediated by the TGF-beta/SMAD pathway that suppresses the transdifferentiation when activated, and the CD44 epidermal growth factor receptor (EGFR) pathway, that promotes transdifferentiation when activated. The stiffness of the matrix needs to be constantly modified to regulate the signaling cascades responsible for the cell functions. This dynamic process is referred to as ECM remodeling. In addition, the process of mechanotransduction wherein mechanical forces are transformed into biochemical signals, are also controlled by the matrix stiffness. *mi*-RNA enhances substrate stiffness function by increasing collagen deposition while those that decrease matrix stiffness enhances the levels of MMPs, which degrade matrix proteins. Development of adequate vasculature is critical to maintain viable and functional skin layers. Several proangiogenic *mi*-RNA have been identified in the dermal layers. Activation of Ras pathway, inhibition of vascular cell adhesion molecule (VCAM) that promotes leukocyte adhesion to endothelial cells, upregulation of GATA2, suppression of the anti-angiogenic factors Spred-1 and PIK3R2 (regulatory subunit 2 of phosphoinositol-3-kinase), and potentiating the proangiogenic growth factors VEGF, IGF, and FGF are the routes through which proangiogenic *mi*-RNA promote neovascularization of skin (Miller et al., 2015).

Incorporation of melanin-producing melanocytes in scaffolds for skin tissue engineering has been in focus lately as melanin provides protection against UV damage and also imparts a native complexion to skin. *mi*-RNA that specifically modulate the activity of microphthalmia-associated transcription factor, the key regulator in melanocytes has been found to enhance melanocyte proliferation. Several *mi*-RNA have also exhibited the potential to prevent melanocytes from undergoing apoptosis by suppressing proapoptotic genes. Another skin appendage that is required in an ideal tissue-engineered skin is the hair follicles, which contain multipotent stem cells at its base referred to as the "bulge." It is also said to maintain skin homeostasis. Several *mi*-RNA have been found to modulate the proliferative (anagen), apoptotic (catagen), shedding (exogen), and resting (telogen) phases of the hair follicles though their integration into scaffolds designed for tissue engineering is yet to be successfully accomplished. The sebaceous glands comprising sebocytes are also regulated through *mi*-RNA that promote sebogenesis. The presence of sebaceous glands in skin is essential to maintain its texture, prevent microbial entry, and eliminate waste through sweat. *mi*-RNA that modulate the functions of biochemical mediators, mainly growth factors, are also of specific interest for skin tissue engineering applications. Table 6.4 lists some of the major *mi*-RNA that regulate the different cells found in skin (Miller et al., 2015).

The levels of *mi*-RNA can be regulated during skin tissue engineering by delivering *mi*-RNA exogenously to enhance its levels while reducing *mi*-RNA levels using antagomiR, an antagonistic oligonucleotide sequence. However, delivery of *mi*-RNA or antagomiR poses several challenges that include site-specific delivery, stability against enzymatic degradation, cell internalization, and controlled release over an extended period of time. Nanocarriers have been able to circumvent most of these problems and a wide range of carriers such as cationic liposomes, dendrimers, poly(L-lysine), poly(ethylene imine), and Gemini surfactants with cationic functional groups has been explored. Viral vector-mediated delivery has been used for delivery of oligonucleotide sequence. Scaffold-based delivery of oligonucleotide sequences has also been attempted. Poly(urethane) scaffolds have been used to deliver small interfering RNA for gene silencing. Similarly, an anti-TGF-beta *si*-RNA was delivered using a chitosan–collagen scaffold that was effective in silencing the expression of TGF-beta for 2 weeks. A *mi*-RNA, miR-29b, involved in the remodeling of the ECM was incorporated in collagen scaffolds and was found to be effective in reducing the levels of collagen I and III for 2 weeks in a fibroblast culture. These scaffolds were also found to be effective in reducing collagen I levels for 2 weeks *in vivo* in a full thickness wound model induced in rats. Hydrogel scaffolds such as alginate, chitosan, agarose, poly(ethylene glycol), gelatin, and cross-linked collagen have been widely explored for oligonucleotide delivery in tissue engineering applications. Though this area is still in its infancy, the potential of *mi*-RNA in regulating the regeneration process can be harnessed through intelligent combination of materials and geometry for development of an ideal bioengineered skin in the near future.

6.3.7 Mechanical Stimulation

The cells and ECM are both responsive to different types of mechanical stress. The "tensional integrity" or "tensegrity" model of the cell describes the regulation of structural organization through mechanical forces at the cellular and tissue level, which is especially applicable to the skin that is organized into epidermal, dermal, and hypodermal layers. Mechanical

TABLE 6.4

mi-RNA Involved in Skin Regeneration

Target	*mi*-RNA	Salient Effects
Keratinocytes	miR-205	Activates Akt signaling pathway and retards apoptosis by acting on SHIP2; essential for keratinocyte migration
	miR-483-3p	Growth inhibitor, especially during re-epithelialization; down-regulates expression of cell cycle proteins MK2, MK167, Yap1, CDC25A phosphatase
	miR-198	Decreases migration by repressing genes involved in migration such as PLAU, DIAPH1, and LAMC2
	miR-21	Promotes keratinocyte migration; acts on TIMP3 and TIAM1 genes
	miR-31	TGF-beta2 regulates levels; targets endotoxin neutralizing protein (ENP)-1 and enhances keratinocyte migration and proliferation
Fibroblasts	miR-125	Decreases cell proliferation
	miR29	Increases cell cycle entry thereby promoting proliferation
	miR-21	Inhibits phosphatase and tensin homolog (PTEN) and inhibits apoptosis while promoting proliferation; found in high levels during scar formation
	miR-22	Enhances proliferation; regulates interferon expression; increases the expression levels of cell cycle specific genes
	miR-152	Induces senescence; modulates cell adhesion and ECM remodeling
	miR-141	Induces senescence
	miR-143	Induces senescence
	miR-519a	Inhibits HuR; induces senescence
	miR-34	Increases epithelial–mesenchymal transition; suppresses SNAIL activity indirectly
	miR-200	Decreases epithelial–mesenchymal transition; suppresses ZEB activity indirectly
	miR-146a	Levels induced by TGF-beta; suppresses SMAD4 and alphaSMA levels thereby decreasing transdifferentiation
	miR-7	Found in high levels in aged cells; decreases CD44 membrane motility; decreases transdifferentiation
	miR-29	Decreases collagen expression thereby decreasing collagen deposition
	miR-150	Decreases ECM deposition; activates TGF-beta signaling
	miR-19a	Decreases collagen expression by suppressing TGF-beta-activated kinase1 binding protein, a negative inhibitor of TIMP-1
	miR-92a	Enhances collagen deposition by decreasing MMP-1 levels
Endothelial cells	miR-132	Pro-angiogenic factor; increases endothelial cell proliferation and migration
	miR-126	Negatively regulates VCAM thereby decreasing vascular inflammation; enhances VEFF and FGF activities
	miR-210	Decreases wound closure and skin proliferation by decreasing E2F3 levels; induced by HIF-1α
	miR-200b	Anti-angiogenic factor; decreases GATA2 and VEGFR2 levels
Melanocytes	miR-17	Decreases apoptosis by targeting the pro-apoptotic gene Bim

(*Continued*)

TABLE 6.4 (*Continued*)

mi-RNA Involved in Skin Regeneration

Target	*mi*-RNA	Salient Effects
	miR-25	Decreases micropthalmia-associated transcription factor, an important melanocyte transcriptional regulator
	miR-203	Decreases micropthalmia-associated transcription factor by suppressing p-cAMP response element-binding protein-1 (CREB-1), increases tyrosinase levels and reduces melanosome transport
	miR-675	Decreases micropthalmia-associated transcription factor by phosphorylating CREB-1, reduces tyrosinase levels, induces N-cadherin during epithelial–mesenchymal transition
Hair follicular cells	miR-199	Enhances development of hair follicle
	miR-31	Increases anagen activity and promotes active hair growth
	miR-200b	Enhances follicle development
	miR-24	Anti-proliferative nature; suppresses hair keratinocyte stemness regulator
	miR-125b	Retards hair growth
Sebaceous gland cells	miR-125b	Involved in the development of the sebaceous gland; modulates vitamin D receptor and Blimp1 expression; induces enlargement of the sebaceous gland
	miR-7	Downregulated during sebogenesis
	miR-203	Increases sebogenesis
	miR-574-3p	Increases lipogenesis and sebogenesis
Antigen presenting cells	miR-142-3p	Decreases immunogenicity by incorporating in to transgene expression cassette and decreasing transgene-directed immunogenicity

forces have been found to elicit different types of responses from keratinocytes, fibroblasts, epithelial, and endothelial cells. Fibroblasts that are at a low mechanical stress have a dendritic morphology and are referred to as "quiescent" due to their low propensity to form ECM components and induce cell migration. In contrast, fibroblasts that experience high levels of mechanical stresses assume a lamellar morphology and actively produce collagen and other ECM components. They also promote cell migration and can transform into myofibroblasts during wound-healing process. Mechanical deformation of ECM can result in exposure of binding domains of proteins that normally remain buried. This can trigger different biochemical pathways thereby altering the cell response. Mechanical forces can also alter the spatial distribution of ligands and cytokines, which can influence cell functions. Exposure to mechanical stress has also been shown to release chemokines such as monocyte chemotactic protein (MCP-1) that are bound to glycosaminoglycans in the ECM under normal stress. During the healing process, leading to formation of new skin, the cells experience a combination of compressive, tensile stresses along with osmotic, shear, and gravitational forces. Intrinsic tensile stresses induce the production of alpha-smooth muscle actin in fibroblasts, favoring contraction of the wound. Fibroblasts have an important role in remodeling the ECM and control wound contraction and scar formation. They are extremely sensitive to mechanical stress and therefore a tight regulation of the stresses experienced by fibroblasts is essential for effective regeneration of skin (Grinnell, 2003). Cells in the ECM experience two types of shear stress: laminar and turbulent. The laminar stresses are more beneficial toward skin regeneration as they upregulate genes encoding for beta-actin, vimentin, actin depolymerizing factor, myosin heavy chain, plectin, and alpha-spectrin that enable cytoskeletal remodeling. Osmotic pressure variations due to fluid accumulation at the wound site have been found to be detrimental to cell proliferation and have to be avoided. Changes in gravitational forces are rarely encountered. However, experiments with microgravity have demonstrated that hypogravity reduces cell proliferation due to reduced cytoskeletal development and inhibition of the release of growth factors from platelets.

Vacuum-assisted wound closure is a method that employs vacuum to stimulate wound healing. The sudden change in mechanical forces acting on the skin results in macrodeformation leading to contraction of the wound, stabilization of the microenvironment of the damaged skin tissue, removal of extracellular fluid, and micro-deformation at the wound interface that promotes cell proliferation and angiogenesis. It has been suggested that the application of vacuum promotes collagen organization and enhances the levels of VEGF and FGF. It is also believed that the application of vacuum results in streaming of ions causing a concentration gradient thereby establishing an electric gradient. The electrical gradient stimulates the migration of keratinocytes leading to formation of new skin.

Skin regeneration and scar formation processes are commonly encountered during the wound-healing process. Scars are nonfunctional tissues characterized by thick collagen deposits and are stiffer when compared to normal skin tissue. Hence, there is an alteration in their response to external stimuli as well as in permeation of sweat. Therefore, the goal of tissue engineering is to promote skin regeneration without scar formation. Hence, it is important to identify factors that induce scar formation and evolve strategies to avoid them. Extrinsic mechanical forces have been found to exert a major influence on scar formation. The wound bed is subjected to several mechanical forces during the normal wound-healing process leading to contraction of the wound. However, when external forces are applied to the wound bed, it stimulates the proliferation of fibroblasts, angiogenesis, nerve growth, and hyper-deposition of collagen resulting in formation of fibrotic scar tissue. Thus, scar formation is due to the disruption of the fragile balance between intrinsic and extrinsic mechanical forces. Abnormal scars characterized by thick deposits that extend beyond the wounded area are referred to as keloids. Hypertropied scars are also abnormal fibrotic tissue that is confined to the wound area. Atrophied scars generally appear as a depression in the injured area unlike hypertrophied and keloid scars that are elevated due to collagen deposits (Agha et al., 2011). Treatment of keloid scars has been accomplished by application of a silicone gel patch that has been found to reduce the tensile stress of the skin, thereby leading credence to the stress theory of scar formation. Creation of scar models in animals can be achieved by subjecting the desired region to tensile stress through extension. Apart from the magnitude of the mechanical force, their mode of application can also have a profound influence on the stimulation of cell proliferation and collagen deposition. Cyclic stresses of the same magnitude as static stresses have been comparatively more effective in triggering angiogenesis and cell proliferation. They also stimulate the production of neuropeptides and growth factors that generate a proinflammatory response that further promote fibrotic tissue formation. The neuropeptides can modify the skin and immune functions such as cytokine production, mast cell degradation, antigen presentation, neurotransmission, vascular permeability, and cell proliferation thereby making the wound region nonfunctional. The external stress alters the mechanotransduction pathway by modifying the mechanoreceptor–mechanosensor/nociceptor responses leading to fibrosis. TGF-beta pathway has been mainly implicated in the proinflammatory trigger leading to scar tissue formation. Efforts to minimize the levels of TGF-beta1, TGF-beta2, tumor necrosis factor (TNF)-alpha, and growth factors like PDGF, FGF, and EGF may reduce scar formation.

Understanding the mechanotransduction pathway leading to fibrosis is essential in designing an effective bioengineered skin, as strategies to suppress the fibrogenic responses can be developed to ensure scar-free skin regeneration. Mechanical stimuli can alter the expression of gene levels in the cells. Early response genes c-fos, c-myc, and nuclear factor (NF)-κB are activated immediately on exposure to mechanical stimuli (Wong et al., 2011). These bind to mechanoresponsive genes initiating a signaling cascade that in turn activates the late response genes such as collagens. The mechanoresponsive genes in a cell can be broadly categorized as ECM-related genes or proinflammatory genes. Table 6.5 summarizes some of the major mechanoresponsive genes and their responses to stress.

Mechanical forces can be transmitted into cells and transformed into biological signals through integrins, cytoskeletal elements, G-protein coupled receptors, stress-activated ion channels, and cell traction forces. Integrins are heterodimeric cell surface receptors that bind to ECM through "RGD" motif found in collagen and fibronectin. Ligand binding leads to conformational changes in integrin forming focal adhesion complexes involving adaptor proteins that activate cell-signaling cascades (Rustad et al., 2013). Integrins comprise alpha and beta peptide chains that associate to form the ligand-binding site. Integrins containing beta1 chains found in fibroblasts stimulate proliferation and collagen deposition. Alpha1beta1 integrins when activated through ligand binding can mediate the transformation of the fibroblasts to myofibroblasts—a key feature of scars (Driskell and

TABLE 6.5

Mechanoresponsive Genes Involved in Skin Repair and Regeneration

Category	Name of the Gene	Response to Mechanical Stress
ECM-related gene	Collagen I	Key component of scar tissue
	Collagen III	Cross-links scar tissue, promotes wound healing
	Collagen XII	Associated with collagen I fibrils
	MMPs (MMP-1, MMP-3, and MMP-13)	Matrix degrading enzymes; aids ECM remodeling
	TIMP-2	Inhibits MMP activity
	TGF-beta1	Mediates stress-induced collagen deposition
	Tenascin-C	Modulates cell adhesion to fibronectin; influences cell proliferation and migration, promotes MMP levels
	Fibronectin	Mediates cell adhesion through interaction with integrin; key player in integrin-mediated mechanotransduction and deposits at site of skin injury
	Connectin	Maintain structural integrity of the cell under mechanical loading
	Cystatin	Inhibit mechanical stress-induced degradation of ECM proteins
	Calmodulin	Modulates activity of myosin light chain kinase; activates calmodulin-dependent protein kinase that activates CREB
Pro-inflammatory gene	COX-2	Promotes matrix remodeling; Releases prostaglandin E $(PGE)_2$
	mPGES-2 (microsomal PGE synthase)	Converts PGH_2 to PGE_2 leading to inflammation
	Interleukin 1beta	Enhances MMP secretion; promotes ECM remodeling

Watt, 2015). Integrin signaling upregulates the levels of Smad protein that increases collagen production. TGF-beta levels are also elevated, which result in increased proliferation of fibroblasts. The focal adhesion complexes activate focal adhesion kinase, integrin-linked kinase, and src kinase that initiate the migration and proliferation of fibroblasts, epithelial cells, and keratinocytes. Activation of mitogen-activated protein kinases (MAPK) such as extracellular signal regulated kinases (ERK), c-Jun N-terminal kinases (JNK), and p38 through integrin-mediated mechanotransduction results in enhanced collagen deposition and release of proinflammatory cytokines (Rustad et al., 2013). Inhibition of focal adhesion kinase activity reduces scar formation confirming its important role in fibrosis. Another signaling pathway activated due to mechanical forces is the PI3 K/Akt cascade that results in the activation of mechanistic target of rapamycin (mTOR). In addition to increased fibroblast proliferation, Akt also inhibits MMP-1 thereby reducing collagen remodeling.

The application of mechanical stress on cells results in formation of stress fibers where bundles of actin filaments assume an oriented morphology with prominent crescent-like appearance. They also interact with the focal adhesion complexes and exhibit additional matrix adhesion. Transmission of mechanical stresses to the cytoskeletal network also occurs through nonintegrin systems such as receptor tyrosine kinases and the cell surface proteoglycans syndecans and CD44. The CD44 binds to hyaluronan and is lysed under stressed conditions to form an intracellular domain (CD44ICD) that serves as a cytokine, leading to calcium influx and activation of phospholipase C and protein kinase C (PKC), which mediate proliferation signals. Syndecans are components of focal adhesion complexes and are intimately associated with the cytoskeletal remodeling process leading to generation of contractile forces. Tensile loads on the cytoskeleton leads to expression of tenascin-C and collagen XII (Wang et al., 2007). Tenascin-C is a mechanoresponsive protein belonging to a unique class of matricellular proteins that also include connective tissue growth factor, tenascin X, and thrombospondin, which can modulate the functions of both the ECM as well as cell. Collagen XII colocalizes with collagen I and is implicated in fibril formation leading to stiffening of the tissue. A strong cross-talk exists between integrin-mediated mechanotransduction and cytoskeletal-mediated responses to mechanical forces. This cross-talk is due to the involvement of Rho-GTPases RhoA, Rac1, and Cdc42. RhoA and Rac1 have been implicated in generating contractile forces in the cell while Cdc42 is involved in the formation of filopodia (Wang et al., 2007). RhoA recruits Rho-dependent kinase (ROCK) that act upon myosin and mediate assembly of stress fibers. Further, activation of Rho results in increased actin polymerization by stimulation of profilin, thereby causing increased cell stiffness. Inhibition of Rho-GTPases results in reduced collagen production that augers well for reduced scar formation.

Stress-activated ion channels respond to mechanical stress resulting in calcium influx into the cells, which in turn activate nitric oxide-mediated oxidative stress and inflammation. The increase in intracellular calcium levels also activates PKC that promotes fibroblast proliferation. PKC also activates transcription factors NF-κB and AP-1 resulting in their translocation. NF-κB binds to the stress-response element and activates cyclooxygenase-2 (COX-2), a key enzyme responsible for inflammation. Inhibition of calcium influx significantly decreased NF-κB translocation and COX-2 activation suggesting that this strategy could be utilized during skin regeneration (Wang et al., 2007). Activation of MAPK signaling cascade through phosphorylation of tyrosine residue in EGF receptor is also triggered by the ionic gradient leading to increased collagen deposition. The stress-activated ion channels also aid the integrin-cytoskeletal interactions leading to transduction of the mechanical stimuli into biochemical signals. Mechanosensitive G-protein coupled receptors are transmembrane proteins that are also activated by stress as well as by the focal adhesion complexes formed during integrin-mediated mechanotransduction. These G-protein-coupled receptors bind to collagen III, an important structural protein found in the granulation tissue and promotes of the wound. They also cause deposition of collagen. Collagen III acts as a cross-linker and hence is an important constituent in wound healing leading to formation of scar tissue (Wang et al., 2007). The traction forces exerted by the interactions of the cytoskeletal elements, especially actin and myosin have also been implicated in the migration, formation of granulation tissue, and contraction of the wound.

An emerging paradigm in harnessing mechanical stimuli for skin tissue engineering is to employ stress to alter the conformation of proteins, thus switching them between active and inactive conformations. Selective exposure of binding sites of proteins can be brought about by mechanical stimulus thereby enabling selective activation of signaling cascades that may be beneficial to tissue regeneration.

6.3.8 Stem Cells for Skin Regeneration

Skin is a complex organ comprising different types of cells. The epidermal layer contains keratinocytes, melanocytes, Merkel cells (nerve cells), and Langerhans cells (immune cells). The dermal layer contains a rich supply of blood vessels that are made of endothelial cells and smooth muscle cells. Fibroblasts are also distributed in the skin layers apart from neurons that serve to transmit signals between the skin and brain. In addition, sebaceous glands to produce sebum, an oily coating that serves to ward off microbial infections and acts as a lubricant, hair follicles and sweat glands are also found in the skin layers. The sweat glands primarily comprise different types of epithelial cells. Therefore, functional skin regeneration cannot be achieved by conventional tissue engineering approaches where only the keratinocytes or fibroblasts are cultured on a scaffold. In this context, use of stem cells that are undifferentiated cells with a capability to differentiate into multiple cell types may be useful in addressing this challenge. The stem cells may be of embryonic origin (embryonic stem cells) or could be isolated from an adult tissue (adult stem cells). Stem cells are characterized by their "potency," the ability to differentiate into different cell types. Unipotent cells are those that can differentiate into single type of cells. Skin epidermal stem cells come under this category as they can form only differentiated epidermal cells. Multipotent stem cells can differentiate into different cell types of a tissue. For instance, hair follicular stem cells can differentiate into hair follicles, neurons, epidermal cells, and sebaceous gland. Pluripotent stem cells such as embryonic stem cells can differentiate into cell types derived from ectoderm, mesoderm, and endoderm germ layers. Totipotent cells such as the fertilized egg can differentiate into any cell type. However, ethical issues have restricted the widespread use of embryonic stem cells for regenerative applications. Moreover, embryonic stem cells are from an allogenic source and hence cannot be employed for skin regeneration due to adverse immune responses. Induced pluripotent stem cells (iPSCs) are derived from an adult differentiated somatic cell through introduction of genes such as Sox-2, c-myc, Oct-4, and Klf4, and hence can circumvent some of the problems associated with embryonic stem cells (Mansbridge, 2009).

MSCs have been the most widely investigated stem cell source for skin regeneration applications. These cells are derived from the stromal cells or connective tissue of umbilical cord blood, placenta, amniotic fluid, muscle, corneal stroma, teeth, or adipose tissue. They are multipotent and can differentiate into different types of cells. In addition, they can also modulate the immune response and regulate the inflammatory cytokines, and hence can play an important role during wound-healing process (Zhang and Fu, 2008). MSCs have been found to suppress tumor necrosis factor and T-cell proliferation, enhance production of interleukins 10 and 4 during the inflammatory phases of wound healing. During the proliferative phase, MSCs have been involved in the recruitment of keratinocytes, dermal fibroblasts, as well as skin stem cells apart from stimulating the production of VEGF, HGF, and PDGF. They also enhance the production of TGF-beta3 and keratinocyte growth factor (KGF), regulate collage deposition and levels of MMPs during the remodeling phase. In the context of skin tissue engineering, direct injection of stem cells at the wound site may not be beneficial as there exist a possibility of migration of the stem cells away from the site of action due to poor immobilization. This will also be reflected as poor proliferation and enhanced cell death. Immobilization of stem cells on a matrix can promote site-specific delivery of the stem cells. In a clinical trial, MSCs seeded collagen sponges were found to accelerate wound healing in 18 out of the 20 patients. Similar positive results were also reported for a formulation of fibrin glue containing suspended MSCs where rapid resurfacing was observed in patients with nonhealing wounds (Chen et al., 2009). Aligned nanofibrous morphology has been found to be useful in promoting the differentiation of MSCs into fibroblast-like cells (Kim et al., 2012). The stiffness of the scaffold or matrix increases levels of Yes-associated proteins and tafazzin (TAZ), a transcriptional factor that promotes stem cell differentiation. This property can be exploited while choosing the scaffold material with appropriate mechanical properties. Currently, Phase I and II clinical trials are underway to explore the potential of MSCs in healing diabetic ulcers and wounds. Human MSC-containing skin substitutes are also being developed for skin regeneration and wound-healing applications. The regenerative ability of MSCs has been attributed to their ability to differentiate into different cell types and fuse with differentiated cells to secrete paracrine factors that regulate the wound-healing process and skin regeneration.

ASCs of mesenchymal origin are isolated from the fat tissue and they express the same type of surface markers like MSCs. ASCs have been found to enhance formation of vascularized epidermal layers and promote proliferation of fibroblasts (Borena et al., 2015). The ASCs also enhance collagen deposition and have been seeded on carboxymethyl cellulose scaffolds to promote wound healing using *in vivo* models. An enhanced proliferation rate and thicker epidermal layer formation was observed in the ASC treated group when compared to the control animals. ASCs seeded in a fibrin matrix have been found to be effective in healing perianal fistula in patients indicating its potential in wound healing and skin-regeneration applications. ASC spheroids were found to be more effective than single cells in enhancing angiogenesis and wound healing in mice models where the wound was also covered with a dressing comprising hyaluronan gel and chitosan sponge (Hsu and Hsieh, 2013). Numerous studies have highlighted the potential of ASCs in scar remodeling, skin rejuvenation, and regeneration applications. A tissue-engineered wound dressing containing cell sheets of adipocytes and ASCs derived from a human donor was found to aid rapid healing in a transgenic mice model through promotion of angiogenesis, matrix protein deposition, and cell migration. Pressure ulcers were healed rapidly and effectively by ASCs in mice models where organized reconstruction of the epidermal and dermal layers was observed along with increased adipogenesis and reduced inflammation (Martin et al., 2015). Similarly, ASCs isolated from the fat pads of mice exhibited promising results in mice models of pressure ulcer (Strong et al., 2015). Enhanced adipogenesis, organized epidermal and dermal layers, rapid wound healing, reduced inflammation and higher expressions of pro-angiogenic, immunomodulatory and reparative mRNAs in the site of application were hallmarks of the ASC mediated therapy.

Hematopoietic stem cells (HSCs) are multipotent cells that are derived from the bone marrow (Shi et al., 2006). Though it has not been explored extensively as MSCs for skin regeneration, recent trials using *in vivo* models have revealed its potential to accelerate wound healing in diabetic mice. Similarly, a collagen matrix seeded with bone marrow suspension was found to promote vascularized tissue formation that was further treated with a skin graft without any adverse effects. The telomere length of HSCs is relatively longer and hence can be more beneficial in regenerating skin layers. It has also been discovered from *in vitro* studies that the human umbilical cord blood stem cells have been able to differentiate into keratinocytes. The ability to regulate epithelial–mesenchymal interactions by HSCs make them promising source for promoting keratinocyte proliferation and differentiation (Fu and Sun, 2009). Endothelial progenitor cells have been employed for improving vasculature in the injured site. In an interesting strategy, PCL scaffolds modified with the peptide sequence RGD were used to deliver EPCs at a wound site that enhanced its survival and function. The discovery of iPSCs from adult differentiated stem cells in the past decade has stimulated great interest among the research community for utilizing these cells for tissue regeneration (Dinella et al., 2014). However, the use of the oncogene *c-myc* for dedifferentiating the cells increases the risk of cancerous growth. Recently, dermal fibroblasts were reprogrammed to form induced pluripotent cells without the introduction of *c-myc*. iPSCs have also been derived from aged patients indicating its potential for tissue regeneration applications. iPSCs have been successfully differentiated to epidermal keratinocytes leading to the formation of a stratified epidermis in mice models. The differentiation was induced by the addition of retinoic acid and bone morphogenic protein (BMP). iPSCs in combination with trichogenic neonatal mouse papilla cells were successfully differentiated to form hair follicles indicating that the potential of stem cell-based therapy for regenerating skin along with its appendages.

Differentiation of a stem cell into a specific cell type can be achieved by using specific cytokines, growth factors, and ECM components in a medium that is known as the "differentiating medium." For example, a cocktail of ECM proteins derived from fibroblasts along with ascorbic acid and BMP-4 has been employed to differentiate MSCs into keratinocytes. However, unless a critical control over the concentration and type of differentiation promoters is available, there exists a risk of undifferentiated cells that may turn tumorigenic. Also, instances of differentiating into other undesired cell type also have been reported. Genetic manipulation of stem cells is another strategy through which differentiation of the stem cells can be achieved. Transfection of a stem cell with genes responsible for activation of signaling cascades leads to the formation of the desired cell type. For instance, transfection of stem cells with c-myc and p63 has been found to promote their differentiation to keratinocytes. c-myc promotes Wnt signaling pathway through modulation of Lef-1/Tcf genes. To avoid uncontrolled expression of proteins in the transfected cells, stimuli-switchable promoters have been employed that respond to light, heat, and chemical stimuli. However, the risk factors associated with the use of genetically modified cells are yet to be thoroughly investigated.

The skin itself is a source of stem cells that have been explored for stem cell-based regeneration (Mohd Hilmi and Halim, 2015). The epidermal stem cells that are unipotent have been isolated from the basal layer of the skin epidermis. These stem cells can produce different adhesion molecules apart from nutritive and regulatory moieties. They exhibit typical self-renewing ability. They are slow cycling cells and proliferate in response to stimuli. The epidermal stem cells have also been stimulated to form sweat glands in the presence of EGF (Borena et al., 2015). The role of MMPs in directing the differentiation of epidermal stem cells is also under investigation. The hair follicle has been a major source of stem cells. Multipotent cells have been isolated from the bulge that are nestin positive and can differentiate into nerve cells, glial cells, keratinocytes, smooth muscle cells, melanocytes, blood cells, follicles, and sebaceous glandular cells. Recent evidences have shown that

TABLE 6.6

Stem Cells from Different Layers of the Skin

Source	Type of Stem Cell	Potency	Type of Differentiated Cells Formed
Basal layer of epidermis	Epidermis stem cell	Unipotent	Epidermal cells
Hair follicle bulge	Follicle stem cell	Multipotent	Hair follicle epithelium, epidermal cells, sebaceous gland cells
Hair follicle bulge	Melanocyte stem cell	Multipotent	Melanocytes
Dermal layer	MSC-like cell	Multipotent	Different types of nerve cells
Dermal sheath of hair follicle	Dermal sheath stem cell	Multipotent	Dermal papilla cells, fibroblasts
Dermal papillae cells from hair follicle	Neural crest stem cell	Multipotent	All types of nerve cells
Dermal papillae cells from hair follicle	HSC	Multipotent	All types of cells from the erythroid and myeloid lineages
Dermal layer	Endothelial stem cell	Multipotent	Endothelial cells

these cells can be employed to reconstruct both epidermal and dermal layers. In addition, a skin-derived progenitor (SKP) cell type has been isolated from the dermal layers that express markers similar to the mesenchymal cells and have the ability to differentiate into nerve cells. Table 6.6 lists the major types of stem cells derived from the skin layers.

Adult hair follicles have also yielded a new type of stem cells, namely, the neural crest stem cells that have the potential to differentiate into keratinocytes, fibroblasts, hair follicle cells, sebaceous gland, smooth muscle cells, neural cells, adipocytes, and melanocytes. These cells have been especially successful in development of a neural network that is essential for the formation of a stimuli-responsive bioengineered skin. Another promising source of stem cells for skin regeneration is the amniotic fluid-derived stem cells (AFS). These cells possess higher expansion capabilities as well as secrete greater quantities of growth factors, chemokines, and cytokines (Ng et al., 2015). A recent report has demonstrated the ability of these stem cells to accelerate wound healing in a mouse model thereby opening up new vistas for the use of AFS for skin regeneration.

The use of scaffolds functionalized with specific molecules has been found to be an effective strategy to regulate the self-renewal and differentiation of stem cells (Wong et al., 2012). Figure 6.6 depicts a representation of the use of scaffolds and stem cells for skin regeneration.

Collagen XVII enables the self-renewal of hair follicle cells through TGF-beta signaling. The protein nephronectin, found in ECM and possessing five EGF-like repeats and an RGD motif, has been found to mediate cell adhesion, spreading, and survival through binding with the alpha8beta1 integrin receptors. Another ECM protein, hyaluronic acid, when embedded in collagen matrix was found to aid keratinocytes to form an organized epidermis. Similarly, collagen IV aided the formation of an epidermal layer from a co-culture of keratinocytes and fibroblasts. A coculture of endothelial cells and MSCs in a fibrin scaffold was found to form new blood vessels through interactions with the integrin receptor alpha-6beta1 and the ECM protein laminin. Coculture of endothelial cells along with adipocyte stem cells (ASCs) on fibrin matrix has been found to promote the differentiation of ASCs without exogenously added differentiating factors. Collagen-based scaffolds have been found to aid the formation of organized layers of epidermis and dermis from a coculture of keratinocytes and MSCs. A 3D patterned hydrogel scaffold was found to induce the expression of genes like Oct4, Klf4, and Sox2 as well as promoted the angiogenic differentiation

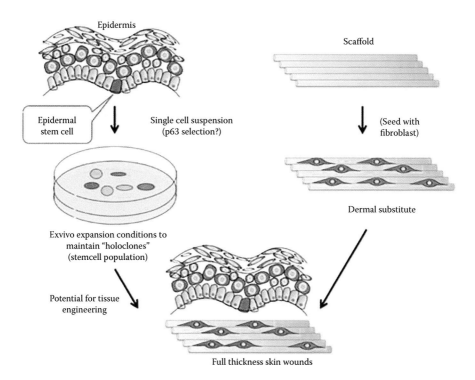

Epidermis

Scaffold

Epidermal
stem cell

Single cell suspension
(p63 selection?)

(Seed with
fibroblast)

Dermal substitute

Exvivo expansion conditions to
maintain "holoclones"
(stemcell population)

Potential for tissue
engineering

Full thickness skin wounds

FIGURE 6.6
Strategy employing scaffolds and stem cells for skin regeneration.

of MSCs. The use of decellularized scaffolds to culture ASCs was found to improve wound healing when compared to gelatin scaffolds. These results reveal the importance of the ECM components in scaffolds to regulate stem cell differentiation and organization into the skin layers. Recently, a novel attempt to differentiate ASCs into keratinocytes was reported wherein the stem cells were seeded in a cell-imprinted scaffold of poly(dimethylsiloxane) (Mashinchian et al., 2014). The stem cells adopted the shape of the imprinted cell, which in this case, was keratinocytes. Analysis of the gene expression levels and phenotype changes with time revealed that the stem cells had differentiated into keratinocytes. This work suggests that cell imprinting might induce differentiation of stem cells into desired phenotype thereby opening up new avenues for regenerative medicine.

6.4 Melanogenesis

One of the major short coming of tissue-engineered skin is the lack of pigmentation. This is due to the lack of melanosome-containing keratinocytes in the epidermal layer. The melanosome contains the skin pigment melanin that not only provides the characteristic color to the skin but also protects the skin from harmful UV radiations. There are two types of melanin, the reddish-yellow pheomelanin and the brownish-black eumelanin. The darker eumelanin has greater photo-protective property than its lighter counterpart. The melanin absorbs UV radiation and scavenges free radicals thereby preventing DNA and cell damage (Gendreau et al., 2013). The melanin synthesis pathway involves tyrosinase enzyme that converts dopamine, tyrosine, and 5,6-dihydroxyindole to melanins through a signaling pathway that also involves tyrosinase-related proteins (TRP-1 and TRP-2) and the melanocyte-stimulating hormone (alpha-MSH). Though use of stem cells has been beneficial in obtaining melanocytes along with other skin cell types, focused attempts to induce generation of melanocytes and a functional pigmented epidermal layer using differentiated cells are also underway. A 3D collagenous gel initially seeded with fibroblasts followed by introduction of keratinocytes and melanocytes after some days, was found to mimic the human skin with a functional pigmentation system. This matrix is currently being employed as a model to study various pigmentation disorders induced by UV irradiation. De-epidermized dermis, which is decellularized ECM from the skin epidermis has also been used to coculture keratinocytes, melanocytes, and fibroblasts to form the epidermal layer with pigmentary system (Gendreau et al., 2013). Several commercial products that employ cell-seeded pigmented scaffolds are listed in Table 6.7.

These pigmented skin products have been primarily employed to test the effects of dermal and cosmetic formulations.

Melanocyte stem cells have also been identified in the bulge of hair follicles. Their expansion and differentiation in murine models has been associated with formation of melanin-producing cells as well as hair growth. Melanocyte stem cells are multipotent, have excellent survival and high proliferation rates, thus making them excellent candidates for use in skin-regeneration applications. In a seminal work, a coculture of epithelial stem cells and melanocyte stem cells was used to investigate the influence of beta-catenin on them. It was found that depletion of beta-catenin affected melanocyte stem cell activity by causing a loss in hair pigmentation (Gendreau et al., 2013). Overexpression of beta-catenin resulted in the differentiation of melanocyte stem cells along with loss of self-renewal ability. In the case of the epithelial stem cells, stable beta-catenin levels enhanced the proliferation of melanocyte stem cells. These data suggest that the melanocyte stem cells are influenced by the Wnt signaling pathway with deactivation of this pathway promoting melanocyte self-renewal while activation of the Wnt signaling induces the differentiation of melanocytes. TGF-beta activity was found to disrupt the cell cycle in melanocytes. Similarly, it has been found that inhibition of Notch signaling also disrupts the self-renewal capacity of melanocyte stem cells and induces apoptosis. Notch1 and Notch 2 receptors in melanocyte stem cells are more significantly affected than the Notch3 and Notch4 receptors. A significant amount of cross-talk exists between epithelial stem cells and melanocyte stem cells (Gendreau et al.,

TABLE 6.7

Commercial Cell-Seeded Scaffolds with Pigmentation

Pigmented Skin Model	Matrix	Salient Features
SkinEthic™	Polycarbonate	Mimics the epidermal layer and is available in different degrees of pigmentation
MelanoDerm™	Collagen gel	Mimics the epidermal layer and is available in different degrees of pigmentation
StratiCell™	Polycarbonate filter	Mimics the epidermal layer and is available with only two different degrees of pigmentation
Melanoma skin model™	Collagen gel	Mimics the dermal layer

2013). The depletion of the ECM protein collagen XVII produced by the epithelial stem cells has been found to induce premature differentiation and dysfunction of melanocyte stem cells. Since collagen XVII is responsible for the architecture of the follicular bulge where the melanocyte stem cells reside, it is evident that employing scaffolds with appropriate topography is essential to exploit the regenerative properties of melanocytes. Recent research has revealed that the stem cell factor, also known as KIT proto-oncogene receptor tyrosine kinase ligand induces the differentiation of melanocyte stem cells. In addition, the transcription factor, nuclear factor IB (NFIB) has been implicated in maintaining the cross-talk between the different stem cell populations in the hair follicle niche including the melanocyte stem cells. These signaling pathways between various stem cell populations are uncoupled if NF1B is targeted by inhibitory molecules like endothelin2. The disruption of the cross-talk results in dysregulated pigmentation and proliferation of the melanocyte stem cells. Currently, concerted efforts are directed to utilize this stem cell source to treat pigmentation disorders and regeneration of other types of tissues including nerves.

6.5 The Conundrum of Vascularization

Oxygen is a major requirement for wound-healing processes as well as skin regeneration. Oxygen is required for the production of adenosine triphosphate (ATP) to meet the energy requirements during new skin formation. It is also required for collagen deposition as well as generation of reactive oxygen species at the site of damaged skin, which serve as cytokines to promote wound healing. Further, bacterial growth is retarded through oxidation reactions mediated by the reactive oxygen species. Hypoxic environment in wound bed has been found to be detrimental to cell survival and proliferation owing to accumulation of lactic acid in the tissue. Therefore, for functional skin regeneration oxygenation of the tissue is essential. This is accomplished through establishment of vasculature that supplies oxygen to the skin. Many efforts to promote angiogenesis have been made to enable effective skin regeneration. These include delivery of pro-angiogenic factors to the wound bed, use of gene delivery systems to deliver angiogenic genes, and use of stem cells that directly differentiate into blood vessels.

6.5.1 Pro-Angiogenic Factors

The growth factors vascular endothelial growth factor (VEGF), PDGF, HGF, FGF, KGF, granulocyte macrophage-colony stimulating factor (GM-CSF), and TGF-beta have been demonstrated to promote formation of blood vessels by stimulating the migration, survival, and proliferation of endothelial cells as well through regulation of sprouting and branching. Recent studies have shown that GM-CSF has great promise in inducing vascularization by inducing the expression of VEGF-A, the main pro-angiogenic factor. The most extensively investigated growth factor is VEGF. It promotes proliferation and migration of endothelial cells, reduces endothelial cell apoptosis, increases vascular permeability, and triggers the release of vasoactive plasma proteins such as fibronectin, vitronectin, and plasminogen by binding to the VEGF receptors vascular endothelial growth factor receptor (VEGFR)-1 and VEGFR-2. There exists different isoforms of VEGF namely VEGF-A, VEGF-B, VEGF-C, VEGF-D, VEGF-E, and VEGF-F, among which VEGF-A has been found to be secreted during skin injuries (Eming et al., 2007). The expression of VEGF is stimulated by hypoxia-inducible factor (HIF) and inflammatory cytokines (Bao et al., 2009). Viral vector-mediated transfection of VEGF-A and related isoforms have been attempted to promote angiogenesis in scaffolds for tissue engineering. VEGF-B is expressed by dermal fibroblasts and has been found to promote angiogenesis during regeneration. VEGF-C is an inducer of lymphangiogenesis. The role of VEGF-D in skin regeneration has not been clearly elucidated while VEGF-E and VEGF-F are derived from nonhuman sources (Eming et al., 2007). However, both these isoforms have been found to promote angiogenesis when delivered through viral vectors at the wound site. Though VEGF is a pro-angiogenic factor, there are also several concerns regarding its use in tissue-engineered scaffolds. The vasculature induced by VEGF is disorganized and leaky with arteriovenous malformations due to poor smooth muscle cell layer. The lymphatic vessels formation stimulated by VEGF is also abnormal and dysfunctional.

Another member of the VEGF family is the placenta growth factor (PlGF) derived from the placenta that exists in four different isoforms and can bind with VEGFR as well as heparin and neuropilins Nrp-1 and Nrp-2 (Eming et al., 2007). This factor has been found to induce the formation of large, mature blood vessels with smooth muscle cell layer. It has been found to potentiate the activity of VEGF and induces angiogenesis though recruitment of monocytes. PlGF is expressed by keratinocytes during the wound-healing process. Studies employing adenoviral-mediated delivery of PlGF gene to the wound site have revealed that PlGF promotes the functions of fibroblasts and also recruit bone marrow-derived progenitor cells at the wound site resulting in rapid wound-healing and blood vessel formation.

Proteolytic processing of VEGF results in several pro-angiogenic factors, the chief among them being VEGF-165. However, the highly inflammatory nature of a wound site results in the degradation of these factors resulting in poor angiogenesis. Another factor involved in the degradation of VEGF and its isoforms is plasmin. Recently, VEGF-165 mutants that are resistant to plasmin degradation have been investigated for their potential in increasing angiogenesis at a wound bed (Eming et al., 2007). It has been found that the VEGF-165 mutant was stable against proteases and recruited pericytes to promote blood vessel formation and maturation.

Another important angiogenic factor that has been used for promoting formation of new blood vessels is Angiopoietin-1 (Ang-1), which activates the receptor Tie-2 that extends the survival of endothelial cells and enables them to respond quickly to cytokine stimuli (Metcalfe and Ferguson, 2007a). Ang-1-stimulated angiogenesis results in the formation of broader, longer blood vessels with greater number of ensheathed pericytes. HGF has also been found to play a major role in angiogenesis (Metcalfe and Ferguson, 2007b). It enhances the survival and migration of epithelial and endothelial cells. However, its short half-life and requirement of high quantities for stimulating angiogenesis limits its use in fabricating bioengineered skin. FGF has also been shown to enhance the proliferation, survival, and migration of endothelial cells. However, its ability to stimulate a wide range of cell types limits its use as a pro-angiogenic factor in skin tissue constructs. PDGF is involved in the recruitment of smooth muscle cells to the endothelial layer thereby promoting maturation of the blood vessels. However, it has been found that high levels of PDGF in the wound bed can destabilize the vasculature. Release of high levels of PDGF has also been implicated in the onset of several diseases.

Several anti-angiogenic factors at the wound site have been found to be detrimental to formation of the vascular network. One of the major anti-angiogenic factors is extracellular adhesion protein (Eap), a 60 kDa protein produced during infections by the bacterium *Staphylococcus aureus* (Eming et al., 2007). Eap suppressed the generation of proinflammatory mediators by inhibiting the interactions between endothelial cells and leukocytes expressing the intercellular cell adhesion molecule (ICAM-1). In addition, it also impairs the integrin-mediated signaling cascade leading to the formation of capillaries. Hence, bacterial infections are detrimental to wound healing and skin regeneration by disrupting neoangiogenesis. Therefore, attempts to maintain a sterile environment during skin regeneration have been made. Other anti-angiogenic factors include the ECM components thrombospondin that activates Akt signaling to suppress vessel formation and proteolytic fragments of collagen XVIII (endostatin) and collagen IV (tumstatin) that inhibit angiogenesis by binding to different integrins thereby suppressing the pro-angiogenic signaling cascades.

The type of cells at the wound site has also been found to be critical in maintaining a stable vascular network. Pericytes, a type of cells that exhibit a large number of contractile proteins like alpha-smooth muscle cell actin, tropomyosin, and myosin, have been associated with the microvasculature present in skin. It has been now recognized that the pericytes maintain the vascular integrity and contribute to the contractile forces responsible for the pumping of blood. These pericytes interact with the endothelial cells through PDGF-mediated signaling. It has been found in diabetic patients that the pericytes detach from their basement membranes and migrate to neighboring regions and transform into nonvascular cells like fibroblasts causing fibrosis. There are different types of pericytes distributed across various tissues. The type II pericytes have been found to display angiogenic properties. In a recent work, pericytes have been shown to exhibit mescenchymal stem cell properties and enhanced the proliferation of epidermal cells through the production of laminin alpha5, a type of ECM protein, thereby paving way for its coculture along with dermal and epidermal cells during skin regeneration for enhanced proliferation as well as promotion of angiogenesis.

Knowledge of the pro-angiogenic factors has resulted in the development of better bioengineered skin constructs that incorporate vector-mediated delivery of the genes encoding these factors to the wound site to promote formation of a blood vessel network. Alternately, attempts to incorporate nano-dimensional delivery systems encapsulating the pro-angiogenic factors to ensure their sustained release at the wound site have also been made (Novosel et al., 2011). In addition, it has been found that the use of a 3D scaffold architecture enhances VEGF secretion and promotes neoangiogenesis. 3D cultures of fibroblasts on scaffolds rather than 2D monolayers have also resulted in enhanced functional activity of the pro-angiogenic factors at the wound site. Another facet that has been identified using *in vitro* studies is that high levels of cellular adhesion on the scaffolds results in tensional forces that impair the ability of the ECM protein fibronectin to bind to alpha5beta1 integrins that is essential to trigger the signaling cascade leading to generation of pro-angiogenic signals (Eming et al., 2007). When compared to synthetic scaffolds, scaffolds made from natural sources such as acellular matrices, amniotic membrane, etc. retain many growth factors and the structural components of the ECM that aid angiogenesis. However, their limited availability poses a challenge in development of tissue-engineered constructs for skin. Hence, nanofibrous scaffolds that mimic the ECM geometry blended with other components and growth factors are being actively investigated. Blending the pro-angiogenic factors with the polymer before fabrication into a porous 3D scaffold has been attempted. However, challenges pertaining to its uniform distribution in the scaffold and loss of activity of the growth factor, limit this strategy. Alternately, encapsulation of the growth factor into nano-dimensional or micron-sized carriers that is incorporated in the scaffold matrix have also been attempted. This strategy ensures sustained release of the growth factor over an extended period of time. Recently, an attempt to integrate both approaches for release of VEGF and PDGF has been reported. VEGF was blended in the nanofibrous scaffold while PDGF encapsulated microspheres were embedded in the matrix (Laschke et al., 2006). This resulted in the release of the growth factors at different time points that augered well for formation of mature blood vessels.

Introduction of endothelial cells along with the other cell types on the scaffold has also been attempted to form a blood vessel network. However, there are several short comings in this approach. Ensuring uniform distribution of the endothelial cells and establishment of endothelial cell communication to form the network was not achieved. Moreover, the absence of other cells such as smooth muscle cells and pericytes in the *in vitro* condition severely impairs the angiogenesis process in the scaffolds. To overcome this lacuna, stem cell-based strategies have been employed. Bone marrow-derived stem cells and EPCs seeded in scaffolds have been found to differentiate into the appropriate cell types—endothelial, smooth muscle cells, and pericytes, required to form a vascular network. Bioreactor-based approaches to maintain a shear stress on the cells to stimulate expression of pro-angiogenic factors have also been investigated (Lovett et al., 2009). Channeled scaffolds that contain patterned micro-dimensional channels mimicking the blood capillaries have also been attempted to ensure rich supply of oxygen deep into the 3D scaffold made from a biodegradable polymer such as PLGA, PCL, or PGS. An alternate approach is to create a scaffold with a gradient of growth factors like VEGF or cell-recognition motifs like RGD to stimulate the migration of endothelial cells in the scaffolds in response to the concentration gradient. Regulation of the blood vessel sprouting and distribution in the scaffold has also been reported through incorporation of a gradient of hyaluronic acid, an anti-angiogenic factor in collagen gels. The endothelial cell spheroid implanted in this gradient scaffold displayed restricted sprouting away from the hyaluronic acid-rich regions. In another interesting attempt, a scaffold-free bilayered cell sheet was designed using a coculture of fibroblasts and endothelial cells over which a layer of epidermal cells were seeded to form the bilayered construct (Liu et al., 2013). Over a period of 3 weeks, a well-defined network of micro-vessels was obtained in the skin mimic. Use of hypoxic conditions to induce angiogenesis and the "hypoxic-preconditioning" method has also been a popular strategy especially in bioreactor-based culture conditions. Hypoxia or oxygen-deficient environment induces the generation of HIF-1. Under normoxic conditions, this factor is degraded but under hypoxic conditions, it remains stable. It triggers the production of VEGF and stromal cell-derived factor (SCDF)-1. SCDF-1 recruits EPCs through binding with the receptor CXCR4 while VEGF induces formation of a vascular network.

Delivery of growth factors to promote angiogenesis has some demerits. Growth factors are expensive and tend to lose their bioactivity with time due to poor stability. In addition, high concentrations of the growth factors can lead to adverse physiological effects. Therefore, alternate strategies to growth factor delivery have been explored. In this context, copper-doped borate bioactive glasses have been recently employed to trigger angiogenesis in wound beds (Zhao et al., 2015). The role of copper ions in promoting angiogenesis is mainly attributed to its ability to stabilize the hypoxia HIF-1 alpha (HIF-1α). This results in recruitment of endothelial cells to form blood vessels. In addition, Cu^{2+} ions also enhance the levels of VEGF and the pro-angiogenic TGF-beta (TGF-β). Hence, copper ions offer a less expensive and effective mediator of angiogenesis when compared to growth factors. Microfibers of bioactive glass with composition $6Na_2O$, $8K_2O$, $8MgO$, $22CaO$, $54B_2O_3$, and $2P_2O_5$ doped with different amounts of CuO (0.5%–3%) were investigated for their potential to promote skin regeneration accompanied by angiogenesis both *in vitro* using endothelial cells and fibroblasts as well as in rodent model of full thickness wounds. The copper-containing borate bioactive glass underwent dissolution over a period of 2 weeks and enhanced angiogenesis marked by enhanced levels of VEGF, PDGF, and basic FGF at the molecular level while endothelial cell migration and an elaborate network of tubule formation was observed *in vivo* confirming the angiogenic property of the copper-doped borate bioactive glass. The re-epithelialization was also pronounced, apparently due to the presence of growth factors that promote migration of epithelial cells, fibroblasts, and follicular progenitor cells to the wound site through chemotactic signals.

Low-level light therapy, also known as photo-biomodulation, is another emerging strategy for promoting angiogenesis at the wound sites. Irradiation of the wound bed with low intensity light in the wavelength between 640 and 680 nm for short durations has been found to be beneficial to skin regeneration. The light irradiation stimulates the migration of stem cells to the wound area and increases the mitochondrial potential of the stem cells. The irradiated light is absorbed by cytochrome *c* oxidase, which in turn releases nitric oxide. Consequently, an increase in cellular ATP and cAMP levels occurs thereby augmenting metabolic pathways leading to differentiation and proliferation of stem cells and promote angiogenesis. This strategy is more effective in cell-based skin regeneration therapies using stem cells. The light source commonly employed is a nonthermal laser or light emitting diodes (LEDs). In an *in vivo* experiment involving human ASCs introduced into the wound bed of a full thickness wound, the wound was irradiated for 10 min each day with red light of wavelength 660 nm and power density 50 mW/cm^2 (Park et al., 2015). The irradiated site resulted in rapid angiogenesis, re-epithelialization, and wound closure with more hair follicles and sebaceous glands when compared with un-irradiated wounds. Increased levels of VEGF, basic FGF, and collagen were also observed. Light irradiation decreases caspase levels and interleukin-6 levels while increasing levels of tissue inhibitors of metalloproteinases (TIMPs). These effects together contribute to skin regeneration and angiogenesis.

6.6 Photosynthetically Activated Wound Healing

The use of stem cells or delivery of pro-angiogenic factors or genes can aid vascularization of the tissue at a later stage but are not available during the initial phases of tissue regeneration. In a novel strategy called *Hyperoxie Unter Licht Konditionierung*, photosynthetic microalgae was entrapped in an Integra® gel for dermal regeneration in a full thickness wound model (Schenck et al., 2015). The photosynthetic algae will be able to provide oxygen to the wounded regions through photosynthesis, which is independent of the vasculature. The photosynthetic microalga used in the study was *Chlamydomonas reinhardtii*. Integra gel consists of a blend of collagen and chondroitin sulfate. The algae were mixed with fibrin and then loaded into the gel. The fibrin reduced immune response against the algae and also ensured uniform distribution of the algae throughout the matrix. The fibrin also prevented the migration of algae to other remote locations and retained them at the site of injury. Irradiation of the injured site with light resulted in production of oxygen by the chlorophyll pigments present in the algae through the photosynthetic pathway. The algae were able to survive in the wound bed for 5 days and no serious adverse effects were observed in the animals due to the presence of the algae. The availability of oxygen in the wound during the early stages aided neoangiogenesis and rapid regeneration of skin.

6.7 Bioprinting Skin

The development of patterning tools and fabrication techniques has resulted in the emergence of 3D bioprinting, a type of additive biofabrication technique, which involves precise positioning of cells in patterns and layers that mimic the organization in native tissues. Laser-, inkjet-, and extrusion-based techniques have been employed to deposit cells in patterned substrates (Ozbolat and Yu, 2013). The precise alignment is regulated through a computer-aided design tool. Bioprinting enables precise regulation of the cells, materials, and signaling molecules required for efficient regeneration. The bioprinted skin may be directly printed on the site or may be matured in a bioreactor before being transplanted in the body. A novel strategy that enables direct printing of the cells on the site (*in situ* printing) is the electrohydrodynamic multineedle system that uses an electric field to deposit polymeric meshes that may be coated with cytokines and growth factors on the injured site (Pereira et al., 2013). Among the other major printing methods, inkjet printing is the most extensively used technique where thermal or acoustic forces are used to deposit the biological material comprising cells, media, and signaling molecules on a prefabricated scaffold. This method is rapid, less expensive, has high resolution, and is compatible with biological entities. However, this technique requires a solidification time as the input is in the form of a liquid. Also, it has been found that biologically relevant cell densities are difficult to achieve in this technique (Guillotin and Guillemot, 2011). Extrusion-based techniques have been mostly employed to fabricate cell-laden constructs for tissue engineering applications. This method uses a dispensing system and a piezoelectric humidifier apart from a light source for illumination and/or photo-activation. The cells are deposited using a computer-aided extrusion process that enables high cell densities. The major drawback of this technique is the alterations that may occur in the viability and function of the cells owing to the shear stresses they are subjected to during the extrusion process (Guillotin and Guillemot, 2011). Laser-assisted bioprinting (LAbP) uses a pulsed laser that is focused on a "ribbon" that is coated with a laser absorbing substance. A bubble is created that pushes the cells to the substrate/scaffold. Though expensive, this method can achieve high cell densities and high resolution without compromising on the cell functions and viability (Koch et al., 2012). However, all types of bioprinting techniques generally employ hydrogel substrates due to their compatibility and water retention capacity that aids nutrient transfer and maintenance of a conducive environment for cells. This compromises the mechanical strength of the system and therefore necessitates cross-linking techniques to improve the mechanical properties. A 3D bioprinted skin was fabricated on a collagen hydrogel using layer-by-layer deposition of keratinocytes and fibroblasts through LAbP. The fabricated construct exhibited normal cell proliferation and expression of adherens junctions and gap junctions as well as formation of the ECM proteins by the cultures' cell layers (Lee et al., 2009). The incorporation of other cell types in the construct could lead to the development of a completely functional bioengineered skin in future.

6.8 Skin-on-a-Chip: An Emerging Paradigm

Bioengineered skin equivalents are also being explored for mimicking diseased skin to test drug molecules, study corrosion and irritation levels of new formulations, as well as understand the mechanisms leading to the onset and progression of skin disorder. In this context, the convergence of microelectromechanical systems and tissue engineering has resulted in the development of a "skin-on-a-chip" that provides a dynamic environment to investigate complex interactions between the skin tissue and the immune components or therapeutic moieties. Such systems are invaluable to understand the underlying mechanisms involved in a diseased condition without ethical issues that arise during the use of animal models. Such disease models have been created for Psoriasis and for evaluation of drug–skin interactions (Eungdamrong et al., 2014). Other disease models that have been developed include infection models, Herpes model, wound-healing model, and melanoma model (Groeber et al., 2011). Recently, a microfluidic device consisting of channels that can facilitate flow of blood-mimicking fluid bifurcated by porous membranes that supports cell layers to mimic the tissue environment has been constructed to understand the interactions between immune components and skin tissue. In another attempt to create a functional model of the skin, microfollicles containing skin tissue equivalent Epiderm®, an epidermal model containing keratinocytes, was cultured on a perfused microfluidic chip. This chip-based system was found to support vascularization and organization of the skin layers was similar to those encountered *in vivo*. An important challenge in developing the skin-on-a-chip system is to ensure an ideal abiotic–biotic interface using an appropriate choice of materials, cells, and fabrication. These skin-on-a-chip models can in future replace the necessity of animal models for drug and cosmetic testing.

6.9 The Road Ahead

Numerous research efforts over several decades have led to advances in developing skin tissue equivalents and strategies to regenerate skin and its appendages. Identification of newer materials, development of strategies to incorporate mechanical and biochemical stimuli, and advances in the fabrication technologies have contributed to the evolution of more advanced constructs for reconstruction and regeneration of skin. There still exist several lacunae in achieving the perfect skin mimic, which will hopefully be circumvented in the near future.

Acknowledgments

I wish to express my gratitude to SASTRA University for the encouragement, infrastructure, and funding. I also wish to thank my colleagues and students at Centre for Nanotechnology & Advanced Biomaterials for their support. I acknowledge the funding support from Department of Science & Technology, Indian Council of Medical Research and Nanomission (SR/FST/LSI-058/2010, 35/21/2010-BMS, SR/S5/NM-07/2006, & SR/NM/PG-16/2007).

References

Agha, R., Ogawa, R., Pietramaggiori, G., Orgill, D.P. 2011. A review of the role of mechanical forces in cutaneous wound healing. *J. Surg. Res.* 171:700–708.
Bao, P., Kodra, A., Tomic-Canic, M. et al. 2009. The role of vascular endothelial growth factor in wound healing. *J. Surg. Res.* 153:347–358.

Bhardwaj, N., Sow, W.T., Devi, D. et al. 2015. Silk fibroin–keratin based 3D scaffolds as a dermal substitute for skin tissue engineering. *Integr. Biol.* 7:53–63.

Bonvallet, P.P., Culpepper, B.K., Bain, J.L. et al. 2014. Microporous dermal-like electrospun scaffolds promote accelerated skin regeneration. *Tissue Eng. A* 20:2434–2445.

Borena, B.M., Martens, A., Broeckx, S.Y. et al. 2015. Regenerative skin wound healing in mammals: State-of-the-art on growth factor and stem cell based treatments. *Cell. Physiol. Biochem.* 36:1–23.

Briquez, P.S., Hubbell, J.A., Martino, M.M. 2015. Extracellular matrix-inspired growth factor delivery systems for skin wound healing. *Adv. Wound Care* 4:479–489.

Chandika, P., Ko, S.-C., Jung, W.-K. 2015. Marine-derived biological macromolecule-based biomaterials for wound healing and skin tissue regeneration. *Int. J. Biol. Macromol.* 77:24–35.

Chen, M., Przyborowski, M., Berthiaume, F. 2009. Stem cells for skin tissue engineering and wound healing. *Crit. Rev. Biomed. Eng.* 37:399–421.

Dinella, J., Koster, M.I., Koch, P.J. 2014. Use of induced pluripotent stem cells in dermatological research. *J. Invest. Dermatol.* 134:e23.

Driskell, R.R., Watt, F.M. 2015. Understanding fibroblast heterogeneity in the skin. *Trends Cell Biol.* 25:92–99.

Eming, S.A., Brachvogel, B., Odorisio, T., Koch, M. 2007. Regulation of angiogenesis: wound healing as a model. *Prog. Histochem. Cytochem.* 42:115–170.

Eungdamrong, N.J., Higgins, C., Guo, Z. et al. 2014. Challenges and promises in modeling dermatologic disorders with bioengineered skin. *Exp. Biol. Med. (Maywood).* 239:1215–1224.

Fu, X., Sun, X. 2009. Can hematopoietic stem cells be an alternative source for skin regeneration? *Ageing Res. Rev.* 8:244–249.

Gainza, G., Villullas, S., Pedraz, J.L., Hernandez, R.M., Igartua, M. 2015. Advances in drug delivery systems (DDSs) to release growth factors for wound healing and skin regeneration. *Nanomedicine* 11:1551–1573.

Gendreau, I., Angers, L., Jean, J., Pouliot, R. 2013. *Pigmented Skin Models: Understand the Mechanisms of Melanocytes.* In *Regenerative Medicine and Tissue Engineering*, J.A. Andrades, ed. (InTech), pp. 759–785.

Grinnell, F. 2003. Fibroblast biology in three-dimensional collagen matrices. *Trends Cell Biol.* 13:264–269.

Groeber, F., Holeiter, M., Hampel, M., Hinderer, S., Schenke-Layland, K. 2011. Skin tissue engineering—*In vivo* and *in vitro* applications. *Adv. Drug Deliv. Rev.* 63:352–366.

Guillotin, B., Guillemot, F. 2011. Cell patterning technologies for organotypic tissue fabrication. *Trends Biotechnol.* 29:183–190.

Hsu, S.-H., Hsieh, P.-S. 2013. Self-assembled adult adipose-derived stem cell spheroids combined with biomaterials promote wound healing in a rat skin repair model. *Wound Repair Regen.* 23:57–64.

Kasetty, G., Kalle, M., Mörgelin, M., Brune, J.C., Schmidtchen, A. 2015. Anti-endotoxic and antibacterial effects of a dermal substitute coated with host defense peptides. *Biomaterials* 53:415–425.

Kim, H.N., Hong, Y., Kim, M.S., Kim, S.M., Suh, K.-Y. 2012. Effect of orientation and density of nanotopography in dermal wound healing. *Biomaterials* 33:8782–8792.

Koch, L., Deiwick, A., Schlie, S. et al. 2012. Skin tissue generation by laser cell printing. *Biotechnol. Bioeng.* 109:1855–1863.

Kuppan, P., Vasanthan, K.S., Sundaramurthi, D., Krishnan, U.M., Sethuraman, S. 2011. Development of poly(3-hydroxybutyrate-co-3-hydroxyvalerate) fibers for skin tissue engineering: Effects of topography, mechanical, and chemical stimuli. *Biomacromolecules* 12:3156–3165.

Laschke, M.W., Elitzsch, A., Vollmar, B., Vajkoczy, P., Menger, M.D. 2006. Combined inhibition of vascular endothelial growth factor (VEGF), fibroblast growth factor and platelet-derived growth factor, but not inhibition of VEGF alone, effectively suppresses angiogenesis and vessel maturation in endometriotic lesions. *Hum. Reprod.* 21:262–268.

Lee, W., Debasitis, J.C., Lee, V.K. et al. 2009. Multi-layered culture of human skin fibroblasts and keratinocytes through three-dimensional freeform fabrication. *Biomaterials* 30:1587–1595.

Li, B., Wang, L., Xu, F. et al. 2015. Hydrosoluble, UV-crosslinkable and injectable chitosan for patterned cell-laden microgel and rapid transdermal curing hydrogel *in vivo*. *Acta Biomater.* 22:59–69.

Liu, Y., Luo, H., Wang, X. et al. 2013. *In vitro* construction of scaffold-free bilayered tissue-engineered skin containing capillary networks. *Biomed. Res. Int.* 2013:561410.

Lovett, M., Lee, K., Edwards, A., Kaplan, D.L. 2009. Vascularization strategies for tissue engineering. *Tissue Eng. B: Rev.* 15:353–370.

Lu, H., Oh, H.H., Kawazoe, N., Yamagishi, K., Chen, G. 2012. PLLA–collagen and PLLA–gelatin hybrid scaffolds with funnel-like porous structure for skin tissue engineering. *Sci. Technol. Adv. Mater.* 13:064210.

MacNeil, S. 2008. Biomaterials for tissue engineering of skin. *Mater. Today* 11:26–35.

Mansbridge, J.N. 2009. Tissue-engineered skin substitutes in regenerative medicine. *Curr. Opin. Biotechnol.* 20:563–567.

Martin, P.M., Maux, A., Laterreur, V. et al. 2015. Enhancing repair of full-thickness excisional wounds in a murine model: Impact of tissue-engineered biological dressings featuring human differentiated adipocytes. *Acta Biomater.* 22:39–49.

Mashinchian, O., Bonakdar, S., Taghinejad, H. et al. 2014. Cell-imprinted substrates act as an artificial niche for skin regeneration. *ACS Appl. Mater. Interfaces* 6:13280–13292.

Metcalfe, A.D., Ferguson, M.W.J. 2007a. Tissue engineering of replacement skin: The crossroads of biomaterials, wound healing, embryonic development, stem cells and regeneration. *J. R. Soc. Interface* 4:413–437.

Metcalfe, A.D., Ferguson, M.W.J. 2007b. Bioengineering skin using mechanisms of regeneration and repair. *Biomaterials* 28:5100–5113.

Meyer, U. 2009. The history of tissue engineering and regenerative medicine in perspective. In *Fundamentals of Tissue Engineering and Regenerative Medicine*, U. Meyer, J. Handschel, H.P. Wiesmann, & T. Meyer, eds. (Springer, Berlin, Heidelberg), pp. 5–12.

Miller, K.J., Brown, D.A., Ibrahim, M.M., Ramchal, T.D., Levinson, H. 2015. MicroRNAs in skin tissue engineering. *Adv. Drug Deliv. Rev.* 88:16–36.

Mohd Hilmi, A.B., Halim, A.S. 2015. Vital roles of stem cells and biomaterials in skin tissue engineering. *World J. Stem Cells* 7:428–436.

Monteiro, I.P., Shukla, A., Marques, A.P., Reis, R.L., Hammond, P.T. 2015. Spray-assisted layer-by-layer assembly on hyaluronic acid scaffolds for skin tissue engineering. *J. Biomed. Mater. Res. A* 103:330–340.

Nayak, S., Dey, S., Kundu, S.C. 2013. Skin equivalent tissue-engineered construct: Co-cultured fibroblasts/keratinocytes on 3D matrices of sericin hope cocoons. *PLoS One* 8:e74779.

Ng, W.L., Yeong, W.Y., Naing, M.W. 2015. Cellular approaches to tissue-engineering of skin: A review. *J. Tissue Sci. Eng.* 6:150.

Nicoletti, G., Brenta, F., Bleve, M. et al. 2015. Long-term *in vivo* assessment of bioengineered skin substitutes: A clinical study. *J. Tissue Eng. Regen. Med.* 9:460–468.

Novosel, E.C., Kleinhans, C., Kluger, P.J. 2011. Vascularization is the key challenge in tissue engineering. *Adv. Drug Deliv. Rev.* 63:300–311.

Oliveira, S.M., Santo, V.E., Gomes, M.E., Reis, R.L., Mano, J.F. 2015. Layer-by-layer assembled cell instructive nanocoatings containing platelet lysate. *Biomaterials* 48:56–65.

Ozbolat, I.T., Yu, Y. 2013. Bioprinting toward organ fabrication: Challenges and future trends. *IEEE Trans. Biomed. Eng.* 60:691–699.

Pardue, E.L., Ibrahim, S., Ramamurthi, A. 2008. Role of hyaluronan in angiogenesis and its utility to angiogenic tissue engineering. *Organogenesis* 4:203–214.

Parenteau-Bareil, R., Gauvin, R., Berthod, F. 2010. Collagen-based biomaterials for tissue engineering applications. *Materials (Basel).* 3:1863–1887.

Park, I.-S., Chung, P.-S., Ahn, J.C. 2015. Adipose-derived stromal cell cluster with light therapy enhance angiogenesis and skin wound healing in mice. *Biochem. Biophys. Res. Commun.* 462:171–177.

Pereira, R.F., Barrias, C.C., Granja, P.L., Bartolo, P.J. 2013. Advanced biofabrication strategies for skin regeneration and repair. *Nanomedicine (Lond).* 8:603–621.

Pezeshki-Modaress, M., Mirzadeh, H., Zandi, M. 2015. Gelatin–GAG electrospun nanofibrous scaffold for skin tissue engineering: Fabrication and modeling of process parameters. *Mater. Sci. Eng. C: Mater. Biol. Appl.* 48:704–712.

Ramanathan, G., Singaravelu, S., Raja, M.D., Sivagnanam, U.T. 2015. Synthesis of highly interconnected 3D scaffold from *Arothron stellatus* skin collagen for tissue engineering application. *Micron* 78:28–32.

Raveendran, S., Dhandayuthapani, B., Nagaoka, Y. et al. 2013. Biocompatible nanofibers based on extremophilic bacterial polysaccharide, Mauran from *Halomonas maura*. *Carbohydr. Polym.* 92:1225–1233.

Rodríguez-Vázquez, M., Vega-Ruiz, B., Ramos-Zúñiga, R., Saldaña-Koppel, D.A., Quiñones-Olvera, L.F. 2015. Chitosan and its potential use as a scaffold for tissue engineering in regenerative medicine. *Biomed. Res. Int.* 2015:821279.

Ru, C., Wang, F., Pang, M. et al. 2015. Suspended, shrinkage-free, electrospun PLGA nanofibrous scaffold for skin tissue engineering. *ACS Appl. Mater. Interfaces* 7:10872–10877.

Rustad, K.C., Wong, V.W., Gurtner, G.C. 2013. The role of focal adhesion complexes in fibroblast mechanotransduction during scar formation. *Differentiation* 86:87–91.

Santoro, M.M., Gaudino, G. 2005. Cellular and molecular facets of keratinocyte reepithelization during wound healing. *Exp. Cell Res.* 304:274–286.

Schenck, T.L., Hopfner, U., Chávez, M.N. et al. 2015. Photosynthetic biomaterials: A pathway towards autotrophic tissue engineering. *Acta Biomater.* 15:39–47.

Schreml, S., Szeimies, R.-M., Prantl, L., Landthaler, M., Babilas, P. 2010. Wound healing in the twenty-first century. *J. Am. Acad. Dermatol.* 63:866–881.

Shi, C., Zhu, Y., Su, Y. et al. 2006. Stem cells and their applications in skin-cell therapy. *Trends Biotechnol.* 24:48–52.

Silva, T.H., Reis, R.L. 2014. Marine inspired biomaterials: From sea up to tissue regeneration approaches. *J. Tissue Eng. Regen. Med.* 8 (Suppl. 1):39–206.

Strong, A.L., Bowles, A.C., MacCrimmon, C.P. et al. 2015. Adipose stromal cells repair pressure ulcers in both young and elderly mice: Potential role of adipogenesis in skin repair. *Stem Cells Transl. Med.* 4:632–642.

Supp, D.M., Boyce, S.T. 2005. Engineered skin substitutes: Practices and potentials. *Clin. Dermatol.* 23:403–412.

Vacanti, C.A. 2006. The history of tissue engineering. *J. Cell. Mol. Med.* 10:569–576.

Vepari, C., Kaplan, D.L. 2007. Silk as a biomaterial. *Prog. Polym. Sci.* 32:991–1007.

Wang, F., Wang, M., She, Z. et al. 2015. Collagen/chitosan based two-compartment and bi-functional dermal scaffolds for skin regeneration. *Mater. Sci. Eng. C: Mater. Biol. Appl.* 52:155–162.

Wang, J.H.-C., Thampatty, B.P., Lin, J.-S., Im, H.-J. 2007. Mechanoregulation of gene expression in fibroblasts. *Gene* 391:1–15.

Willard, J.J., Drexler, J.W., Das, A. et al. 2013. Plant-derived human collagen scaffolds for skin tissue engineering. *Tissue Eng. A* 19:1507–1518.

Wong, V.W., Akaishi, S., Longaker, M.T., Gurtner, G.C. 2011. Pushing back: Wound mechanotransduction in repair and regeneration. *J. Invest. Dermatol.* 131:2186–2196.

Wong, V.W., Levi, B., Rajadas, J., Longaker, M.T., Gurtner, G.C. 2012. Stem cell niches for skin regeneration. *Int. J. Biomater.* 2012:926059.

Xie, Z., Paras, C.B., Weng, H. et al. 2013. Dual growth factor releasing multi-functional nanofibers for wound healing. *Acta Biomater.* 9:9351–9359.

Yamaguchi, Y., Hearing, V.J., Itami, S., Yoshikawa, K., Katayama, I. 2005. Mesenchymal–epithelial interactions in the skin: Aiming for site-specific tissue regeneration. *J. Dermatol. Sci.* 40:1–9.

Yang, Y., Xia, T., Chen, F. et al. 2012. Electrospun fibers with plasmid bFGF polyplex loadings promote skin wound healing in diabetic rats. *Mol. Pharm.* 9:48–58.

Zhang, C., Fu, X. 2008. Therapeutic potential of stem cells in skin repair and regeneration. *Chin. J. Traumatol.* 11:209–221.

Zhang, Z., Michniak-Kohn, B.B. 2012. Tissue engineered human skin equivalents. *Pharmaceutics* 4:26–41.

Zhao, S., Li, L., Wang, H. et al. 2015. Wound dressings composed of copper-doped borate bioactive glass microfibers stimulate angiogenesis and heal full-thickness skin defects in a rodent model. *Biomaterials* 53:379–391.

7

Biomaterials and Nanotechnology for Tissue Engineering: Neural Regeneration

Wei Chang*, Munish Shah*, Paul Lee, Rachel Rosa, Karen
Kong, Matthew Kandl, and Xiaojun Yu

CONTENTS

---

* These authors contributed equally to this work.

7.1 Introduction

7.1.1 Function of the Central Nervous System and Peripheral Nervous System

The central nervous system (CNS) is responsible for the regulation of the body's processes and systems to remain homeostatic (Zhong and Bellamkonda, 2008). The peripheral nervous system (PNS) provides a pathway for messages to and from the CNS, which allows the brain, spine, and the entire body to communicate (Daly et al., 2012).

7.1.1.1 Central Nervous System

The CNS has three major components: the brain, brain stem, and spinal cord. The brain and spinal cord, covered by membranes and meninges, are contained within the cerebrospinal fluid. The CNS is made up of numerous neurons that are supported by the neuroglia and is divided into gray and white matter. Gray matter houses nerve cells that are confined in neuroglia and the white matter contains nerve fibers that are confined in the neuroglia as well. Synapses serve as a bridge to the neurons in the body with the neurons in the brain (Zhong and Bellamkonda, 2008). The brain coordinates higher-level functions and the spine serves as a pathway for communication between the brain and the body, specifically in bilaterally symmetric animals. The CNS is mostly located within the dorsal body, however, the brain is nested in the cranial cavity.

7.1.1.2 Peripheral Nervous System

The PNS is made up of nerves and ganglia outside of the CNS. Nerves are a bundle of axons and connective tissue that are protected within an epineurium, an outer of layer of fibrous connective tissue. There are blood vessels and fascicles within the epineurium, all of which are contained within the perineurium, also a layer of connective tissue (Daly et al., 2012). Fascicles are bundles of axons and each axon is wrapped with a connective tissue called the endoneurium. The nerves of the PNS are classified either as cranial or spinal.

7.1.2 Biomaterials and Nanotechnology for Neural Regeneration

There have been numerous efforts made to use tissue engineering strategies to treat injuries to the CNS and PNS. The goal of these strategies is to mimic the characteristics of natural tissue. Tissue engineering strategies include biomaterial-based strategies and cell-based delivery, which are introduced into the body to aid in self-repair. Biomaterial-based strategies use either natural or synthetic materials as scaffolds, which can be a therapeutic drug carrier and a substrate for cells to attach to and proliferate to encourage tissue regrowth, in this case neural regeneration (Orive et al., 2009). These scaffolds need to meet a certain criteria such as providing adequate mechanical strength, having certain cues, and facilitating new tissue integration. The nanotechnology aspect of these biomaterials allows close and direct connection to cells that can affect development and cellular response.

The scaffolds are molded to a certain shape to conform to the requirements of the injury. For example, injectable hydrogels are a common tissue engineering strategy to treat traumatic brain injury or spinal cord injury. The hydrogels are introduced in liquid form into the site of injury and provide the opportunity for growth factors and cell delivery to yield a favorable environment for regeneration. Several biomaterials have been studied such as agarose, methylcellulose, poly(N-isopropylacrylamide), and poly(ethylene glycol) (PEG)-poly(lactic acid)-PEG tri-block polymer (Zhong and Bellamkonda, 2008; Kubinová and Syková, 2010). These biomaterials have been observed to encourage cell infiltration, reduce scar tissue infiltration, and aid neurite extension for functional recovery in experimental models.

Unlike injectable hydrogel systems, solid polymer-based nerve guidance conduits (NGCs) are used as bioactive scaffolds for peripheral nerve injury. These scaffolds are alternatives to autografts and allografts, and are intended to provide a favorable environment for nerve regeneration. While there are commercial scaffolds available, there is still an ongoing effort to develop new scaffolds that can better mimic the native nerve and further improve recovery.

7.2 Neural Regeneration in the CNS

7.2.1 Introduction

The full effect of CNS trauma and the impact on cellular responses is not yet fully understood, especially in terms of cellular responses. Since the gray matter is located on the outer layer of the brain, any traumatic impact can result in a large degree of cell body damage. The impact can be continuous regardless of the area of the impact (Valmikinathan et al., 2010). The primary effect of trauma leads to a chain of harmful events that affect the cell body and the function of axons. This may be lead to impaired function and degeneration of the affected nerve(s) (Shoichet et al., 2008).

7.2.2 Challenge

Since the CNS has a lower potential to regenerate by itself than the PNS, an alternative is needed. Tissue engineering approaches such as cell delivery and drug delivery have been investigated by researchers and have shown promise based on animal study results, however, this has yet to be successfully transitioned to a clinical setting. The inability to successfully transplant cells, ensuring cell survival, and circumventing the blood brain barrier have hindered the diffusion of therapeutic molecules (Shoichet et al., 2008).

7.2.2.1 Blood–Brain Barrier and Blood–Spinal Cord Barrier

The blood–brain barrier and the blood–spinal cord barrier house the components of the brain and spinal cord. Both barriers are developed from endothelial cells held closely together. Endothelial cells have electrical resistivity to protect the spinal cord and brain. The blood–brain barrier and the blood–spinal cord barrier are obstructed and release macrophages, molecules, and fibroblasts during times of trauma (Johnson et al., 2010; Conova et al., 2011). This feature, which serves to protect the brain and spinal cord, also serves as a challenge to deliver the therapeutic components to the CNS.

7.2.2.2 The Role of Inflammation in CNS Injury

Inflammation is the localized swelling or pooling of liquid that follows injury, which usually creates a cascade of events from healing to further damage. There is a lot of controversy about the benefits of inflammation following trauma to the brain and spinal cord. Over time, the proinflammatory cytokines have overall positive effects; however, short-term effects are mostly harmful including dysfunction and promotion of death in the neurons (Tam et al., 2014). Most of the immune cells brought to the site have dual roles. Because there are two opposing roles, treatments for brain and spinal cord trauma are very difficult. Therefore, biomaterials must be passive to the resident cells' immune response (Khaing et al., 2014).

7.2.2.3 Glial Scar Limits Regeneration

Glial scarring is a tight network of glial cells formed around the injury site. Much like the immune cells involved in inflammation, the glial scaring has both positive and negative effects. Immediate effects of the glial cells are overall beneficial. These cells help to repair blood brain barrier (BBB) and blood–spinal cord barrier (BSCB), and isolate the injury off from the rest of the CNS (Shoichet et al., 2008). Long-term effects are opposite, however, the glial cells limit the axonal regeneration along with myelin-associated glycoprotein. To degrade the glial scar has become one of major challenge in spinal cord injury (SCI) and traumatic brain injury (TBI) repair (Tam et al., 2014).

7.2.3 Neuroprotection and Neuroregeneration Treatment Strategies

Neuroprotection and neuroregeneration are the two classifications for CNS treatment. Neuroprotection focuses on reducing the effect of secondary events, which cause cell damage and death and neuroregeneration focuses on plasticity and axonal growth (Bradbury and McMahon, 2006). Axonal growth is necessary at the site of spinal cord injury for proper neuroregeneration to take place. Since the impact following CNS injury can lead to progressive cell death, a therapy for neuroprotective treatment is necessary to reduce disability while also permitting the damaged area of the CNS to be more susceptible to regenerative treatments (Owen et al., 2013).

7.2.4 Cell-Based Treatment for Tissue Engineering Strategies

Transplantation of new cells into areas of the CNS is a viable option to replenish the dead or injured tissue. There are three points related to transplantation that must be addressed: cell distribution, cell survival, and biocompatibility (Straley et al., 2010). The immune system as well as other barriers may stop transplantation from being viable (Pfeifer et al., 2006; Matsuse et al., 2011). Using hydrogels as a cell delivery system is a possible method to deliver the cells and nutrients and oxygen as they keep the cells together during transport in a minimally invasive surgery. Hydrogels can support the viability of the cells by including prosurvival factors and providing certain signals that would allow for the optimal usage of the stem cell (Evans and Kaufman, 1981; Kolb et al., 2007; Bozkurt et al., 2010).

7.2.4.1 NGCs for Cell-Based Treatment

The purpose of NGCs is to provide a favorable environment for regeneration. NGCs provide a physical surface, referred to as contact-mediated guidance, for neurons to travel from the proximal end to the distal end (Kubinová and Syková, 2010). Simultaneously, an NGC is expected to prevent surrounding scar tissue infiltration and create an environment in which neurotrophins can accumulate to aid nerve regeneration (Shoichet et al., 2008). The size, materials used, and additives can affect the regenerative capability of an NGC

(Straley et al., 2010). NGC application has mostly been limited to PNS but there is a potential that CNS injuries may be able to be treated using NGCs.

Many factors are essential to the design of NGC, including material, structure, and incorporation of bioactive components (Flemming et al., 1999). Current research focuses on using synthetic or natural materials for NGC, such as biodegradable polymers or polysaccharides. Degradable materials have an advantage over nondegradable materials in that the implant does not require a second surgery. Currently, natural materials are widely utilized, but they have a disadvantage in greater variability when being harvested and fabricated. They also have a greater potential to cause an adverse immune response in comparison to synthetic materials (Schnell et al., 2007, Bozkurt et al., 2010). However, synthetic materials also have their drawbacks. One main drawback is the potential for toxic degradation products that can cause more damage to the nerve injury. Because of this, synthetic polymers are being closely studied to determine possible adverse effect from degradation products (Jiang et al., 2007).

The main reason that this technology is currently only primarily utilized in PNS regeneration is because SCI develop glial scars that block communication. The use of scaffolds can assist with preventing the scarring, but it is currently still difficult to regain proper functionality of the spinal cord due to its anatomy. With the advent of nanofibers, it has been proven to assist in regeneration of the proper architecture of the CNS (Tam et al., 2014). The most common method presently used to create nanofiber is electrospinning. Studies have shown that these nanofibers are effective at assisting with the growth of align nervous tissue because it creates a favorable environment with structural cues for the cells to grow and proliferate on (Straley et al., 2010).

The performance of NGC has been further enhanced with attempts to mimic the native nerve and provide contact-mediated guidance for regeneration. Cell attachment onto materials occurs using two methods: nonspecific adsorption and specific adhesion. Nonspecific adsorption is affected by roughness and surface topography (Tam et al., 2014).

Most research of NGC has focused on specific adhesion. It is thought that channels modified with proteins or peptides derived from the extracellular matrix will more closely mimic the environment in peripheral nerve grafts and result in similar regeneration success. There are two approaches to achieve specific adhesion on NGC: inclusion of proteins and linkage of shorter active peptide sequences to the surface of the material (Straley et al., 2010). Precoating materials with proteins has shown significant improvement in neural cell affinity and functional recovery (Cheng et al., 2013).

7.2.4.2 Injectable Hydrogel for Cell-Based Treatment

Hydrogels can also be used in cell delivery and transplantation. Currently, there are many issues with cell delivery and transplantation without the use of hydrogels; the two main issues are low cell viability after transplantation as well as uncontrolled cell differentiation. Studies have shown that the use of hydrogels can mitigate some of these problems by acting as the delivery vehicle for the cell (Nakaguchi et al., 2012). There is data demonstrating that the use of hydrogels significantly increases transplanted cell viability in comparison and reduces inflammation at the site of the injury. A combination of the right hydrogel scaffold, growth factors, and the appropriate cells is necessary to effectively repair injured tissue. The cells that are usually transplanted are not typically mature nervous cells, but rather neural stem and progenitor cells (NPCs). These can then be differentiated into the specific cell types that will aid in recovery. In order for proper differentiation to occur, the right growth factors must be present and the hydrogel must be able to provide structural guidance (Tam et al., 2014).

7.2.4.2.1 Brain

Current research shows the positive effect that biomaterials can have on transplanted cells and its interaction with the host tissue. Hyaluronan (HA), a natural polysaccharide, is located in the extracellular matrix (ECM) of the CNS contributes to the cell by having antiinflammatory characteristics and supporting cell attachment and cell survival (Ellis-Behnke et al., 2006). Researchers used HA, gelatin, and heparin to transport neural stem/progenitor cells (NSPCs) into the brains of stroke-injured mice and found better cell survival and better immune response than cells delivered without a hydrogel (Nakaguchi et al., 2012). Use of bioactive molecules has also been shown to enable better differentiation and survival. Researchers created a hydrogel with peptides that allowed for better differentiation and tissue regeneration than with cells in only saline (Emerich et al., 2010). The usage of polycaprolactone (PCL) scaffolds has also shown to increase the survival and reproduction of these cells. Vascular growth on grafts has also been supported by bioactive molecules and biomaterials. These advances show that the ability for these cells to repair the damaged CNS and then continue to survive in the CNS is greatly enhanced with biomaterials and bioactive molecules.

7.2.4.2.2 Spinal Cord

Transplantation of many types has been attempted to repair damage in the spinal cord but the cells have not survived well. They have contributed to some increase in function. Certain stem cells differentiated incorrectly, which led to complications (Tam et al., 2014). Using hydrogels will hopefully enable better cell survival and encourage correct differentiation by including peptides and/or growth factors (Hejčl et al., 2010). Research has been conducted that shows that cells delivered via hydrogels into rat spinal cord lesions have survived longer and helped with recovery more than cells in only saline solution (Piantino et al., 2006). Research has also been conducted, which shows that cells delivered using fibrin scaffolds with heparin-binding peptides allow heparin and heparin-binding proteins to bind. Cell survival and correct differentiation occurred better in only 2 weeks with this combination of cells and growth factors. Unfortunately, tumors formed from the stem cells that were delivered after 8 weeks (Tam et al., 2014). This can be fixed by using a more specific population of stem cells. A combination of synthetic hydrogels and synthetic peptides has been used for cell transplantation into the spinal cord. One experiment used this combination to transplant mesenchymal stromal cells into rats with injuries to the spinal cord. The outcome from this experiment yielded better functional repair in the rats with this transplantation showing reduced tissue degeneration, improved cell migration, and axonal elongation inside the NGC, and development of new blood vessels than rats that were not treated after the injury but not compared to rats with only hydrogel implants (Menon et al., 2012). This experiment and others show that natural and synthetic polymers along with bioactive molecules work as well to transplant cells and supports functions such as cell survival and differentiation (Jain et al., 2006; Conova et al., 2011).

Repair of the spinal cord has been enabled very well by hydrogels with nanofiber design. One example is the self-assembling peptide nanofiber scaffolds (SAPNS) that guide neurites at the site of the lesion (Goldsmith and de la Torre, 1992). One experiment used SAPNS to transplant Schwann cells and NSPCs, which lived for up to 6 weeks following the delivery and showed the best axonal growth, host cell assimilation, and blood vessel incorporation in both motor and sensory neurons. Predifferentiation of NSPCs to neurons has displayed better cell viability, synapse formation, and functional and behavioral repair.

7.2.4.2.3 Retina

Retinal cell transplantation in solution has experienced issues including cell reflux, grouping of cells, apoptosis, and inability to assimilate into the host tissue. Better results have come from transplantation of full sheets instead of cell suspensions. The cell sheets have an uninterrupted adherence to the matrix protecting the cells from anoikis (anchorage-dependent cell death), constant cell polarity, and better immune tolerance (Tam et al., 2014). Another option is using biomaterials for transplantation. This creates a surface for adhesion that enables better cell survival, more evenly spread cells, and the ability to include useful factors (Royo and Quay, 1959). Biomaterials for retinal transplantation need to have certain characteristics to avoid damage and provide the best repair. One experiment combined poly(lactic-*co*-glycolic acid) (PLGA) and polylactic acid (PLA), which created a scaffold that could perfectly bend to match the retinal structure that minimizes damage and keeps the scaffolds safe during transplantation (Wongpichedchai et al., 1992). Unfortunately, this transplantation of mouse retinal progenitor cells (RPCs) in PLGA/PLA scaffolds did not exhibit photoreceptor or neuronal differentiation. The researchers advise to add chemical factors to the scaffolds to encourage differentiation (Chaitin and Brun-Zinkernagel, 1998). Cell survival has been shown to improve with biomaterials usage over bolus injections. Using biomaterials allows for precise placement of transplanted cells. Several issues of PLGA/PLA scaffolds are that the surgery is highly invasive and the biomaterials remain present for over 4 weeks, which could hurt the retina (Ghosh et al., 2008).

One of the major steps in a successful transplantation is moving the cells from the biomaterial to the host tissue. One experiment used a PLGA scaffold with metalloproteinase-2 (MMP2), which degrades a protein that forms a matrix in the degrading cell hindering neurite extension (Bhatt et al., 1994; Tao et al., 2007). RPCs delivered with this scaffold had better migration than cells in PLGA–bovine serum albumin scaffolds and differentiated into photoreceptors. Another method has been shown in research that transplanted cells on micron scale sheets with or without pores (Lavik et al., 2005). The porous sheets had better results of surviving cells, which was due to a better retention of cells during transplantation (Lewis and Fisher, 2003; Ballios et al., 2010). The porous sheets showed successful cell migration and differentiation. The goal in retinal transplantation is to limit damage to the eye (Pastor et al., 2002; Moon et al., 2003). The biomaterials in these experiments require a 5-mm incision, which can cause damage. Research has been conducted using even smaller scaffolds transplanted using injection that uses a much small 1–2 mm incision. Cells using these scaffolds have migrated well with some differentiation. The use of less-invasive techniques is definitely a viable and possibly better alternative (Yamanaka et al., 1984; Giordano et al., 1995).

7.2.5 Drug/Biological-Based Treatment for Tissue Engineering Strategies

In the case of TBI, drug delivery is used to reduce swelling in an attempt to minimize further brain damage. Methods to accomplish this include hypocapnia, mannitol, moderate hypothermia, and decompressed craniotomy (Shoichet et al., 2008). Tissue engineering approaches have been investigated by researchers for several years; however, none have yet been successfully applied in a clinical setting. In the spinal cord, the goal for drug delivery is not only to reduce inflammation, but also to preserve the functionality of the axons (Jimenez Hamann et al., 2005). The only approved method to date is the use of an antiinflammatory steroid called methylprednisolone (Straley et al., 2010); however, current research has shown promise of developing new drugs. Delivering the drugs to the

CNS and the brain is a separate matter entirely. The molecules are most successfully being administered by local injections. These injections are done either via epidural, intrathecal, or intramedullary routes (Hauben et al., 2000; Chan, 2008; Kang et al., 2010). Epidural delivery provides a more localized delivery that is minimally invasive; however, a lot of the drug is lost as the molecules injected need to travel through the dura mater, arachnoid mater, pia mater, and the fluid-filled intrathecal space. Intrathecal delivery resolves this issue, however, is more invasive. During intrathecal delivery, the dura matter is punctured, thus the injected molecules need only to travel through the pia mater before reaching the damaged tissue. Although this seems more desirable, long-time use of the intrathecal system can cause inflammation, scarring, increase the possibility of infection, and may cause compression in the spinal cord. Intramedullary injection is not typically used because it causes tissue damage. Besides injects, drugs may be delivered to the site of trauma systematically. This method, although easier to administer, requires a higher dose of the drug, which can have harmful side effects (Zuo et al., 1998; Chen et al., 2000).

7.2.5.1 Injectable Hydrogel for Drug/Biological-Based Treatment

Delivering therapeutic agents to the CNS is a promising method in enhancing neuroprotection, controlling inflammation, and encouraging stem cell reproduction and movement to the injured tissue (Straley et al., 2010). CNS treatment is difficult because the issues that are being treated normally cause many diverse symptoms that complicates the possibility of treating with drugs and the blood–brain/spinal cord barrier limits the ability for proper treatment to reach the necessary location. Several methods have been developed to solve these problems (Straley et al., 2010; Rossi et al., 2013; Tam et al., 2014). One method is injection of high doses of medicines that fail because of unpredictable exposure to the area (Tam et al., 2014). Injections into the brain are too invasive and risky. Recent advances have been made in bypassing the barrier to deliver the necessary compounds. Using biomaterials instead allow a precise delivery and necessary protection of the compounds in scaffolds or other protective materials. These biomaterials can be crafted to perform certain tasks in specific ways including controlling the release rate.

The major challenges in drug delivery to the CNS are the BBB and BSCB, in addition to the unique immune response of the CNS (Pakulska et al., 2012). Hydrogels designed to emulate the mechanical properties of nervous tissue overcome these obstacles by being used (in combination with) in direct intrathecal injection, which is a direct injection into the spinal canal. The direct injection allows the hydrogel to bypass the BBB and the BSCB, and the hydrogel's similarity to the host tissue reduces the immune response (Straley et al., 2010; Kubinová and Syková, 2010; Tam et al., 2014).

Both natural and synthetic polymers are currently being researched to investigate their effectiveness in drug delivery in the CNS. The major natural polymers being utilized are fibrin, hyaluronan–methylcellulose blend, hyaluronic acid, agarose, and chitosan (Straley et al., 2010). Chitosan is particularly noteworthy in its potential for nasal delivery, which could be a less-invasive and more easily accessible alternative to intrathecal injections. In addition, the nasal passage is an ideal location due to its porous endothelial membrane, high surface area, high blood flow, and ability to bypass the BBB through trigeminal and olfactory pathways (Wang et al., 2009; Wei et al., 2010). Chitosan is an ideal candidate for nasal delivery because of its mucoadhesive property, allowing the desired products to adhere longer and release a higher concentration of the product (Shoichet et al., 2008).

Some synthetic polymers that are currently being studied for drug delivery include poly-L-lactic acid (PLLA), PLGA, and PEG (Erlandsson et al., 2011). In comparison to natural polymers, synthetic polymers allow for better control over degradation rates and bulk properties because modifications can be made while synthesizing them.

However, both natural and synthetic polymers have drawbacks in their incorporation into hydrogels. The effects of the degradation products of many of these polymers are largely unknown and have the potential to be bioactive. While these products could be either beneficial or detrimental to the regeneration of the CNS, the fact is that the effects largely untested contributes a degree of variability that is undesirable when dealing with the CNS.

7.2.5.1.1 Brain

The proliferation, migration, differentiation, and functional recovery ability of stem cells can be improved with growth factors. Many drug carriers can be delivered using systemic delivery (Sun et al., 2003; Teramoto et al., 2003; Popa-Wagner et al., 2010; Erlandsson et al., 2011). One of the methods to deliver drugs is by performing epi-cortical implant with growth factors in a hydrogel (Popa-Wagner et al., 2010). This combination and location of the implant allows drugs to be delivered into the brain without needing the blood–brain barrier or by risking damage to the brain. An important step in nerve injury recovery and a return of function is regenerating the tissue coupled with revascularization (Liu et al., 2013). One experiment used an injection of a polymer that made the brain return to its correct shape. The addition of a growth factor greatly improved the cell density in the NGC. The results from this experiment also showed that continuous release of the growth factor encouraged improved functional recovery.

7.2.5.1.2 Spinal Cord

Drug delivery into the cerebrospinal fluid can be performed using intrathecal delivery via minipumps but the drug is not circulated well and many complications could occur. Recent research has used nanoparticles (NPs) in hydrogels to deliver drugs to the spinal cord (Shoichet et al., 2008; Straley et al., 2010; Khaing et al., 2014). This can be improved by focusing on a localized delivery instead. Regenerating the axons to improve motor function repair can be performed using localized drug delivery (Tester et al., 2007). Research has been conducted showing that hydrogel scaffolds with proteins and growth factors have encouraged growth of dense bundles of neurites. Research is also being conducted in finding methods to support neuroprotection with saving as much tissue as possible. Solutions containing growth factors have shown ability to spare white matter and cell regeneration but no functional benefits were observed (Straley et al., 2010; Khaing et al., 2014; Tam et al., 2014)

An important effect of spinal cord injury, inflammatory response can have positive and negative effects on recovery based on several factors (Freund et al., 2006; Hawryluk et al., 2008). Beneficial effects of inflammatory response following the hydrogel implantation include sufficient blood vessel formation and an increase of axonal growth and a decrease in macrophage infiltration and loss of ECM proteins (Lee et al., 2010). Two well-known and research regenerative agents are chondroitinase ABC (ChABC) and anti-neurite outgrowth inhibitor (NOGO) antibodies. ChABC encourages growth by degrading growth inhibitory factors and works best in sustained delivery. ChABC needs to be protected *in vivo*. One experiment showed that ChABC delivered in hydrogels survived longer and degraded more growth inhibitory factors than ChABC delivered through normal injections (Pakulska et al., 2013). Functional recovery improved in animal models with the presence of more antibodies to prevent the effect of the myelin inhibitory NOGO-A (anti-NOGO-A) (Freund et al., 2006). Research has shown that anti-NOGO-A delivered continuously can encourage more axonal regeneration.

7.2.5.2 NPs for Drug/Biological-Based Treatment

The use of biocompatible polymers is a strategy being applied to overcome this challenge (Baratchi et al., 2009). The advantage is that drugs are exposed to target areas in doses and reduce any side effects. This approach has been applied in the surgery of recurring malignant brain tumors (Lee et al., 2010). Systemic drug delivery is when a drug is regularly applied as needed and is an alternative approach. Targeting the areas of interest can reduce the systemic side effects, however, exposure to the drug is inevitable (Tam et al., 2014). Due to these drawbacks, the choice of the drug delivery carrier depends on the type and affected area of the disease (Schäbitz et al., 2007).

7.2.5.2.1 Systemic Drug Delivery Systems

Polymeric NPs can be delivered through systemic delivery, which can be made of natural or synthetic polymers (Drake et al., 1988; Amsalem et al., 2007; Tester et al., 2007). These polymers have a better chance to penetrate the BBB to deliver the therapeutic agents to the target area(s). Polymeric NPs and liposomes have been extensively applied for drug delivery (Tester et al., 2007). Systemic drug delivery has been successfully completed with intravenous injection (Amsalem et al., 2007). Active targeting may lead to a potential solution. Any brain delivery system must have the long-circulating properties of the carrier and sufficient surface characteristics to allow contact with the endothelial cells (Drake et al., 1988).

7.2.5.2.2 Liposomes

Liposomes are commonly used to treat CNS ailments. The BBB at the tumor can be compromised if newly formed blood vessels at the tumor site have leaky vasculature. Liposome penetration through the BBB can be improved through active targeting, which is used to change the tissue distribution of liposomes (Hall et al., 2005). Coupling liposomes with hydrophilic polymers like poly(ethylene glycol) and targeting vectors is an efficient strategy to extend its circulation time in the blood and improve its penetration through the BBB to reach its target. Active targeting is also used to promote binding of liposomes to specific cells (Ginsberg et al., 2000; Tester et al., 2007).

7.2.5.2.3 Polymeric NPs

Polymeric NPs are stable when they are in contact with biological fluids and their polymeric nature allows its use for them to have controlled drug release (Tam et al., 2014). Drug release from NPs is regulated through diffusion through an NP matrix. The polymers applied for NP fabrication are polyacetates, polysaccharides, and copolymers (Straley et al., 2010; Erlandsson et al., 2011; Tam et al., 2014).

The delivery of NPs through the BBB is believed to be regulated by receptor-mediated endocytosis or passive diffusion (Wohlfart et al., 2012). Polybutylcyanoacrylate NPs covered with polysorbate-80 have been passed through the BBB (Zhong and Bellamkonda, 2008; Kim et al., 2009). Dalargin, loperamide, tubocurarine, and doxorubicin have so far been delivered successfully to the CNS using polybutyl cyanoacrylate (PBCA) NPs (Benfey and Aguayo, 1982; Guan et al., 2008; Henrich-Noack et al., 2012; Pakulska et al., 2013).

7.2.5.2.4 Local Delivery Systems

Delivery of drugs from a biocompatible delivery system implanted at the target site has been hypothesized to be a viable strategy to alleviate systemic side effects. This strategy is useful for malignant gliomas. Drug delivery using polymeric implants in the CNS circumvents the challenge of passing through the BBB and systemic side effects and toxicity (Whalen et al., 1999; Guan et al., 2008; Erlandsson et al., 2011). The drawbacks are that the dosage cannot be changed after implantation, the rate of drug release reduces with time, repeated implantation could be required for long-term release, and the implantation surgery is invasive.

7.2.6 Combination Treatment Strategies

Cells, growth factors, and biomaterials have been used separately and in combination to improve cell survival and compatibility after cell transplantation (Whalen et al., 1999; Straley et al., 2010; Tam et al., 2014). This approach has overcome the challenge of entering the BBB and systemic side effects. Biomaterials have the potential to transport therapeutic molecules, which can yield sustained and tunable drug release. Biomaterials can also be used to deliver cells as well as provide physical support for cells to ensure their survival and proliferation (Verma, 2000). Hydrogels are water swollen materials and are capable of achieving the same mechanical properties as natural tissue. Finally, biomaterials are noncytotoxic, allow cell migration, and allow for biomolecules to diffuse from the scaffold at the same time retaining their physical structure (Kubinová and Syková, 2010; Pakulska et al., 2013; Khaing et al., 2014).

7.3 Neural Regeneration in the PNS

7.3.1 Introduction

Peripheral nerve injury is defined as any injury to the nerves or surrounding tissue of PNS. Severe nerve injuries are significant clinical problem and can require surgical intervention or otherwise may lead to paralysis. The PNS has higher potential to regenerate than the CNS after injury. In gaps up to 5 mm, the injured nerve stumps are directly sutured together, a technique known as neuroanastomosis, but for injuries greater than 5 mm an autograft is applied. These techniques are the current gold standard in the treatment of segmented peripheral nerves. The use of an autograft requires harvesting a nerve from a secondary location on the patient and suturing it to the primary site of injury. The use of the autologous nerve graft has numerous drawbacks: loss of function at the donor site, limited availability, and neuroma formation (Belkas et al., 2004). These injuries result in approximately $150 billion in annual healthcare expenditure in the United States alone (Corso et al., 2006).

Neuromas are a growth that can occur on nerves following nerve injury and can cause certain segments of the nerve to lose function. Nerve degeneration occurs in several stages following injury. In the proximal end, the axons degenerate at least as far as a nodes of Ranvier. This degenerated stump then prepares for regeneration. The distal end undergoes Wallerian degeneration, in which the axons degenerate. This starts following the injury and last for 24–48 h. Schwann cells in the distal end break down the myelin sheath. Macrophages contribute to the degeneration and break down the degenerated matter.

There are several factors that affect nerve repair, such as the type of nerve that is injured. Nerves that have a mixture of motor and sensory fascicles have a complicated method of repair. The proximal and distal fascicle groups need to be matched to allow the function to return completely. Motor and sensory nerves undergo an easier repair since the two ends can be reattached without needing to match fascicular groups. The age of the patient affects outcome as well since recovery occurs faster and better for younger patients. There is faster degeneration in the distal end, which allows for better axon growth as well as a stronger metabolic biosynthesis that allows for faster growth (Bawa et al., 2009). Finally, the extent of the injury affects recovery. Neuromas or other growths along the nerve as well as small discontinuities have a better chance of recovery than nerves with long discontinuities or excessively long issues along the nerve (Kleinman et al., 1986).

7.3.2 Current Gold Standard and Alternative

A viable alternative for autologous nerve grafts is NGC, which are tubular guidance channels sutured to the ends of the injured nerve stumps to provide a favorable environment for nerves to regenerate from the proximal stump to the distal stump. Initially, silicone NGC were applied to bridge the gaps, however, these devices were either biodegradable or permeable and required a second surgery for removal. The current commercialized NGC are generally developed using either natural or synthetic. Numerous devices developed from a variety of natural and synthetic biomaterials have been produced from numerous research groups. Favorable conduits must be biocompatible, biodegradable, permeable, have sufficient mechanical properties that the conduit does not collapse, and be able to limit infiltration from surrounding tissue. The choice of biomaterial can have a significant impact on the outcome of regeneration (Jiang et al., 2010).

7.3.3 Mechanism of Nerve Regeneration within NGC

The mechanism of nerve regeneration within a hollow NGC has been outlined in the following five phases, which occur in a sequence: (i) the fluid phase; (ii) the matrix phase; (iii) the cellular migration phase; (iv) the axonal phase; and (v) the myelination phase. For the fluid phase, plasma is released from the proximal and distal nerve stumps. The plasma contains neurotrophins and extracellular matrix molecules (Siemionow et al., 2010). A acellular fibrin cable is then formed within 1 week between the proximal stump and the distal stump from the ECM precursor molecules released from the fluid phase. During the second week, Schwann cells from both stumps travel along the newly formed fibrin cable. These cells then proliferate and align to form the Bands of Büngner, which provides a topographical tissue cable for the axonal phase of repair (Liu et al., 2002; Daly et al., 2012). In the axonal phase, regenerative axonal sprouts, use this cable as a guidance cue to reach their target. Schwann cells, which mature to become a myelinating phenotype, envelop the regenerated axons to create the myelin sheath for functional repair (Ribeiro-Resende et al., 2009).

7.3.4 Tissue Engineering Strategies to Fabricate Conduits and Improve Regeneration

Any tissue engineering approach must support cells in a three-dimensional (3D) space to allow for cellular communication for successful nerve regeneration (Pabari et al., 2014). The structures of the extracellular matrix proteins range from 50 to 500 nm in diameter, which is why nanotechnology is a potential strategy for the treatment of severe peripheral nerve injury. Aligned nanofibers are used to aid cell orientation, migration, and in turn enhance neurite growth direction (Zhang et al., 1995; Branco et al., 2009).

It is common practice in laboratories to improve the efficacy of conduits in an effort to aid nerve regeneration by incorporating chemotactic and haptoactic cues. Approaches include cell therapy, incorporation of growth factors and proteins, and sometimes applying these techniques in combination (Mukhatyar et al., 2009). Finally, research groups often modify the structure of a conduit by often providing conduits with a greater cross-sectional sur-face area, known as multichannel conduits, than is achieved with a standard tubular struc-ture (Brenner et al., 2006). Current commercial conduits have a tubular structure, which also leads to nerve dispersion and can only treat up to a 3 cm nerve gap (Cunha et al., 2011).

7.3.4.1 Natural and Synthetic Materials

Natural materials generally have greater biocompatibility than other materials since they exhibit properties similar to the tissues they are replacing. Collagen is a preferred polymer since it is one of the major constituents of the extracellular matrix and is nested in the con-nective tissues (Wang et al., 2008). The drawback with natural materials is cost as well as the fact that they are difficult to modify compared to synthetic materials (McKenzie et al., 2004; Griffin et al., 2010).

The compositions of synthetic materials are better known than that of natural materi-als and can be modified to better suit the needs of nerve regeneration. PLGA and PCL are popular synthetic materials and have been preapproved by the Food and Drug Administration for use in and as biological devices. The disadvantage of the synthetic materials is that they are not as biocompatible as natural polymers, which is reflected in their lack of cell recognition signals (Woodruff and Hutmacher, 2010; Doubra et al., 2015).

Innovative nanotechnology has focused on providing and enhancing such character-istics in the conduits to better mimic the native nerve and yield a more favorable envi-ronment for regeneration. The focus has been to aid and improve cellular migration, proliferation, and differentiation through the development of nanoscale biomaterials (Sachlos and Czernuszka, 2003).

7.3.4.2 The Use of Structural Guidance Cues

Longitudinally aligned nanofibers on the inner surface, neurotrophins, cell therapy, and extracellular proteins are the additives that have been used to enhance an NGC's ability to aid nerve regeneration (Madaghiele et al., 2008).

The rat sciatic nerve is the animal model and anatomical site commonly used to assess the efficacy of conduits, both for laboratory settings and preclinical testing for commer-cialization purposes. A 1.5 cm gap is noted as a critical gap length, as it is difficult to bridge using a bare tubular conduit. For this critical gap length, a tubular structure has to be coupled with chemotactic and haptotactic cues as identified above or a multichannel conduit must be used. As such, a 1.5 cm gap length is used to assess the efficacy of various techniques of incorporating haptotactic and chemotactic cues and the efficacy of multi-channel conduits (Liu and Cao, 2007; Deumens et al., 2010).

Several physical features have been altered and added at the micrometer scale and bio-mimetic nanoscale of conduits, which include incorporating longitudinal microchannels on the inner surface of a conduit and fabricating nanofibers since it mimics the physical structure of the native extracellular matrix. The methods to develop nanofibers are elec-trospinning and self-assembly, and sometimes the incorporation of nanofibers on these channels (Siemionow and Brzezicki, 2009). These features are useful in guiding neurites of a regenerating nerve. The neurites have a diameter 2–5 or 15–20 μm depending on the location and type of nerve. These alternations are particularly useful for large gap length injuries (Desai, 2000; Deumens et al., 2010).

The incorporation of structural intraluminal guidance cues aides Schwann cell migration and proliferation as well as provides topographical guidance cues to regenerating axons. Their purpose is to mimic fibrin cable mentioned above (Madduri et al., 2010). A popular technique is the incorporation of electrospun nanofibers into the NGC. Studies have shown that the orientation of these cues is critical as well. It has been observed in numerous studies that longitudinally aligned nanofibers on the inner surface of a conduit significantly improve nerve regeneration. In addition to aligned nanofibers, intraluminal guidance cues include gels, sponges, and films (Chiono et al., 2009).

Electrospinning is the technique of applying an electrical charge to fabricate fine fibers from a liquid solution in a syringe. Electrospinning allows for variation in the thickness of the fibers and porosity of the meshes of the fibers (Ma and Zhang, 1999; Lyons et al., 2004). The drawbacks of electrospinning are that the range of fiber thickness can vary, it can be a challenge to collect the nanofibers, and the resultant fibers have low mechanical properties (Nguyen-Vu et al., 2006). Self-assembly works similar to extracellular matrix assembly from the bottom up (Martins et al., 2008; Kyle et al., 2009). The resulting material is similar to the natural extracellular matrix in structure and function. Self-assembly has potential in fabricating novel scaffolds that can have potential in efficient nerve regeneration (Tan et al., 2005; Chew et al., 2008).

Cells live in the pores and fibers at the nanometer scale. For this reason, NGC must be designed and fabricated to accommodate this requirement. Macroscopic pores (~100 nm in diameter) and pore interconnectivity are useful for uniform cell distribution and cell migration in a 3D space (Chen et al., 2006). Both features are critical aspects of successful nerve regeneration. Pores can impact the size of the regenerated nerve as well as allow for nutrient exchange. Finally, biomaterials at the nanoscale may be applied for controlled release of drug delivery and cell therapy. This is due to the fact that the structure, size, morphology, and surface properties can be altered to suit the needs of nerve regeneration.

7.3.4.3 The Incorporation of Additives through Surface Modification

Neurotrophins include growth factors neurotrophins 3, 6, and 7, nerve growth factor, and brain-derived neurotrophic factor. These are critical for the formation, repair, and continuous maintenance of the nervous system (Bhang et al., 2007; Madduri et al., 2010). Controlled release of neurotrophins is preferred since it yields better results than burst release. The therapeutic drug is blended with the substances of the material used to develop an NGC and the drug is released as the device degrades (Hoehn et al., 2007). In addition, the target drug is mixed with the material used to electrospin longitudinally aligned nanofibers on the inner surface, which are used to achieve controlled release (Jendelová et al., 2003). The same method is also used to incorporate extracellular matrix proteins. In some applications, extracellular matrix proteins and neurotrophins have been coblended to further improve the capability of the NGC (Wang et al., 2008).

As aforementioned, the structure of the NGC could be crucial in the rate of nerve regeneration. NGC with multiple channels offer a greater surface area for cellular attachment and migration. In applications for cell therapy, multiple channels offer the opportunity to include more cells to attach. An array of cell types have been studied so far in assessing their ability to further aid nerve regeneration and have yielded successful results.

Acknowledgments

The work was supported by the Office of the Assistant Secretary of Defense for Health Affairs through the Peer Reviewed Orthopaedic Research Program under Award No. W81XWH-13-1-0320 and NIH-R15 NS074404.

References

Amsalem, Y., Mardor, Y., Feinberg, M.S. et al. 2007. Iron-oxide labeling and outcome of transplanted mesenchymal stem cells in the infarcted myocardium. *Circulation*. 116: I38–I45.

Ballios, B.G., Cooke, M.J., van der Kooy, D., and Shoichet, M.S. 2010. A hydrogel-based stem cell delivery system to treat retinal degenerative diseases. *Biomaterials*. 31: 2555–2564.

Baratchi, S., Kanwar, R.K., Khoshmanesh, K. et al. 2009. Promises of nanotechnology for drug delivery to brain in neurodegenerative diseases. *Curr Nanosci*. 5: 15–25.

Bawa, P., Pillay, V., Choonara, Y.E., and Du Toit, L.C. 2009. Stimuli-responsive polymers and their applications in drug delivery. *Biomed Mater*. 4: 022001.

Beck, K.D., Nguyen, H.X., Galvan, M.D., Salazar, D.L., Woodruff, T.M., and Anderson, A.J. 2010. Quantitative analysis of cellular inflammation after traumatic spinal cord injury: Evidence for a multiphasic inflammatory response in the acute to chronic environment. *Brain*. 133: 433–447.

Belkas, J.S., Shoichet, M.S., and Midha, R. 2004. Peripheral nerve regeneration through guidance tubes. *Neurol Res*. 26: 151–160.

Benfey, M., and Aguayo, A.J. 1982. Extensive elongation of axons from rat brain into peripheral nerve grafts. *Nature*. 296: 150–152.

Bhatt, N.S., Newsome, D.A., Fenech, T., Hessburg, T.P., Diamond, J.G., Miceli, M.V., Kratz, K.E., and Oliver, P.D. 1994. Experimental transplantation of human retinal pigment epithelial cells on collagen substrates. *Am J Ophthalmol*. 117: 214–221.

Bhang S.H., Lim, J.S., Choi, C.Y., Kwon, Y.K., and Kim, B.S., 2007. The behavior of neural stem cells on biodegradable synthetic polymers. *J. Biomater. Sci. Polym. Ed.*, 18(2): 222–239.

Bozkurt, A., Deumens, R., Beckmann, C. et al. 2010. *In vitro* cell alignment obtained with a Schwann cell enriched microstructured nerve guide with longitudinal guidance channels. *Biomaterials*. 30: 169–179.

Bradbury, E.J. and McMahon, S.B. 2006. Spinal cord repair strategies: Why do they work? *Nat Rev Neurosci*. 7: 644–653.

Branco, M.C., Pochan, D.J., Wagner, N.J., and Schneider, J.P. 2009. Macromolecular diffusion and release from self-assembled β-hairpin peptide hydrogels. *Biomaterials*. 30: 1339–1347.

Brenner, M.J., Hess, J.R., Myckatyn, T.M., Hayashi, A., Hunter, D.A., and Mackinnon, S.E. 2006. Repair of motor nerve gaps with sensory nerve inhibits regeneration in rats. *Laryngoscope*. 116: 1685–1692.

Chaitin, M.H. and Brun-Zinkernagel, A.M. 1998. Immunolocalization of CD44 in the dystrophic rat retina. *Exp Eye Res*. 67: 283–292.

Chan, C. 2008. Inflammation: Beneficial or detrimental after spinal cord injury? *Recent Pat. CNS Drug Discov*. 3: 189–199.

Chen, M.S., Huber, A.B., van der Haar, M.E., Frank, M., Schnell, L., Spillmann, A.A., Christ, F., and Schwab, M.E. 2000. Nogo-A is a myelin-associated neurite outgrowth inhibitor and an antigen for monoclonal antibody IN-1. *Nature*. 403: 434–439.

Chen, Y.W., Chiou, S.H., Wong, T.T., Ku, H.H., Lin, H.T., Chung, C.F., Yen, S.H., and Kao, C.L. 2006. Using gelatin scaffold with coated basic fibroblast growth factor as a transfer system for transplantation of human neural stem cells. *Transplant Proc*. 38: 1616–1617, June.

Cheng, T.Y., Chen, M.H., Chang, W.H., Huang, M.Y., and Wang, T.W. 2013. Neural stem cells encapsulated in a functionalized self-assembling peptide hydrogel for brain tissue engineering. *Biomaterials.* 34: 2005–2016.

Chew, S.Y., Mi, R., Hoke, A., and Leong, K.W. 2008. The effect of the alignment of electrospun fibrous scaffolds on Schwann cell maturation. *Biomaterials.* 29: 653–661.

Chiono, V., Tonda-Turo, C., and Ciardelli, G. 2009. Artificial scaffolds for peripheral nerve reconstruction. *Int Rev Neurobiol.* 87: 173–198.

Conova, L., Vernengo, J., Jin, Y. et al. 2011. A pilot study of poly (N-isopropylacrylamide)-g-polyethylene glycol and poly(N-isopropylacrylamide)-g-methylcellulose branched copolymers as injectable scaffolds for local delivery of neurotrophins and cellular transplants into the injured spinal cord: Laboratory investigation. *J Neurosurg Spine.* 15: 594–604.

Corso, P., Finkelstein, E., Miller, T., Fiebelkorn, I., and Zaloshnja, E. 2006. Incidence and lifetime costs of injuries in the United States. *Inj Prev.* 12: 212–218.

Cunha, C., Panseri, S., and Antonini, S. 2011. Emerging nanotechnology approaches in tissue engineering for peripheral nerve regeneration. *Nanomed Nanotechnol.* 7: 50–59.

Daly, W., Yao, L., Zeugolis, D., Windebank, A., and Pandit, A. 2012. A biomaterials approach to peripheral nerve regeneration: Bridging the peripheral nerve gap and enhancing functional recovery. *J R Soc Interface.* 9: 202–221.

Desai, T.A. 2000. Micro- and nanoscale structures for tissue engineering constructs. *Med Eng Phys.* 22: 595–606.

Deumens, R., Bozkurt, A., Meek, M.F., Marcus, M.A., Joosten, E.A., Weis, J., and Brook, G.A. 2010. Repairing injured peripheral nerves: Bridging the gap. *Prog Neurobiol.* 92: 245–276.

Doubra, N., Amiri, A., Jamalpoor, Z., Fooladi, A.A.I., and Nourani, M.R. 2015. Fabrication of PLGA conduit for peripheral nerve regeneration. *J Appl Tissue Eng.* 1(1): 13–19.

Drake, K.L., Wise, K.D., Farraye, J., Anderson, D.J., and BeMent, S.L. 1988. Performance of planar multisite microprobes in recording extracellular single-unit intracortical activity. *Biomed Eng.* 35: 719–732.

Ellis-Behnke, R.G., Liang, Y.X., You, S.W., Tay, D.K., Zhang, S., So, K.F., and Schneider, G.E. 2006. Nano neuro knitting: Peptide nanofiber scaffold for brain repair and axon regeneration with functional return of vision. *Proc Natl Acad Sci USA.* 103: 5054–5059.

Emerich, D.F., Silva, E., Ali, O., Mooney, D., Bell, W., Yu, S.J., Kaneko, Y., and Borlongan, C. 2010. Injectable VEGF hydrogels produce near complete neurological and anatomical protection following cerebral ischemia in rats. *Cell Transplant.* 19: 1063–1071.

Erlandsson, A., Lin, C.H.A., Yu, F., and Morshead, C.M. 2011. Immunosuppression promotes endogenous neural stem and progenitor cell migration and tissue regeneration after ischemic injury. *Exp Neurol.* 230: 48–57.

Evans, M.J. and Kaufman, M.H. 1981. Establishment in culture of pluripotential cells from mouse embryos. *Nature.* 292: 154–156.

Flemming, R.G., Murphy, C.J., Abrams, G.A., Goodman, S.L., and Nealey, P.F. 1999. Effects of synthetic micro- and nano-structured surfaces on cell behavior. *Biomaterials.* 20(6):573–588.

Freund, P., Schmidlin, E., Wannier, T., Bloch, J., Mir, A., Schwab, M.E., and Rouiller, E.M. 2006. Nogo-A-specific antibody treatment enhances sprouting and functional recovery after cervical lesion in adult primates. *Nat Med.* 12: 790–792.

Ghosh, F., Rauer, O., and Arnér, K. 2008. Neuroretinal xenotransplantation to immunocompetent hosts in a discordant species combination. *Neuroscience.* 152: 526–533.

Ginsberg, H.J., Sum, A., Drake, J.M., and Cobbold, R.S. 2000. Ventriculoperitoneal shunt flow dependency on the number of patent holes in a ventricular catheter. *Pediatr Neurosurg.* 33: 7–11.

Giordano, G.G., Chevez-Barrios, P., Refojo, M.F., and Garcia, C.A. 1995. Biodegradation and tissue reaction to intravitreous biodegradable poly (D,L-lactic-co-glycolic) acid microspheres. *Curr Eye Res.* 14: 761–768.

Goldsmith, H.S. and De La Torre, J.C. 1992. Axonal regeneration after spinal cord transection and reconstruction. *Brain Res.* 589: 217–224.

Griffin, J., Carbone, A., Delgado-Rivera, R., Meiners, S., and Uhrich, K.E. 2010. Design and evaluation of novel polyanhydride blends as nerve guidance conduits. *Acta Biomater*. 6: 1917–1924.

Guan, Y., Johanek, L.M., Hartke, T.V., Shim, B., Tao, Y.X., Ringkamp, M., Meyer, R.A., and Raja, S.N. 2008. Peripherally acting mu-opioid receptor agonist attenuates neuropathic pain in rats after L5 spinal nerve injury. *Pain*. 138: 318–329.

Hall, E.D., Sullivan, P.G., Gibson, T.R., Pavel, K.M., Thompson, B.M., and Scheff, S.W. 2005. Spatial and temporal characteristics of neurodegeneration after controlled cortical impact in mice: More than a focal brain injury. *J Neurotrauma*. 22: 252–265.

Hamann, M.C.J., Tator, C.H., and Shoichet, M.S. 2005. Injectable intrathecal delivery system for localized administration of EGF and FGF-2 to the injured rat spinal cord. *Exp Neurol*. 194: 106–119.

Hauben, E., Butovsky, O., Nevo, U. et al. 2000. Passive or active immunization with myelin basic protein promotes recovery from spinal cord contusion. *J Neurosci*. 20: 6421–6430.

Hawryluk, G.W., Rowland, J., Kwon, B.K., and Fehlings, M.G. 2008. Protection and repair of the injured spinal cord: A review of completed, ongoing, and planned clinical trials for acute spinal cord injury: A review. *Neurosurg Focus*. 25: E14.

Hejčl, A., Šedý, J., Kapcalová, M. et al. 2010. HPMA-RGD hydrogels seeded with mesenchymal stem cells improve functional outcome in chronic spinal cord injury. *Stem Cells Dev*. 19: 1535–1546.

Henrich-Noack, P., Prilloff, S., Voigt, N., Jin, J., Hintz, W., Tomas, J., and Sabel, B.A. 2012. *In vivo* visualisation of nanoparticle entry into central nervous system tissue. *Arch Toxicol*. 86: 1099–1105.

Hoehn, M., Wiedermann, D., Justicia, C., Ramos-Cabrer, P., Kruttwig, K., Farr, T., and Himmelreich, U. 2007. Cell tracking using magnetic resonance imaging. *J Physiol*. 584: 25–30.

Jain, A., Kim, Y.T., McKeon, R.J., and Bellamkonda, R.V. 2006. *In situ* gelling hydrogels for conformal repair of spinal cord defects, and local delivery of BDNF after spinal cord injury. *Biomaterials*. 27: 497–504.

Jendelová, P., Herynek, V., DeCroos, J., Glogarová, K., Andersson, B., Hájek, M., and Syková, E. 2003. Imaging the fate of implanted bone marrow stromal cells labeled with superparamagnetic nanoparticles. *Magn Reson Med*. 50: 767–776.

Jiang, D., Liang, J., and Noble, P.W. 2007. Hyaluronan in tissue injury and repair. *Annu Rev Cell Dev Biol*. 23: 435–461.

Jiang, X., Lim, S.H., Mao, H.Q., and Chew, S.Y. 2010. Current applications and future perspectives of artificial nerve conduits. *Exp Neurol*. 223: 86–101.

Johnson, P.J., Tatara, A., Shiu, A., and Sakiyama-Elbert, S.E. 2010. Controlled release of neurotrophin-3 and platelet derived growth factor from fibrin scaffolds containing neural progenitor cells enhances survival and differentiation into neurons in a subacute model of SCI. *Cell Transplant*. 19: 89.

Kang, Y.M., Hwang, D.H., Kim, B.G., Go, D.H., and Park, K.D. 2010. Thermosensitive polymer-based hydrogel mixed with the anti-inflammatory agent minocycline induces axonal regeneration in hemisected spinal cord. *Macromol Res*. 18: 399–403.

Khaing, Z.Z., Thomas, R.C., Geissler, S.A., and Schmidt, C.E. 2014. Advanced biomaterials for repairing the nervous system: What can hydrogels do for the brain? *Mater Today*. 17: 332–340.

Kim, Y.T., Caldwell, J.M., and Bellamkonda, R.V. 2009. Nanoparticle-mediated local delivery of methylprednisolone after spinal cord injury. *Biomaterials*. 30: 2582–2590.

Kleinman, H.K., McGarvey, M.L., Hassell, J.R., Star, V.L., Cannon, F.B., Laurie, G.W., and Martin, G.R. 1986. Basement membrane complexes with biological activity. *Biochemistry*. 25: 312–318.

Kolb, B., Morshead, C., Gonzalez, C., Kim, M., Gregg, C., Shingo, T., and Weiss, S. 2007. Growth factor-stimulated generation of new cortical tissue and functional recovery after stroke damage to the motor cortex of rats. *J Cerebr Blood F Met*. 27: 983–997.

Kubinová, Š. and Syková, E. 2010. Nanotechnology for treatment of stroke and spinal cord injury. *Nanomedicine*. 5: 99–108.

Kyle, S., Aggeli, A., Ingham, E., and McPherson, M.J. 2009. Production of self-assembling biomaterials for tissue engineering. *Trends Biotechnol*. 27: 423–433.

Lavik, E.B., Klassen, H., Warfvinge, K., Langer, R., and Young, M.J. 2005. Fabrication of degradable polymer scaffolds to direct the integration and differentiation of retinal progenitors. *Biomaterials*. 26: 3187–3196.

Lee, H., McKeon, R.J., and Bellamkonda, R.V. 2010. Sustained delivery of thermostabilized chABC enhances axonal sprouting and functional recovery after spinal cord injury. *Proc Natl Acad Sci USA*. 107: 3340–3345.

Lewis, G.P. and Fisher, S.K. 2003. Up-regulation of glial fibrillary acidic protein in response to retinal injury: Its potential role in glial remodeling and a comparison to vimentin expression. *Int Rev Cytol*. 230: 263–290.

Liu, B.P., Fournier, A., GrandPré, T., and Strittmatter, S.M. 2002. Myelin-associated glycoprotein as a functional ligand for the Nogo-66 receptor. *Science*. 297: 1190–1193.

Liu, W. and Cao, Y. 2007. Application of scaffold materials in tissue reconstruction in immunocompetent mammals: Our experience and future requirements. *Biomaterials*. 28: 5078–5086.

Liu, Z., Gao, X., Kang, T. et al. 2013. B6 peptide-modified PEG–PLA nanoparticles for enhanced brain delivery of neuroprotective peptide. *Bioconjugate Chem*. 24: 997–1007.

Lyons, J., Li, C., and Ko, F. 2004. Melt-electrospinning part I: Processing parameters and geometric properties. *Polymer*. 45: 7597–7603.

Ma, P.X. and Zhang, R. 1999. Synthetic nano-scale fibrous extracellular matrix. *J. Biomed. Mater. Res.* 46(1): 60–72.

Madaghiele, M., Sannino, A., Yannas, I.V., and Spector, M. 2008. Collagen-based matrices with axially oriented pores. *J Biomed Mater Res A*. 85: 757–767.

Madduri, S., di Summa, P., Papaloïzos, M., Kalbermatten, D., and Gander, B. 2010. Effect of controlled co-delivery of synergistic neurotrophic factors on early nerve regeneration in rats. *Biomaterials*. 31: 8402–8409.

Madduri, S., Papaloizos, M., and Gander, B. 2010. Trophically and topographically functionalized silk fibroin nerve conduits for guided peripheral nerve regeneration. *Biomaterials*. 31: 2323–2334.

Martins, A., Reis, R.L., and Neves, L.M. 2008. Electrospinning: Processing technique for tissue engineering scaffolding. *Int Mater Rev*. 53: 257–274.

Matsuse, D., Kitada, M., Ogura, F., Wakao, S., Kohama, M., Kira, J.I., Tabata, Y., and Dezawa, M. 2011. Combined transplantation of bone marrow stromal cell-derived neural progenitor cells with a collagen sponge and basic fibroblast growth factor releasing microspheres enhances recovery after cerebral ischemia in rats. *Tissue Eng A*. 17: 1993–2004.

McKenzie, J.L., Waid, M.C., Shi, R., and Webster, T.J. 2004. Decreased functions of astrocytes on carbon nanofiber materials. *Biomaterials*. 25: 1309–1317.

Menon, P.K., Muresanu, D.F., Sharma, A., Mossler, H., and Sharma, H.S. 2012. Cerebrolysin, a mixture of neurotrophic factors induces marked neuroprotection in spinal cord injury following intoxication of engineered nanoparticles from metals. *CNS Neurol Disord Drug Targets (Formerly Current Drug Targets-CNS & Neurological Disorders)*. 11: 40–49.

Moon, L.D., Asher, R.A., and Fawcett, J.W. 2003. Limited growth of severed CNS axons after treatment of adult rat brain with hyaluronidase. *J Neurosci Res*. 71: 23–37.

Mukhatyar, V., Karumbaiah, L., Yeh, J., and Bellamkonda, R. 2009. Tissue engineering strategies designed to realize the endogenous regenerative potential of peripheral nerves. *Adv Mater*. 21: 4670–4679.

Nakaguchi, K., Jinnou, H., Kaneko, N., Sawada, M., Hikita, T., Saitoh, S., Tabata, Y., and Sawamoto, K. 2012. Growth factors released from gelatin hydrogel microspheres increase new neurons in the adult mouse brain. *Stem Cells Int*. 915160.

Nguyen-Vu, T.D., Chen, H., Cassell, A.M., Andrews, R., Meyyappan, M., and Li, J. 2006. Vertically aligned carbon nanofiber arrays: An advance toward electrical–neural interfaces. *Small*. 2: 89–94.

Orive, G., Anitua, E., Pedraz, J.L., and Emerich, D.F. 2009. Biomaterials for promoting brain protection, repair and regeneration. *Nat Rev Neurosci*. 10: 682–692.

Owen, S.C., Fisher, S.A., Tam, R.Y., Nimmo, C.M., and Shoichet, M.S. 2013. Hyaluronic acid click hydrogels emulate the extracellular matrix. *Langmuir*. 29: 7393–7400.

Pabari, A., Lloyd-Hughes, H., Seifalian, A.M., and Mosahebi, A. 2014. Nerve conduits for peripheral nerve surgery. *Plast Reconstr Surg.* 133: 1420–1430.

Pakulska, M.M., Ballios, B.G., and Shoichet, M.S. 2012. Injectable hydrogels for central nervous system therapy. *Biomed Mater.* 7: 024101.

Pakulska, M.M., Vulic, K., and Shoichet, M.S. 2013. Affinity-based release of chondroitinase ABC from a modified methylcellulose hydrogel. *J Control Release.* 171: 11–16.

Pastor, J.C., de la Rúa, E.R., and Martín, F. 2002. Proliferative vitreoretinopathy: Risk factors and pathobiology. *Prog Retin Eye Res.* 21: 127–144.

Pfeifer, K., Vroemen, M., Caioni, M., Aigner, L., Bogdahn, U., and Weidner, N. 2006. Autologous adult rodent neural progenitor cell transplantation represents a feasible strategy to promote structural repair in the chronically injured spinal cord. *Regen Med.* 1(2): 255–266.

Piantino, J., Burdick, J.A., Goldberg, D., Langer, R., and Benowitz, L.I. 2006. An injectable, biodegradable hydrogel for trophic factor delivery enhances axonal rewiring and improves performance after spinal cord injury. *Exp Neurol.* 201: 359–367.

Popa-Wagner, A., Stöcker, K., Balseanu, A.T., Rogalewski, A., Diederich, K., Minnerup, J., Margaritescu, C., and Schäbitz, W.R. 2010. Effects of granulocyte-colony stimulating factor after stroke in aged rats. *Stroke.* 41: 1027–1031.

Ribeiro-Resende, V.T., Koenig, B., Nichterwitz, S., Oberhoffner, S., and Schlosshauer, B. 2009. Strategies for inducing the formation of bands of Büngner in peripheral nerve regeneration. *Biomaterials.* 30: 5251–5259.

Rossi, F., Perale, G., Papa, S., Forloni, G., and Veglianese, P. 2013. Current options for drug delivery to the spinal cord. *Expert Opin Drug Del.* 10: 385–396.

Royo, P.E. and Quay, W.B. 1959. Retinal transplantation from fetal to maternal mammalian eye. *Growth.* 23: 313–336.

Sachlos, E. and Czernuszka, J.T. 2003. Making tissue engineering scaffolds work. Review: The application of solid freeform fabrication technology to the production of tissue engineering scaffolds. *Eur Cell Mater.* 5: 39–40.

Schäbitz, W.R., Steigleder, T., Cooper-Kuhn, C.M., Schwab, S., Sommer, C., Schneider, A., and Kuhn, H.G. 2007. Intravenous brain-derived neurotrophic factor enhances poststroke sensorimotor recovery and stimulates neurogenesis. *Stroke.* 38: 2165–2172.

Schnell, E., Klinkhammer, K., Balzer, S., Brook, G., Klee, D., Dalton, P., and Mey, J. 2007. Guidance of glial cell migration and axonal growth on electrospun nanofibers of poly-ε-caprolactone and a collagen/poly-ε-caprolactone blend. *Biomaterials.* 28: 3012–3025.

Shoichet, M.S., Tate, C.C., Baumann, M.D., and LaPlaca, M.C. 2008. Strategies for regeneration and repair in the injured central nervous system. In: Reichert, W.M. (ed.), *Indwelling Neural Implants: Strategies for Contending with the In Vivo Environment.* Boca Raton, Florida: CRC Press/Taylor & Francis.

Siemionow, M. and Brzezicki, G. 2009. Current techniques and concepts in peripheral nerve repair. *Int Rev Neurobiol.* 87: 141–172.

Siemionow, M., Bozkurt, M., and Zor, F. 2010. Regeneration and repair of peripheral nerves with different biomaterials: Review. *Microsurgery.* 30: 574–588.

Straley, K.S., Foo, C.W.P., and Heilshorn, S.C. 2010. Biomaterial design strategies for the treatment of spinal cord injuries. *J Neurotrauma.* 27: 1–19.

Sun, Y., Jin, K., Xie, L., Childs, J., Mao, X.O., Logvinova, A., and Greenberg, D.A. 2003. VEGF-induced neuroprotection, neurogenesis, and angiogenesis after focal cerebral ischemia. *J Clin Invest.* 111: 1843.

Tam, R.Y., Fuehrmann, T., Mitrousis, N., and Shoichet, M.S. 2014. Regenerative therapies for central nervous system diseases: A biomaterials approach. *Neuropsychopharmacology.* 39: 169–188.

Tan, S.H., Inai, R., Kotaki, M., and Ramakrishna, S. 2005. Systematic parameter study for ultra-fine fiber fabrication via electrospinning process. *Polymer.* 46: 6128–6134.

Tao, S., Young, C., Redenti, S., Zhang, Y., Klassen, H., Desai, T., and Young, M.J. 2007. Survival, migration and differentiation of retinal progenitor cells transplanted on micro-machined poly (methyl methacrylate) scaffolds to the subretinal space. *Lab Chip.* 7: 695–701.

Teramoto, T., Qiu, J., Plumier, J.C., and Moskowitz, M.A. 2003. EGF amplifies the replacement of parvalbumin-expressing striatal interneurons after ischemia. *J Clin Invest.* 111: 1125.

Tester, N.J., Plaas, A.H., and Howland, D.R. 2007. Effect of body temperature on chondroitinase ABC's ability to cleave chondroitin sulfate glycosaminoglycans. *J Neurosci Res.* 85: 1110–1118.

Valmikinathan, C.M., Bawa, H.K., Junka, R., and Yu, X. 2010. Nanotechnologies for peripheral nerve regeneration. *Nanotechnology in Tissue Engineering and Regenerative Medicine.* Boca Raton, Florida: CRC Press, pp. 1–24.

Verma, A. 2000. Opportunities for neuroprotection in traumatic brain injury. *J Head Trauma Rehab.* 15: 1149–1161.

Wang, J., Valmikinathan, C.M., and Yu, X. 2009. Nanostructures for bypassing blood brain barrier. *Curr Bioactive Compd.* 5: 195–205.

Wang, W., Itoh, S., Matsuda, A., Aizawa, T., Demura, M., Ichinose, S., Shinomiya, K., and Tanaka, J. 2008. Enhanced nerve regeneration through a bilayered chitosan tube: The effect of introduction of glycine spacer into the CYIGSR sequence. *J Biomed Mater Res A.* 85: 919–928.

Wang, W., Itoh, S., Matsuda, A., Ichinose, S., Shinomiya, K., Hata, Y., and Tanaka, J. 2008. Influences of mechanical properties and permeability on chitosan nano/microfiber mesh tubes as a scaffold for nerve regeneration. *J Biomed Mater Res A.* 84: 557–566.

Wei, Y.T., He, Y., Xu, C.L., Wang, Y., Liu, B.F., Wang, X.M., Sun, X.D., Cui, F.Z., and Xu, Q.Y. 2010. Hyaluronic acid hydrogel modified with nogo-66 receptor antibody and poly-L-lysine to promote axon regrowth after spinal cord injury. *J Biomed Mater Res B.* 95: 110–117.

Whalen, M.J., Clark, R.S., Dixon, C.E. et al. 1999. Reduction of cognitive and motor deficits after traumatic brain injury in mice deficient in poly(ADP-ribose) polymerase. *J Cerebr Blood F Met.* 19: 835–842.

Wohlfart, S., Gelperina, S., and Kreuter, J. 2012. Transport of drugs across the blood–brain barrier by nanoparticles. *J Control Release.* 161: 264–273.

Wongpichedchai, S., Weiter, J.J., Weber, P., and Dorey, C.K. 1992. Comparison of external and internal approaches for transplantation of autologous retinal pigment epithelium. *Invest Ophthalmol Vis Sci.* 33: 3341–3352.

Woodruff, M.A. and Hutmacher, D.W. 2010. The return of a forgotten polymer—Polycaprolactone in the twenty-first century. *Prog Polym Sci.* 35: 1217–1256.

Yamanaka, A., Nakamae, K., Takeuchi, M., Momose, A., Fukado, Y., Oshima, K., and Goto, H. 1984. Scanning electron microscope study on the biodegradation of IOL and suturing materials. *Trans. Ophthalmol. Soc UK.* 104: 517–521.

Zhang, S., Holmes, T.C., DiPersio, C.M., Hynes, R.O., Su, X., and Rich, A. 1995. Self-complementary oligopeptide matrices support mammalian cell attachment. *Biomaterials.* 16: 1385–1393.

Zhong, Y. and Bellamkonda, R.V. 2008. Biomaterials for the central nervous system. *J R Soc Interface.* 5: 957–975.

Zuo, J., Neubauer, D., Dyess, K., Ferguson, T.A., and Muir, D. 1998. Degradation of chondroitin sulfate proteoglycan enhances the neurite-promoting potential of spinal cord tissue. *Exp Neurol.* 154: 654–662.

8

Tissue Engineering Therapies for Ocular Regeneration

Yogendra Pratap Singh, Shreya Mehrotra, Jadi Praveen Kumar, Bibhas Kumar Bhunia, Nandana Bhardwaj, and Biman B. Mandal

CONTENTS

8.1 Introduction

The term *Tissue Engineering* was coined at the National Science Foundation in the late 1980s, and since then the notes of tissue engineering and regenerative medicine started reverberating in the entire world. It is unfolding as a significant potential alternative to address tissue and organ failure by implanting synthetic, natural, or semisynthetic tissue that are fully functional and mimic the native structure. The general approach of tissue engineering is to use biomaterials as temporary scaffolds to support and direct the growth of cells to form new tissue. However, in order to engineer complex tissues, observation of the smallest cues present in a cell's microenvironment and the extracellular matrix (ECM) is required (Atala et al., 2012).

Ocular tissues offer great opportunity to display tissue engineering possibilities in a less complex environment. Most ocular structures such as cornea, lens, retina, and vitreous are avascular; moreover, corneal and retinal structures are easy to mimic, being intrinsically simple stacked sheets of cells. Basically avascular in nature, oxygen and nutrient transfer in these tissues is mainly by diffusion, which reduces the chances of immune reaction with respect to the material used as an implant. This bonus of immune privilege provides a wider range to choose as materials and cells for developing a suitable tissue construct. More than two decades of research in tissue engineering has shown progress toward regeneration of several tissues such as skin, bone, cartilage, and myocardial tissue. Applications of tissue engineering in some of these fields have reached clinical trials and even commercialization; however, in ophthalmology progress is markedly slow. This is majorly due to the challenges of creating a tissue-engineered construct that is biocompatible, optically transparent, and mechanically strong along with obstacles of graft rejection, infection, and inflammation. Notwithstanding the tremendous medical progress in ophthalmology, prevalence of vision impairment has magnified. Thus, there is an urgent need for suitable strategies to overcome the challenges.

Vision needs light to enter through the cornea, traverse the lens and vitreous reaching the retina so that neural stimulation is sent from the brain via the optic nerve and any disturbance in this light path would results in vision loss or blindness. According to WHO, an estimated 285 million people are visually impaired worldwide of which 39 million are blind and 246 have low vision (WHO, 2012). The major causes of impaired vision being refractive errors and cataract followed by glaucoma, diabetic retinopathy, and age-related macular degeneration (AMD). With more awareness and better healthcare services, tissue engineering offers appreciable indices of success in this field. The opportunity and incentive for the development of novel implant material to treat all kinds of eye aberrations and age-related tissue deterioration is under-utilized or least explored.

With these perspectives, in this chapter, we aim to present an overview of ocular tissue engineering with recent progress, development, and major steps taken toward the generation of functional ocular tissue. This chapter deals with a variety of materials used in different formats to tissue engineer different parts of the eye from the thinnest layer of retina and cornea to the whole of lens or complete vitreous fluid replacement. Finally, we focus on recent innovations, and future prospects of ocular tissue engineering.

8.2 Anatomy and Physiology of the Eye

It is important to understand the different parts of the eye and the diseases associated with each of them before going into the intricate depth of ocular tissue engineering. The structure of the mammalian eye can be broadly divided into two regions: the extraocular region comprising parts adjacent to but outside the eyeballs and ocular region, which comprises the eyeball and the parts within it (Figure 8.1). The structures that form the extraocular region are (1) orbit, (2) extraocular muscle, (3) the conjunctiva lacrimal system, and (4) the eyelids. The major functions associated with these parts include lubrication and protection. However, the intraocular regions are more complex and can be broadly classified as (1) tunica fibrosa, which comprises the sclera and cornea, (2) tunica vasculosa, which comprises the choroid, ciliary body, and iris, (3) lens, (4) aqueous humor, (5) vitreous humor (VH), and (6) retina.

Each part of the eye has its unique function in maintaining the integrity and functionality of the organ. The orbit is a pear-shaped structure, which protects the eye from physical injuries while the eyelids are designed not only to protect, but also nourish and sustain the cornea and the anterior sclera. The extraocular muscles as the name indicates control the movement of the eye. A fine mucous membrane called conjunctiva is present in the inner lining of eyelids covering the sclera and functions to lubricate the eye with mucus and tears, along with lacrimal glands. The lacrimal glands are paired glands, which are

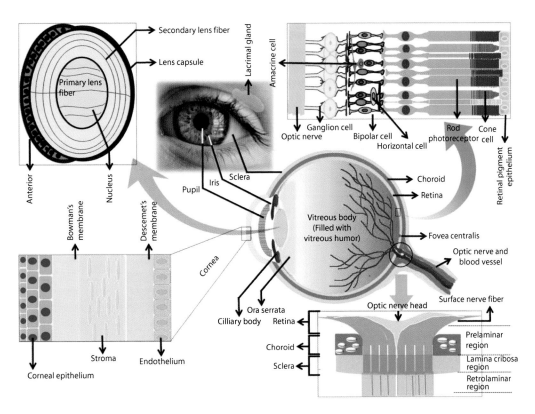

FIGURE 8.1
Detailed cross-sectional view of human eye.

present within the fossa of the frontal bone and play an important function of homeostatic maintenance for disease-free ocular surfaces through tear secretion. The sclera and cornea form the outer tunic of the eye and are protective in function. The sclera, also known as the white of the eye is a fibrous outermost layer of the eye made of mainly collagen and elastin fibers. It is a nonuniform layer ranging from 0.3 to 1 mm in thickness. Separated by corneal limbus lies the cornea, which is the front transparent part of the eye and focuses light into the eye. It acts as a barrier between the eye and the environment thereby protecting it from dryness and pathogens. It covers iris and pupil and is in continuation with the sclera. The cornea is composed of five layers (from anterior to posterior): corneal epithelium, Bowman's membrane, stroma, Descemet's membrane, and corneal endothelium. The three major layers (epithelium, stroma, and endothelium) are cellular parts while Bowman's layer and Descemet membrane are acellular. The native cornea renders three fundamental functions to the intraocular contents: protection, transmission, and refraction of light to the retina. Below the tunica fibrosa is tunica vasculosa comprising the ciliary body and iris. They are the most visible part of the eye. The ciliary body is the thickest part with iris forming the central part of the uvea. The aqueous humor is watery fluid that fills the space between cornea and lens. The lens is avascular and derives it nutrients from the aqueous humor. It is elastic and transparent and held in place by suspensory ligament or zonule. The vitreous body is a clear, transparent gel that fills the space between the retina and the lens that adheres to the retina, and function to maintain the shape and turgidity of the eye and to permit passage of light rays to the retina. The retina is the innermost layer of the eyeball, which is composed of photoreceptor cells, and is the neurosensory organ of the eye. Its outer part is protected by a tough scleral layer and blood is supplied from the choroid layer. There are as many as 10 different layers present in retina of which only the photoreceptor layer is light sensitive and takes part in photo-transduction. The optic disc (also called "the blind spot") is a part of the retina that is deprived of photoreceptors and is located at the optic papilla (zone where the optic nerve fibers leave the eye). A small pigmented area called as macula is present at the center of the retina, and has a central rich in cone cells called as fovea. This is responsible for central high resolution vision. The optic nerve extends from the optic disc and transmits visual information from the retina to the brain.

8.3 Tissue Engineering of the Ocular Parts

8.3.1 Cornea

Cornea is the front transparent part of the eye having a complex structure with three major cellular layers; an outer stratified squamous epithelium, a middle stroma with corneal keratocytes, and an inner endothelial layer (Griffith et al., 1999). Corneal transparency is a result of avascularity, regular and smooth epithelium, and the arrangement of collagen fibers with cellular components in the stroma. The endothelium is a monolayer, which is crucial in maintaining stromal hydration. The cornea and sclera meet at the limbus, which houses stem cells used to replace damaged cells in all three cellular layers. The detail will be discussed in respective sections in this chapter. Corneal blindness arising from malfunction, infection, degeneration, dystrophy, inflammation, and collateral damage during ocular surface disease alters the corneal transparency, leading to corneal scarring and ultimately blindness (Tan et al., 2012). Currently, the single common restorative treatment is corneal grafting, where damaged or diseased cornea is surgically replaced in part (lamellar keratoplasty) or whole (penetrating keratoplasty) by donated corneal tissue, called the graft. The magnitude of corneal blindness ranks cornea first among tissues transplanted worldwide with 70,000–80,000 performed annually in the United States alone, of which about 50% are penetrating keratoplasty (Eye Bank Association of America, 2014). The material used in corneal grafting can either be allogenic or synthetic. Currently, the preferred choice of allogenic tissue from donors is severely constrained by acute donor shortage and high immune rejection. An initial postimplantation below 10% rejection rate rises dramatically to 25% after 4–5 years and continues throughout the patient's lifetime (George and Larkin, 2004; Nishida et al., 2004b).

Wherever, cornea transplant is not feasible, the alternative is to use artificial cornea, through the procedure called keratoprosthesis. Although many artificial corneas (keratoprosthesis) have been developed, only four are in commercial use: the Boston keratoprosthesis (BKpro), osteo-odonto-keratoprosthesis, alphaCor, and the keraKlear. The BKpro is the most commonly used artificial cornea, and is of two main types: type I BKpro (more commonly used) and the type II BKpro (used in severe cases). The BKpro is made of poly(methyl methacrylate) (PMMA), a plastic that allows for excellent tissue tolerance and has excellent optical properties (Al Arfaj, 2015). This alternate procedure of keratoprosthesis is also affected by relatively high host rejection rate. In this chapter, we will discuss the various strategies and approaches adopted in corneal tissue engineering to formulate a construct, which is a viable native cornea equivalent.

The cornea demands effective and compatible techniques to construct its constituent cell types (epithelial, keratocyte, and endothelial) and main functional locus (highly organized, central complex stromal ECM). The challenges in creating successful corneal constructs are being addressed through state-of-the-art expertise in cellular behavior and matrix structure. Accordingly, tissue engineering uses the following two main strategies: (1) cell-based approach, where cells are manipulated before transplanting to the host and (2) scaffold-based approach, where an ECM is developed to mimic *in vivo* conditions.

8.3.1.1 Cell-Based Approach

The first crucial step in reconstructing a tissue by engineering is isolation and culture of high-quality cells, which defines the quality of the engineered construct. The cell source should provide cells with extensive proliferation properties and appropriate differentiation abilities making self-renewable stem cells an ideal cell source. Corneal stem cells and progenitor cells already committed to a cell lineage may be more suitable because they differentiate to produce only the tissue of origin unlike the multiple cell lineages from multipotent stem cells. Once the appropriate source of stem cells has been located, isolation and culture under suitable conditions is vital to maintain its functional and regenerative capacities.

8.3.1.1.1 Corneal Epithelium Cells

The corneal epithelium is an area of persistent cell renewal and regeneration with continuous sloughing from the uppermost layer surface and vital replacement by cell proliferation limited to basal cells (Hanna and O'Brien, 1960). Only cells in contact with the basement membrane retain mitotic ability while cells displaced into the supra-basal layers become postmitotic losing capability for cell division (Lavker et al., 1991). Several studies have shown that the limbal region of the cornea is rich in corneal epithelial stem cells (Kruse, 1994). Limbal cells exhibit better growth, longer lifetime, and higher proliferative potential in culture compared to cells from central cornea (Ebrahimi et al., 2009). The first clinical success of using cultured limbal stem cells (LSCs) was reported in 1997 in two patients with complete loss of corneal limbal epithelium of one eye (Pellegrini et al., 1997). Cells were isolated from a small limbus biopsy of the healthy eye and cultured for 19 days. The sheets stained positive for cytokeratin 3, a specific marker of corneal lineage (Schermer et al., 1986) following which they were released from the culture plastic using protease Dispase II and transplanted into the affected eye of the patients. On receiving graft, both patients developed a stable and transparent corneal epithelium without vascularization. Although this attempt was a success, the area that needed immediate attention was use of proteases to remove cultured sheets. Enzymes can disrupt tight cell junctions and the form ECM proteins, thus severely compromising the cell adhesion property of the cultured sheets. Although protective, postoperational soft contact lenses guard epithelial cell sheets from shearing action of eyelids during blinking; the high probability of easy cell sloughing from poor adherence and integration in the exposed corneal surface cannot be ruled out. Therefore, new culture techniques without the use of enzymes were investigated. Temperature responsive polymer surfaces showed promising results for construction of epithelial cell sheets, without the use of any enzyme (Nishida et al., 2004a). The study used a polymer poly(N-isoproplyacrylamide) (PNIPA), which is hydrophobic at 37°C and facilitates cell attachment and proliferation. When temperature is lowered to 20°C, the polymer becomes hydrophilic and results in rapid expansion that leads to cell detachment. Therefore, this method allows harvesting intact sheets of cultured cells with deposited ECM differing from enzymatic methods (Yang et al., 2006).

8.3.1.1.2 Corneal Stromal Keratocytes

Corneal keratocytes (fibroblasts) are mesenchymal-derived cells (neural crest origin) of the corneal stroma that have a slow turnover rate. These cells are sparsely distributed in the stroma and are interconnected through their own dendritic processes (Müller et al., 1995). On replication, corneal keratocytes readily differentiate into fibroblasts, losing their phenotype and native morphology, hindering their capacity to secrete transparent connective tissue (Long et al., 2000). Originally it was assumed that fibroblastic transformation was irreversible, but recently early passage stromal cells with the capacity to re-express differentiated characteristics, have been observed (Ren et al., 2008). Currently, focus has shifted to the potential of stem cells derived from bone marrow, as certain specific stem cells of the stroma, called the "wandering cells" are bone marrow derived (Nakamura et al., 2001). In addition, adult stroma also contains other cell types that express stem cell markers (Pax6 gene—expressed in early development by ocular precursor cells) and have the potential to divide extensively, generate adult keratocytes thereby maintain the cellular pool (Du et al., 2005). An interesting behavior of keratocytes is the tendency of its subpopulation to undergo apoptosis, following injury (Wilson et al., 2003). In case of corneal epithelium injury, the epithelial cells are scraped off the outer surface of the cornea with an intact underlying basement membrane. In such a situation, the keratocytes immediately underneath the basement membrane undergo apoptosis. Shortly thereafter, the dead cells are replaced by division of adjacent cells. This apoptotic behavior of keratocytes is a benign response that must have originated to protect the cornea from further inflammation and subsequently the loss of corneal transparency.

8.3.1.1.3 Corneal Endothelium Cells

In a native cornea, the primary task of endothelium is to pump excess fluid leaked from inside of the eye, out of the stroma (Maurice, 1957). In the absence of this pumping action, the stroma would swell and turn opaque. A perfect balance between the fluid moving in and out of the cornea is very essential for a healthy eye. As the endothelial cells do not have the capacity to regenerate, their excessive destruction can result in corneal edema and blindness. The central and peripheral corneal endothelial cells, in spite of retaining the proliferative potency, do not multiply *in vivo* (Konomi et al., 2005). However, some researchers indicate the peripheral area to be more favorable (Mimura and Joyce, 2006). Sphere-forming assays have been used to isolate human corneal endothelial progenitor cells (Yamagami et al., 2007). Peripheral cells formed a higher number of spheres. These studies attested that the peripheral region (same as in epithelial cells) is the best anatomic site to isolate corneal endothelial cells for tissue reconstruction.

However, temperature responsive culture surfaces have been exploited to engineer endothelial cell sheet. The resulting cell morphology, cellular interconnections, and the monolayer architecture have been found to mimic the natural corneal endothelium (Sumide et al., 2006).

8.3.1.2 Scaffold-Based Approach

The other major approach is to design a substrate, suitable for cell growth. Recent interest in engineering cornea equivalents has generated a number of biomaterials for regeneration of the three corneal layers, which will be discussed here.

8.3.1.2.1 Corneal Epithelium

Amniotic membrane (AM) is the innermost layer of fetal membranes and is widely used substrate for corneal reconstruction. AM acts as antimicrobial barrier and subdues both inflammation and scarring (Tosi et al., 2005). The successful transplantation of human AM to the damaged cornea of rabbit has been reported (Kim and Tsenq, 1995). The use of AM as a cell carrier was advantageous in improved handling of the constructs, but clinically disadvantageous due to development of severe eye threatening complications in patients after AM transplantation (Schechter et al., 2005). Therefore, various other methods to culture epithelial sheets without a carrier were investigated.

The continued search for a suitable scaffold that is biocompatible, transparent, and mechanically stable led to the exploration of many natural and synthetic polymers (SPs). Collagen, a natural protein has become a widely used biomaterial. Humans have as many as 22 types of collagens of which type I collagen is the major component of human cornea. Collagen is fabricated into sheets of variable thickness, either in its native fibrillar form or after denaturation (Cen et al., 2008). The collagen scaffold provides environment that mimic the physiological conditions for cell growth and proliferation (Nakayasu et al., 1986). Collagen as a natural polymer can promote cell adhesion and proliferation superior to SPs. Orwin et al. cultured human epithelial cells on collagen sponges (pore size of 0.1 mm). H&E staining showed that epithelial cells form a monolayer of cells on the sponge surface. Scanning electron microscope (SEM) images of the surface in these cultures showed that the cells have migrated from the center to the entire peripheral area. Coculturing epithelial cells with endothelial cells showed an increment in epithelial cell layers on sponge surface as compared to culturing epithelial cells only. Histological studies of these cultures showed that within 14 days of culture, three to four layers of epithelial cells developed covering the entire surface of the sponge (Orwin and Hubel, 2000). To meet the requirements such as increased functionality and mechanical properties and mimicking the natural ECM conditions; collagen was blended with glycosaminoglycan (GAG) and chondroitin sulfate (CS) using 1-ethyl-3-(3-dimethyl aminopropyl) carbodiimide (EDC) as coupling reagent. The sectioning results showed a thin, differentiated, and stratified layer on the surface. The immunohistochemical affinities were confirmed by positive cytokeratin 3 staining for corneal epithelium and collagen type IV-positive staining for basal lamina deposition (Vrana et al., 2008). In another fabrication technique, human corneal limbal epithelial cells were encapsulated in collagen hydrogels to form stratified epithelial layers (Mi et al., 2010). Unfortunately, collagen gels have reduced mechanical properties and show rapid degradation *in vivo*. Various cross-linking reagents were explored to enhance the strength of collagen gels. Doillon et al. investigated the properties of type I collagen in combination with CS cross-linked with various concentrations of glutaraldehyde (0%–0.08%); further treated with a glycine to reduce the cytotoxic effects of glutaraldehyde (Doillon et al., 2003). The results showed that cross-linking strengthened the matrix and concurrently permitted cell growth with addition of CS increasing transparency. This suitability of exogenous collagen in ophthalmology is handicapped by antigenic and immunogenic response *in vivo* (Lynn et al., 2004) due to its helical structure along with central and terminal amino acid sequences.

Fibrin, a combination of fibrinogen and thrombin is another common protein material useful in synthesizing a gel, which physiologically resembles human blood clots. Their ability to be isolated from autologous plasma makes it an ideal tissue engineering material. Fibrin gel was used as a scaffold material for the growth of corneal epithelium (Han et al., 2002). The suspended cells showed proliferation in the gel and developed confluence colonies in 15 days of culture. Immunostaining gels for keratin 3 (AE5) and keratin 19 showed positive response indicating differentiation along the corneal epithelium lineage. Grafting of cultured autologous limbal cells on fibrin gels showed repair of the corneal epithelium (Talbot et al., 2006).

Chitin is the hallmark polysaccharide of crustacean-exoskeleton and fungal cell wall. Deacetylation of chitin generates chitosan, a linear polysaccharide with the building blocks of β-(1-4)-linked D-glucosamine and N-acetyl-D-glucosamine. The outstanding properties of biocompatibility and biodegradability of chitosan have conferred a special niche to it in the domain of regenerative medicine. These features are attributed to the primary amines in its backbone. In the quest for corneal tissue engineering, hydroxypropyl cellulose, collagen, polycaprolactone (PCL), and elastin blends have been fabricated with chitosan (Grolik et al., 2012). A synergy of properties often emanates as a consequence of blending different polymers. A complex of collagen–chitosan–sodium hyaluronate (Col–Chi–NaHA) has been used as a substrate for culturing cells (Chen et al., 2005). The results showed that this complex is biocompatible, biodegradable, and suitable substrate for the culture of rabbit corneal epithelial cells, stromal keratocytes, and endothelial cells. Chitosan films are transparent, strong, and have high water absorption ability. However, much research is to be done in terms of their properties and scaffolds formulation.

Silk fibroin is a widely studied protein polymer obtained from the cocoon of the domesticated silk worm *Bombyx mori* (Altman et al., 2003). Silk fibroin as a biomaterial has remarkable properties such as biocompatibility, transparency, tunable biodegradability, aqueous processing, robust mechanical properties, and ability to be fabricated into film, scaffold, hydrogels, etc. (Gil et al., 2010). Silk films support cellular attachment and proliferation producing results similar to tissue culture plastic (Lawrence et al., 2009). In addition, patterned silk film surfaces promote cell growth directionality and the orientation of their ECM (Gupta et al., 2007). Transparency of silk films has also recently been established over the full range of optical wavelengths (Perry et al., 2008).

Culturing of human epithelial cell on silk and subsequent functional organization has instigated tremendous research interest. In this context, the topographical influence of silk film on the attachment, proliferation, and growth of human epithelial cell has been documented (Lawrence et al., 2012a). Optimal contact guidance could be exploited for dictating the migration of epithelial cell in a collective manner or the direction of tissue epithelialization on silk surfaces (Lawrence et al., 2012b). In a recent study, a membrane was fabricated with a blend of silk fibroin and poly(ethylene glycol) (PEG) and was further cross-linked with genipin (Suzuki et al., 2015). The membrane was used to culture human corneal epithelial cell line and primary cultures of human limbal epithelial cells. The results showed that the addition of PEG had substantial effect on certain structural properties of the membrane but not very effective as cell growth substratum. Also, the cross-linking with genipin did not improve the mechanical properties significantly. Therefore, although the unique properties of silk make it a promising substrate for corneal wound repair, much research is to be done toward producing a fully functional construct.

Gelatin is obtained by hydrolysis of collagen. It has various advantages, when compared to the widely used collagen, including lower immunogenicity (de la Mata et al., 2013), better water solubility, and gelation transition at 30°C (Zhu et al., 2006). Gelatin can be cross-linked with other materials thereby altering its mechanical and biochemical properties. In one study, gelatin was blended with chitosan and cross-linked with glutaraldehyde to be further reduced with sodium borohydride (de la Mata et al., 2013). In comparison to tissue culture plate, the limbal epithelial stem cells maintained a more stem-like phenotype at 20:80 (chitosan:gelatin) optimal ratio.

8.3.1.2.2 Corneal Stroma

Tissue engineering of corneal stroma is challenging due to its requirements in assembling a fibrous ECM with sporadically populated keratocytes and nerve fibers, into a transparent and mechanically strong construct (Mimura et al., 2011). SPs have been used for corneal stromal substrate due of their tunable mechanical properties and ability to be processed into nanosized fiber forms for organization and differentiation of stromal cells. Human stromal stem cells, when cultured on poly(ester urethane) urea substratum, differentiated toward keratocyte lineages (Wu et al., 2013), an indication of its potential in engineering stroma, but is limited by its low transparency. The amalgamation of synthetic and natural materials showed better transparency and other biological responses. Hydrogels and films of chitosan blended with PEG and polylactic acid (PLA) nanofibers grouped with type I collagen exhibited improved optical, mechanical, and biological properties, when compared to synthetic fibers alone (Ozcelik et al., 2013). Encapsulating cells using type I collagen have been reported to have additive advantage as it is an integral part of stroma (Ghezzi et al., 2011). However, certain drawbacks such as degradation, relatively poor mechanical properties, and liability to cell-mediated remodeling led to the use of chemical cross-linkers with type I collagen for stromal regeneration (Duncan et al., 2010). Alternatively, electrospun nanofibers of type I collagen have shown great promise in spatial guidance to fibroblasts but the construct showed optical limitations (Phu et al., 2010).

Acellular matrices are ideal implants for donors and suitable scaffolds for tissue engineering (Zhou et al., 2011). Acellular corneal stroma from allogeneic or autologous graft lacks lipid membrane and membrane-associated antigen, thereby suppressing undesirable immune response. Acellular corneal matrix from porcine (ACMP) has been used as a corneal cell sheet frame and transferred to rabbit corneal stroma (Xu et al., 2008). On culturing rabbit corneal cells (epithelial cells, keratocytes, and endothelial cells) on ACMP, a confluent cell sheet is reported. Thus, use of ACMP as a cell sheet frame has immense potential in this particular field.

Groove-patterned surface silk fibroin films when coupled with arginine–glycine–aspartic acid (RGD) peptide cell-receptor motif, efficiently support corneal fibroblast attachment, orientation, proliferation, increased stromal gene expression, and deposition of aligned fibrillar collagen (Lawrence et al., 2009). RGD-coupled silk films also improve attachment and differentiation of mesenchymal stem cells (Chen et al., 2003a). Further, Gil et al. used a RGD-coupled fibroin lamellar structure to culture human corneal fibroblasts. This lamellar structure showed integration of stromal tissue with helicoidally aligned ECM, as evident from histological studies (Figure 8.2a) (Gil et al., 2010). Keratocytes are native resident cells of the corneal stroma and are chiefly responsible for the maintenance of the transparent stroma by secretion of various matrix molecules (Long et al., 2000). The *in vitro* culture of keratocytes leads to their differentiation into corneal fibroblasts that exhibit a wound-healing phenotype and secrete disorganized ECM typically found in corneal scars (Beales et al., 1999).

Hydrogels formed by covalently linking gelatin with hydroxypropyl chitosan have also been investigated as replacement for corneal stroma (Wang et al., 2009). Further addition of CS improved the biocompatibility as shown by cell adhesion and proliferation studies. Later, Lai et al. demonstrated that increasing CS in the scaffold cultured with rabbit corneal keratocytes enhanced the total collagen and GAG production, without evoking IL-6 expression (Lai et al., 2012). However, the use of high CS reduced the level of an important biomarker of the keratocyte phenotype called keratocan.

8.3.1.2.3 Corneal Endothelium

The corneal endothelium plays a major role in maintaining corneal transparency, thickness, and hydration (Peh et al., 2011). Corneal endothelium dysfunction is the second leading cause of corneal blindness, and human corneal endothelial cells being nonregenerative

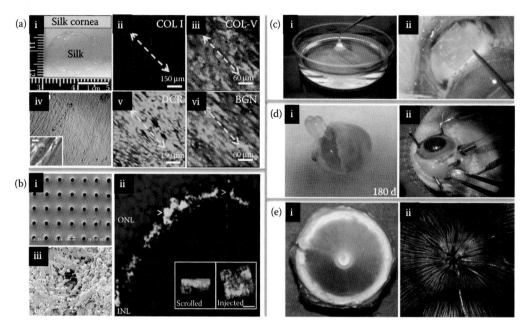

FIGURE 8.2

(a) *Corneal tissue engineering*; stacked transparent silk constructs (i), confocal image of human cornea fibroblasts (hCFs) after 6 days in culture on RGD-coupled patterned/porous silk films and immunostained with collagen type I (Col I) (ii), collagen type V (Col V) (iii), phase contrast image of hCFs grown on RGD modified patterned silk film (iv), decorin (DCR) (v), and biglycan (BGN) (vi). (Reprinted from *Biomaterials*, 31, Gil, E.S. et al., Helicoidal multi-lamellar features of RGD-functionalized silk biomaterials for corneal tissue engineering, 8953–8963, Copyright 2010, with permission from Elsevier.) (b) *Retinal tissue engineering*; SEM of PGS topology (i), RPC adhesion (iii) and attachment, proliferation, and migration of green fluorescent protein (GFP) labeled RPC cells (ii). (Reprinted from *Biomaterials*, 30, Redenti, S. et al., Engineering retinal progenitor cell and scrollable poly(glycerol-sebacate) composites for expansion and subretinal transplantation, 3405–3414, Copyright 2009, with permission from Elsevier.) (c) *Conjunctival surface reconstruction*; developed hydrated AM (i) and implantation into the eye (ii). (Reprinted from *Prog Retin Eye Res.*, Nakamura, T. et al., Ocular surface reconstruction using stem cell and tissue engineering, Copyright 2015, with permission from Elsevier.) (d) *Vitrous tissue engineering*; the FCVB-PVA hydrogel supported retina operates perfectly in the vitreous cavity after 180 days (i) its implantation into vitreous cavity (ii). (Reproduced under a Creative Commons Attribution-Non Commercial-NoDerivs 3.0 Unported License. (Adapted from Feng, S. et al. 2013., *Sci Rep.*, 3: 1838.) (e) *Tissue engineering of nerve fiber*; electrospun radial scaffold (i) and labeled neuronal b3-tubulin showing the radial direction of axons extending to the optic nerve head in rat retinal explant. (Reprinted from *Biomaterials*, 34, Kador, K.E. et al., Tissue engineering the retinal ganglion cell nerve fiber layer, 4242–4250, Copyright 2013, with permission from Elsevier.)

makes its preservation and maintenance imperative. Natural polymers such as chitosan, gelatin, type I collagen, and decellularized tissues are used in the engineering of functional endothelium (Honda et al., 2009; Liang et al., 2011; Watanabe et al., 2011). Decellularized AM along with human corneal endothelial cells were assessed in a lamellar keratoplasty model (where endothelium and part of Descemet's membrane were removed) and the replacement subsequently functioned as a corneal endothelium equivalent (Fan et al., 2013). The handling and transportation of cell sheet was a major challenge. Lai et al. used endothelialized gelatin carrier for *in vivo* endothelial sheet delivery. An intact cell sheet was formed by culturing primary human corneal endothelial cells on PNIPA substrates, which was transferred to a gelatin carrier. The developed constructs were then transported to a de-endothelialized rabbit cornea and studied for 6 months. The results showed that gelatin could be used successfully for this application (Lai et al., 2006, 2007).

8.3.2 Conjunctiva

The conjunctiva, along with cornea, the limbus, and the tear film constitutes the ocular surface that protects the eye from injury, infection, and drying (Schrader et al., 2009b). It is a thin transparent mucous membrane comprising a nonkeratinized stratified epithelium (three to five cell layers thick) containing goblet cells and a vascularized stroma. The conjunctival surface is mainly divided into three regions: bulbar (covering the eye surface), palpebral (lining the under surface of eyelids), and a middle forniceal region. The conjunctival epithelium consists of a population of goblet and nongoblet epithelial cells. The goblet cells produce mucins, which is vital for the tear film. The limbal epithelium physically separates the corneal epithelium and the conjunctival epithelium and acts as a barrier between the central clear avascular cornea and the peripheral opaque vascularized conjunctiva. Also, the limbal epithelium contains the LSCs, which are essential for regeneration of corneal epithelium (Ahmad et al., 2006). The conjunctival stroma provides a mechanically stable and elastic matrix for the conjunctival epithelium. In addition, it contains organized lymphoid tissue (conjunctiva-associated lymphoid tissue), which together with lacrimal gland and efferent tear duct system form part of the antimicrobial defense of the outer eye surface (Knop and Knop, 2003; Paulsen, 2008). The conjunctival epithelium cells have a rapid turnover and its stem cells are believed to be present within the tissue (Lavker and Sun, 2003). The exact location of conjunctival stem cells is debated, but they are thought to be distributed at various locations including the limbus (Pe'er et al., 1996), fornix (Wei et al., 1995), bulbar conjunctiva (Pellegrini et al., 1999), palpebral conjunctiva (Chen et al., 2003b), and mucocutaneous junction on the eyelid margin (Wirtschafter et al., 1999). On further investigation, when bovine conjunctival epithelial cells were cultured on a corneal basement membrane, there was expression of corneal-specific keratins (Kawasaki et al., 2006). Further, grafting of conjunctival epithelial cells in rabbits showed expression of corneal CK-3/12, which is a differentiation marker expressed by central corneal epithelium but excluded from LSCs (Tanioka et al., 2006). The results indicate the possibility of interchanging ability of human conjunctival and limbal epithelia, and holds great promise for tissue-engineered alternatives that may be used in the treatment of conjunctival disorders.

The conjunctiva secretes the mucin component of the tear film, forms a mechanical barrier against pathogens and contributes to the immune defense of the eye surface. The conjunctival epithelia itself is susceptible to a varied range of diseases from injuries such as chemical burns to inflammatory diseases including mucous membrane pemphigoid and Stevens–Johnson syndrome, which results in visual impairment. The prolonged inflammation results in depletion of the limbal epithelial stem cells, leading to corneal conjunctivalization and neovascularization, in growth of subepithelial fibrous tissue and stromal scarring (Jhagta and Jain, 2015). Current treatment methods include conjunctival autografting, which has been used successfully to cover small conjunctival defects (Vastine et al., 1982). The drawbacks of autografting method include its size limitation and possibilities of occurrence of autoimmune-mediated inflammations, such as Stevens–Johnson syndrome or ocular cicatricial pemphigoid. There are different treatment methods, which are used as a therapy for LSC deficiency (LSCD) (He and Yiu, 2014). However, there are limited approaches for developing conjunctival epithelial constructs for scarred conjunctival diseases (Ang et al., 2010). This demands need to develop other alternative techniques, which are easy to perform with good functional results and also support the functional anatomy of the conjunctiva.

An ideal conjunctival substitute construct should be a thin, biocompatible, stable, and elastic matrix. Various materials ranging from natural biopolymers to synthetic matrices have been proposed for corneal surface transplantation and could possibly be adapted for conjunctival reconstruction strategies. The use of synthetic matrices composed of fibrin, keratin, silk fibroin, collagen, and poly(lactide-*co*-glycolide) (PLGA) are briefly discussed here as a potential scaffold material. So far, the most widely accepted substitute for the optimization of culture and transfer of epithelium onto the eye is human AM (Selvam et al., 2006). It promotes rapid epithelialization, reduces inflammation and vascularization, and concomitantly suppresses fibrosis (Shimazaki et al., 1997). AM has been successfully used as a substrate in ocular surface reconstruction (Nakamura et al., 2015) (Figure 8.2c). However, the limited supply of membranes, cost, and standardization in the preparation of AM needs to be addressed. Recently, keratin films fabricated from human hair keratin have been utilized as an interesting alternative, and supported cellular attachment and proliferation (Reichl et al., 2011). The resultant film was found to be stronger and transparent as compared to AM. In addition, the keratin films supported similar cellular behavior like AM. Thus, keratin films maybe a promising alternative for conjunctival reconstruction.

There are several treatment approaches available for LSCD. Limbal epithelium derived stem cells were cultured onto a fibrin substrate for treatment (Rama et al., 2001). Within a month, the corneal surface was covered by a transparent normal looking epithelium with improved visual acuity. Also, the transparency of the cornea was maintained during the observation period of 14 months along with further improvement in visual acuity. These promising results are compromised by bovine serum and animal feeder cells used for confluence of oral mucosal cells. Recently, research has been focused on growth of corneal epithelial cells under serum-free conditions. The use of acrylic acid polymer-coated surfaces has been successful as a dermal epithelial cell culture substrate in serum-free settings (Bullock et al., 2006). In one study, researchers used an acrylic acid plasma polymerized coated contact lens as a carrier for limbal epithelial cells, which are grown directly on the surface of contact lens (Deshpande et al., 2009). This method provided a suitable carrier and also a culture surface for cells of the eye.

Later, the use of some acellular polymers was also investigated as matrix substitution and to address conjunctival scarring. Severe conjunctival scarring and contraction is a major problem of chronic inflammatory ocular surface disease. Hsu et al. studied the use of collagen-GAG (CG) copolymer matrix. The porous matrix of 8 mm diameter full thickness was grafted into the conjunctival wounds in a rabbit model. Fornix depth was measured regularly at an interval of 7 days up to a month and compared to an ungrafted full thickness wound on the same eye. In comparison to an ungrafted group, the presence of the CG copolymer reduced fornix shortening significantly (Hsu et al., 2000). This method may be useful in small conjunctival defects. However, it lacked an epithelium and took 14 days to epithelialize compared to 7 days for an ungrafted wound and unviable in clinical situations, which require donor epithelium. In addition, the elasticity and degradability of the graft needs to be further investigated.

In another scaffold-based approach, porous biodegradable PLGA scaffolds for conjunctival tissue regeneration were fabricated using particulate-leaching method and was further modified with collagen type I, hyaluronic acid (HA), and human AM (Lee et al., 2003). The growth of epithelial cells and stromal fibroblasts on scaffolds was assessed. All the modified PLGA scaffolds demonstrated enhanced cell adhesion and proliferation as compared to PLGA untreated scaffolds. The results showed that the modified PLGA graft may be used to repair damaged conjunctival tissue with less scar formation and contraction.

Further, silk fibroin was also investigated for its capacity to function as a substratum for the attachment and growth of corneal stem/progenitor cells harvested from the corneoscleral limbus of donor human corneal tissue (Chirila et al., 2007). The human limbal epithelial cells were seeded and cultured onto fibroin membranes. Post 5 days of culture, cells showed high density of attachment and proliferation, making it a suitable substratum for repairing conjunctiva.

Recently, vitrified collagen membranes for the culture of conjunctival epithelial cells were developed (Zhou et al., 2014). The gel produced by the vitrification of collagen had superior mechanical and optical properties, with its unique fibrillar structure supporting the growth and phenotype of conjunctival epithelial cell. Further, grafting in a rabbit, it enhanced conjunctival regeneration with rapid re-epithelization and adequate repopulation of goblet cells as shown by gene expression studies and histological staining. The obtained results demonstrated the potential of vitrified collagen as a carrier for epithelial cell transplantation for the reconstruction of damaged conjunctiva. All the above-mentioned substrates have potential advantages and disadvantages therefore; further careful investigation is again needed before treating patients with severe conjunctival dysfunction using these substrates.

8.3.3 Lacrimal Gland

The lacrimal gland is an exocrine tubuloalveolar gland, which is composed of small lobules made up of many fine tubules. This gland lies in the superior lateral corner of the orbit just behind the orbital rim within the lacrimal fossa of the frontal bone. Each tubule of the gland is composed of a layer of cylindrical cells, which outline the lumen and a layer of flat basal cells (myoepithelial) lying on a basement membrane. Along with the main lacrimal gland, the small accessory lacrimal glands of Krause and Wolfring helps in secretion of aqueous tears, consisting of water and various tear proteins such as lactoferrin. The tear films afford functional support that includes moisturizing and antimicrobial activity, thereby protecting the epithelial surface and visual function (Sweeney et al., 2013). Tear secretion by the lacrimal glands is essential for maintaining the physiological function and homeostasis of the ocular surface microenvironment. The decline in the quality or quantity of tears causes a chronic condition called keratoconjunctivitis sicca, also known as dry eye syndrome (DES). DES arises due to lacrimal gland dysfunction resulting from systemic diseases and environmental exposures such as Sjogren's syndrome and ocular cicatricial pemphigoid (Mantelli et al., 2013). The symptoms of DES include damage of ocular surface epithelial causing ocular discomfort and significant loss of vision. Currently, therapies such as artificial tear solutions are palliative and are not a complete substitute for normal tear complexes, which contain water, salts, hydrocarbons, lipids, and proteins (Messmer, 2015). Therefore, an alternative therapeutic approach using regenerative medicine and tissue engineering is required to treat DES and restore the function of lacrimal gland.

Transplantation of the lacrimal gland is challenging due to the short ischemia time of the tissue (<6 h). Also, unavailability of suitable lacrimal gland transplant led to the use of salivary glands for treatment of dry eye (Geerling et al., 1998). However, the electrolyte and protein composition of tears and saliva differ greatly and results in persistent ocular surface disease. Therefore, engineered lacrimal gland construct may provide a suitable alternative. However, it is a challenging task and the construct must meet several criterions before treatment. Also, the construct should have sufficient functional lacrimal gland cells (acinar cells) to produce an adequate amount of tear fluid along with a suitable matrix for its delivery. The use of a progenitor cell population is very crucial for long-term success of a tissue-engineered lacrimal gland constructs.

Tissue regeneration using adult stem cells to restore lacrimal gland function is an area of intense research because of its potential clinical advantages (Purnell, 2008). Several studies on salivary and mammary glands have indicated the presence of stem/progenitor cells in these tissues (Shackleton et al., 2006; Lombaert et al., 2008). For stem cell therapy of the lacrimal glands, Zoukhri et al. showed the presence of stem/progenitor cells in murine lacrimal glands, which increased in number after interleukin-1-induced inflammation. Following inflammation, the acinar cells are lost (by apoptosis and autophagy) during gland repair and followed by an increase in the number of stem/progenitor cells and upregulation of the BMP7 pathway (Zoukhri et al., 2008). Various potential stem cells expressing markers such as c-kit, ABCG2, and ALDH1 have been found in human lacrimal gland cells (Tiwari et al., 2014).

The engineering of lacrimal gland requires two main components: differentiated cells and a scaffold to maintain the morphological and physiological properties of the cells. At present, the main cell source for a tissue-engineered lacrimal gland is lacrimal gland derived acinar cells, which are successfully isolated from species such as rabbit, rat, and also humans (Yoshino et al., 1995). Cellular morphology, proliferation, and differentiation largely depend on the cell culture conditions and the type of scaffold used.

Later, Baum et al. developed a fluid-secreting device for the construction of an artificial salivary gland. A combination of porous blind-end tubes made into a single unit was used to make the device later useful for clinical transplantation. The tubes could be made of a biocompatible, biodegradable/nonbiodegradable substrate material with two major components: an ECM component (peptides or macromolecules) to promote formation of a polarized epithelial cell monolayer and a cellular component consisting of allogeneic epithelial cells that can be genetically engineered to transport water and salt in one direction. The physiologic similarity between salivary gland and the lacrimal gland enabled the use of same strategy to develop a bioartificial lacrimal gland device (Baum et al., 1999).

In another study, Yoshino used a thin layer of Matrigel® for the proliferation and differentiation of human lacrimal gland epithelial cells (Yoshino, 2000). Matrigel is a solubilized preparation made from basement membranes isolated from the Engelbreth–Holm–Swarm (EHS) mouse sarcoma line rich in ECM molecules such as laminin, collagen IV, entactin, perlecan, proteoglycans, and nidogen along with additional growth factors (Kleinman and Martin, 2005).

Furthermore, investigating polymer as scaffold material, Selvam et al. studied the growth of purified rabbit lacrimal gland acinar cells on matrix protein-coated polymers such as silicone, collagen I, copolymers of poly-D,L-lactide-*co*-glycolide (PLGA; 85:15 and 50:50), poly-L-lactic acid (PLLA), and cell culture plastic coverslips. Monolayers of acinar cell were found on all the different types of polymeric substrates. Beta-hexosaminidase activity in the supernatant medium showed significant increases in protein secretion after stimulation with 100 µM carbachol on matrix protein-coated and uncoated polymers such as silicone, PLGA 85:15, and PLLA. The study showed PLLA to be more favorable compared to other polymers (Selvam et al., 2007).

AM is a widely used matrix, and supported adhesion, migration, and proliferation of epithelial cells in various studies. In a study by Schrader et al., they observed the growth pattern and the secretory function of lacrimal gland acinar cells on AM. The seeding of acinar cells on AM resulted in small cell clusters, which increased in size and established a coating of several cell layers in patches. The cells maintained their histotypic features for up to 28 days of culture; however, there was no notable necrosis in the center of the clusters (Schrader et al., 2007).

A three-dimensional (3D) lacrimal gland construct with acinar cells, which are not directly exposed to the ocular surface might mimic the physiological situation. In 1996, Hatfill et al. (1996) developed 3D tissue construct using rotary cell culture systems. Further, Schrader et al. used the above-mentioned system to develop spheroidal aggregates (mean diameter of 384.6 ± 111.8 μm) after 7 days. The spheroids consisted of organized acinar cell aggregates with fine granulation in their cytoplasm, which is characteristic of secreting cells; however, an apoptotic region was observed in the center of spheroids (Schrader et al., 2009a).

Recently, a bioengineered organ germ technique was developed, which involves compartmentalization of high cell density of epithelial and mesenchymal cells in a type I collagen gel matrix to reconstruct bioengineered organ germs *in vitro* (Oshima et al., 2011). Orthotropic transplantation of the bioengineered lacrimal gland germs into an adult mice bearing an extra-orbital lacrimal gland defect (a mouse model that mimics the corneal epithelial damage caused by lacrimal gland dysfunction), resulted in the development of both the bioengineered lacrimal and harderian gland germs with sufficient physiological functionality. This study supports the potential for bioengineered lacrimal gland replacement to restore lacrimal gland function (Hirayama et al., 2013).

8.3.4 Lens

Lens is a transparent biconvex structure of the eye, which refracts light to the retina along with cornea (Remington and Meyer, 2007). It is an avascular and aneural tissue composed of three main parts: lens capsule, lens epithelium, and lens fibers (Dhamodaran et al., 2014). Lens capsule is a specialized basement membrane, which encloses the lens and protects it from bacterial and viral infection (Danysh and Duncan, 2009). Major components of lens capsule are fibronectin, collagen type IV, laminin, entactin, and heparin sulfate. The component of capsule contributes to the shaping of lens (Sharma and Santhoshkumar, 2009). The lens epithelium is a simple cuboidal epithelium and is divided into two regions; the central nondividing region and the germinative (dividing) region. Cells in the dividing regions differentiate into fiber cells (Sharma and Santhoshkumar, 2009). Lens fibers form bulk of the lens and their tightly packed layers are referred to as laminae.

The transparency of lens allows light to travel through the ocular media without any impediment and reach its target (Petrash, 2013). Clear vision of eye deteriorates when the lens loses its transparency (cataract) or diminishes its ability to change shape (presbyopia) (Petrash, 2013). Cataract is the major cause of eye blindness worldwide. Studies show that there is no proven medical treatment for age-related cataract. To restore the function of lens, cataract is surgically removed and replaced with artificial intraocular lenses (IOL) (Francis et al., 1999). PMMA was the first material of choice used as IOL in the 1990s (Burk et al., 1986; Hofmeister et al., 1988). Sir Harold Ridely was the first person to implant PMMA as an IOL in 1950. Since then, various potential materials were investigated for manufacturing IOL. These materials can be divided into three groups: hydrophobic acrylics (phenylethylmethacrylate and phenylethylacrylate), hydrophilic acrylics (predominantly polyhydroxyethylmethacrylate (pHEMA), and silicone (polydimethylsiloxane) (Lace et al., 2015). The correction of cataract surgically has been successful to some extent. However, the residues of lens epithelium postsurgery grow on the capsule causing haziness and opacification, ultimately leading to posterior capsule opacification (PCO) (Karamichos,

2015). Therefore, patients need to come back for second surgery in order to remove the PCO. Several studies have shown that the residue of lens epithelial cells remaining after cataract surgery can differentiate into fiber cells, only if integrity of the capsule is maintained (Milliot, 1872; Gwon et al., 1993). Further, Gwon et al. had reported the regeneration of crystalline lens by biodegradable scaffolds (Gwon and Gruber, 2010). Cross-linked HA or cohesive HA, SP, and HA/SP were separately injected into capsule bags (which was used to seal capsulotomy) to investigate regeneration ability of the polymers. Lens regenerated on the HA scaffolds were spherical with excellent cortical structure and spherical nucleus with transparency. However, lens regenerated on SP scaffold were opacified while the HA/SP combination showed a mixed effect with HA surface being transparent and polymer surface being opacified. HA scaffold supported the growth of lens epithelial cells and regenerated into lens without opacification (Gwon and Gruber, 2010). Miura et al. had reported the lens regeneration by poly(vinylpyrrolidone) (PVP) hydrogel (Miura et al., 2009). PVP hydrogels injected into capsule had supported lens epithelial cells' growth, and regenerated lens was transparent for 12 months without opacification.

Few urodeles and teleost can regenerate their lens throughout their adult life (Tsonis et al., 2001). Post lensectomy of the newt eye, the pigmented dorsal iris epithelial cells undergoes dedifferentiation, proliferation, and finally redifferentiate into lens cells (Kodama and Eguchi, 1995). Studies of wolffian lens regeneration in the newt showed that only dorsal iris can regenerate into new lens, whereas this property was not showed by ventral iris (Yamada, 1977). Ito et al. (1990) had also reported that the lens regeneration was from the dorsal iris of newt. Dorsal and ventral iris cells were isolated from the singly dissociated pigment epithelial cells of iris. These cells were cultured to dedifferentiate and reaggregate. Reaggregated cells were implanted into the blastema of the forelimb in the newt to study the ability of lens regeneration. Thereafter, only dorsal cells of iris redifferentiated into lens, whereas the ventral cells showed an inhibitory effect on the lens formation (Ito et al., 1999).

Extracellular signals play an important role in lens development. It is well known that the members of fibroblast growth factors (FGF) family of protein have a crucial role in normal lens development (Lang, 1999). Hayashi et al. (2002) had reported the role of FGF *in vitro* lens regeneration from the dorsal iris cells. Dorsal and ventral iris cells cultured on cell culture dish did not show lens development even in the presence of FGF-2/4, whereas dorsal iris cells cultured on collagen gel, supplemented with 100 ng/mL of FGF 2/4 had shown depigmentation, reaggregation, and formation of lens. Three subclasses (α, b, and γ) crystallin protein was detected at different stages of lens development. Depigmentation, reaggregation, and crystallin were not seen by the ventral iris cells cultured on the collagen gel (Hayashi et al., 2002). Other factors that play an important role during lens regeneration are Hox gene (Jung et al., 1998), Prox-1 (Del Rio-Tsonis et al., 1999), retinoic acid receptors (Tsonis et al., 2000), cyclin-dependent kinases (Tsonis et al., 2004), and complement components (Kimura et al., 2003).

Pigment epithelium cells (PECs) of iris also show lens regeneration in higher species, including human (Eguchi, 1993, 1998). Tsonis et al. had reported redifferentiation of human dedifferentiated PECs (H80HrPE-6 cells) into lens on Matrigel (an ECM derived from EHS mouse sarcoma) (Tsonis et al., 2001). Under *in vitro* condition, H80HrPE-6 cells cultured on cell culture dish had shown aggregation, but they did not redifferentiated into lens cells. In contrast, H80HrPE-6 cells cultured on Matrigel had shown better redifferentiation and transparency than the cells cultured on the hard agar. Cells cultured on Matrigel had shown synthesis of crystalline protein, which is a characteristic property of lens cells. Gene expression studies also show that the Matrigel had supported the redifferentiation of human dedifferentiated PECs into lens, which can be used for *in vivo* implantation (Tsonis et al., 2001).

Hoffmann et al. had reported comparative intrinsic regeneration potential of newt dorsal iris pigment epithelial (IPE) cells versus mouse lens epithelial (MLE) cells (Hoffmann et al., 2013). Dorsal IPE cells cultured in basic medium on Matrigel had shown complete cell aggregation and lens was formed within 17 days. In contrast, MLE cells showed incomplete cell aggregation with defined-size lentoids with partial optical transparency. Complete transparent lens formation was seen by the MLE cells cultured on Matrigel in medium supplemented with basic FGF (bFGF). Fiber cells of lens formed by the dorsal IPE cells show positive αA-crystallin and lens formation by the MLE (in the presence of bFGF) had also shown the increased βA-crystallin. This study shows that an intrinsic regeneration property of lens in newt and mice varies with their supplementation of growth factors (Hoffmann et al., 2013). There is no systemic approach to study the cataract due to the lack of appropriate animal models and various limitations of human primary lens cultures. Later, Yang et al. had reported the development of *in vitro* lentoids by using human embryonic stem cells (hESCs), which can be used to study the lens formation and mechanisms of cataractogenesis (Yang et al., 2010).

8.3.5 Vitreous Humor

As discussed in earlier sections, VH is a transparent gel (Chirila and Hong, 1998), rich in HA and unbranched collagen type II fibrils (Scott, 2003), which fills the posterior cavity of the eye. The hyaluronan content in the VH is higher than the protein content and plays an integral role in maintaining the internal tension (Kummer et al., 2007) of VH by a process called Donnan swelling (Kleinberg et al., 2011). Structurally, VH is nonuniform in density and is firmly attached to the anterior retina at the vitreous base. At the base, collagen fibers penetrate the retina, attach to the basement membrane of the ciliary epithelium and peripheral retinal pigment epithelium (RPE). Several materials have been tested as substitutes for VH, each of them serving either of the main purposes as described. The implants may either be used to replace a dysfunctional VH, when opacification or when physical collapse of the original structure has occurred or they may have other applications during retinal surgery. Since, both the applications require implantation of the material within the patients' eyes it is important for them to be transparent, gel-like, viscous, and highly biocompatible (Kummer et al., 2007; Foster, 2008). The density, shear modulus, and the refractive index of the implanted materials should also be close to that of VH in order to maintain its true functionality (Kummer et al., 2007).

As hypothesized, the main goal behind vitreous tissue engineering is liquefaction (Los et al., 2003). It is not only important to maintain the structure of VH via tissue engineering, but also it is equally important that the implants separate the vitreous from the retina and destabilize the network without damaging the adjacent tissues. In order to hold retina in its place, several substitutes are used after vitrectomy, which includes gases (such as sulfur hexafluoride or n-perfluoropropane), hydrocarbons and blends of oils and hydrocarbons, and some natural polymers. Silicone oils mainly have applications during retinal surgery due to their mechanical and flow properties. They must be removed postsurgery as they may result in ocular side effects such as corneal decompression (Foster, 2008) and glaucoma. However, it is very difficult to remove the silicon oils completely. Other substitutes include poly(2-hydroxyethyl acrylate) (Chan et al., 1984), polymethyl-3,3,3-trifluoropropylsiloxane-*co*-dimethylsiloxane (Doi and Refojo, 1994), semi-fluorinated alkanes (Zeana et al., 1999), methylated collagen (Liang et al., 1998), and collagen/HA mixtures (Nakagawa et al., 1997). The other recently discovered group of vitreal substitutes are magnetic fluids (Foster, 2008). Their application is not independent but requires a magnetic buckle around the sclera. The magnetic field, which results from the band would then assist in maintaining the vitreous substitute in contact with the retinal tear that lies beneath the magnetic portion (Foster, 2008).

However, smart hydrogels have set the vitreous substitute class apart. Not only do they mimic the biofunctionality, but also respond to external physical stimulus and environment really well. Some of the hydrogels that have been under consideration so far for vitreous tissue engineering include poly(1-vinyl-2-pyrrolidone) (PVP), poly(vinyl alcohol) (PVA), and poly(acrylic acid) (PAA). PVP is the first studied polymer for vitreous replacement (Hong et al., 1998). However, opacification of vitreous, inflammation due to the presence of vacuoles and granules (Swindle-Reilly et al., 2009), and intraocular reactivity are the main issues that prevents its use alone for vitreous replacement. Many other blends with this polymer are underway in research as the material has density and viscosity similar to vitreous. PVA has good optical and rheological properties making it a suitable biomaterial for this application. Maruoka et al. added trisodium–triphosphate as a cross-linking agent to PVA. The addition of this molecule improved the material properties such as rheological characteristics and diffusion behavior when compared to PVA alone (Maruoka et al., 2006). Another blend of the polymer PVA-methacrylate (MA) has also laid its ground in vitreal tissue engineering (Cavalieri et al., 2004). This polymer contains a photo-initiator, which forms a gel network after being irradiated. The degree of gelification can be delimited by polymer concentration and light intensity. However, there is still a need of PVA-MA properties to be tested *in vitro* as well as *in vivo* to evaluate vitreous biomimicry and biocompatibility. PAA is another class of biomaterial that is highly stable, biocompatible, and presents similar density and viscosity to the vitreous. However, studies regarding its implantation are underway. Copoly(acrylamide) is a variant of PAA, which exhibits no significant ocular toxicity upon implantation as compared to the other polymers (Swindle et al., 2006). It is a clinically stable molecule with better gel properties as compared to PAA with same refractive index and viscoelastic properties of vitreous. Hydroxypropyl methylcellulose is another polymer that exhibits good physicochemical properties as well as biocompatibility (Robert et al., 1988). Different experimental polymers have been studied, varying the molecular weight (Fernandez-Vigo et al., 1990b). One of the challenges faced with this polymer is the intraocular degradation time. Researchers are working hard on that interface but as of now this product is yet not available for VH (Fernandez-Vigo et al., 1990a). Other polymers, which have been employed for vitreal tissue engineering include poly(glyceryl methacrylate) (Hogen-Esch et al., 1976), poly(2-hydroxyethyl methacrylate) (PHEMA) (Swindle et al., 2006), and poly(2-hydroxyethylacrylate) (Baino, 2011). However, each of these polymers faced some kind of biocompatibility issues resulting in inflammation or had rheological issues. There also exists report on the use of Pluronic F127 (p-F127), a thermo reversible gelatin (Davidorf et al., 1990). It could easily form a gel at 21°C but on implantation as a biomaterial it exhibited severe retinal toxicity retarding its suitability for clinical use.

With respect to implants, bioengineering has thrown some light on the use of artificial capsular bodies made by Gao and coworkers. These capsular bodies were made out of silicone rubber elastomer and filled with a saline solution, silicone oil and were controlled using a valve system (Gao et al., 2008). This foldable capsular vitreous body (FCVB) was biocompatible and offered good optical, mechanical, and rheological properties. It has been found to be effective as a vitreous substitute to treat severe retinal detachment. Recently, researchers have focused on the use of PVA as a filling molecule implanted in rabbits (Feng et al., 2013). It was found that 3% concentration of PVA showed the best results in rheological, physical, and cytotoxicity tests. It was also found that using PVA in this manner would reduce its degradation time, which was earlier faced as a problem, when PVA was used as a hydrogel alone. In the PVA-FCVB rabbit implanted eyes, the structure of the retina could be maintained intact up to 90 days postsurgery. However, when the implant was placed for 180 days, retinal disorders were reported due to long-term capsule-induced mechanical pressure to the retina (Feng et al., 2013) (Figure 8.2d).

Vitreous regeneration is another recent area of investigation. The challenge to create a completely new 3D vitreous structure requires a vigorous study of the materials. In a recent research, the researchers have taken into account the controlled proliferation of hyalocytes along with specific growth factors (bFGF stimulates and transforming growth factor (TGF)-β1 inhibits) (Sommer et al., 2008) and with the properties of the material. The production of HA with related components was also evaluated (Nishitsuka et al., 2007) apart from other related biocompatibility and mechanical properties.

8.3.6 Retina

The retina consists of highly sophisticated and multilayered, light-sensitive neural tissues located at the back of the eye. It receives visual stimuli, which is converted into chemical and electrical signals and finally inferred by the brain for sight (Inoue et al., 2010; Karl and Reh, 2010). Retinitis pigmentosa (RP) and AMD are two major retina-related diseases, which involve degeneration of photoreceptor cells and normally result in clinically apparent visual loss. The estimated prevalence of AMD in the United States and other developed countries is 1 in 2000 persons. It is projected that approximately 8.7% of all blindness accounts for AMD and is predicted to affect 196 million people by 2020 globally. It is also reported that populations of European descent are more susceptible to AMD than those of Asian or African descent (Wong et al., 2014). RP is the heterogeneous group of inherited retinal disorders and more than 1.5 million patients suffer from this disorder with the prevalence of 1 in 3000–7000 individuals worldwide (Ferrari et al., 2011; Ikeda et al., 2014). Current therapies for AMD consist of photodynamic approaches, which employs photosensitizing dye verteporfin (Visudynes®, Novartis), laser photocoagulation, and some pharmacological treatments like anti-angiogenic therapy using the oligonucleotide antagonist pegaptanib (Macugens®, Eyetech Pharmaceuticals and Pfizer) (Bylsma and Guymer, 2005; Ishibashi and Group, 2013), the vascular endothelial growth factor (VEGF), antibody fragment ranibizumab (Lucentis™, Genentech), and the VEGF antibody bevacizumab (Avastin™, Genentech) (Thorell et al., 2014). In some cases like diabetic retinopathy, bioactive molecules such as advanced glycation end-product inhibitors or antioxidants are applied (Comer and Ciulla et al., 2005). The intake of diet that are rich in omega-3 fatty acids with low doses of vitamin E (400 IU/day) and vitamin A palmitate supplements (15,000 IU/day) has been suggested to be effective preventative measures for RP treatment (Berson et al., 1993, 2004). However, at best, all these therapies do not provide complete recovery and only slow down the disease progressions or may temporarily protect the photoreceptors from dying. Therefore, there is a need of a suitable approach, which can restore the lost vision by transplanting photoreceptors (Taylor et al., 2013) or replace the photoreceptor with electronic visual implants (Zrenner, 2002; Shoval et al., 2009).

In the past few decades, researchers have developed photoreceptors' replacement strategies to overcome a numbers of obstacles. Several findings suggest that the fate of the transplanted cells to integrate into nonautologous retina depends not only on developmental stage of host, but also on stage of donor cells (Van Hoffelen et al., 2003; Pearson et al.,

2010; Barber et al., 2013). In earlier studies, postmitotic photoreceptor precursor cells were used to avoid the possible threats associated with tumor formation (Arnhold et al., 2004). Moreover, restricted supply of these tissues due to ethical concern was another limiting factor. Therefore, scientists need a suitable and reproducible source of photoreceptor precursor cells, which is remunerated by stem cells.

To date, embryonic stem (ES) cells have shown promising results to generate retinal cell types. Several convincing studies have already been done to generate retinal cells from mouse, monkey, and human with or without growth factors or by genetic modifications (Lamba et al., 2009; Osakada et al., 2009). One study showed that ES cells have the abilities to self-organize and mimic the morphological development of the retina, when cultured in a 3D system (Eiraku et al., 2011). However, the introduction and utilization of induced pluripotent stem cells (iPSCs) alleviates many of the shortcomings of ES cells including its ethical concern, restricted availability, low efficiency of isolation, and potential immune rejection to nonmatched tissue (West et al., 2010). Several reports suggest that iPSCs are similar to ES cells and have the proficiency to differentiate into retinal fate. Though, there are some conflicts about its potential of retinal differentiation to retinal lineages. Several reports suggest that iPSCs are similar to ES cells and have the proficiency to differentiate into retinal fate, however, there are some conflicts about its potential of retinal differentiation to retinal lineages (Lamba et al., 2006, 2010; Hirami et al., 2009; Osakada et al., 2009). Retinal stem cells (RSCs) are another renewable cell source for retinal cell implantations. Generally, retinal stem cells are isolated from fetal or postnatal retina (Klassen et al., 2008), muller glial cells (Das et al., 2006), or from the ciliary epithelium of the retina. Ramachandran et al. (2010, 2012) showed that muller glial cells in zebrafish functioned as multipotent RSCs that respond to the lost photoreceptors. Several earlier reports showed that cilliary epithelium (CE) comprises stem-like cells that have self-renewal activity and multipotentiality, when cultured *in vitro* (Ahmad et al., 2000). However, few groups have recently questioned the full multipotentiality of CE cells (Cicero et al., 2009; Gualdoni et al., 2010), and showed that ciliary epithelial cells derived from neural retina leucine zipper (NRL)–GFP mice failed to differentiate into rod photoreceptors (Gualdoni et al., 2010).

Cellular transplantation therapy helps to restore lost vision in patients with retinal degeneration and to ensure the success of this approach; the transplanted cells must be integrated to the host. The various types of retinal tissues that are grafted include RPE cells for AMD treatment (Alqvere, 1996; Alqvere et al., 1998) and neural retinal cells for RP patients (Das et al., 1999). Although neural retinal cells have the capability to differentiate into different types of cells of retina, they however fail to undergo complete differentiation. Young et al. showed that retinal progenitor cells (RPCs) are not only predisposed to differentiate into retinal neurons, but also exhibited integrative abilities similar to those of brain-derived stem cells (Klassen et al., 2004). Therefore, RPCs have advantage over the neural retinal cells for photoreceptor replacement therapy in retinal diseases. In this approach, cells suspension prepared in saline is typically, delivered by injection into the subretinal space or into the vitreous cavity (Young, 2005). However, this technique suffers from limitations such as improper localization of cells, cellular aggregation, loss of cellular viability, and leakage of cells from injection site due to shearing force at the time of injection. On the other hand, delivering of cells with scaffolds, hydrogel, or membrane-based retinal sheet reduces these formidable challenges and restores damaged retina. The polymers, which are being utilized for subretinal delivery purposes should be biocompatible, nonimmunogenic, and biodegradable so that it slowly disintegrates through hydrolysis without altering the extracellular milieu of retina (Redenti et al., 2009). In addition, the fabricated scaffolds must be thin (<50 µm), porous, and robust enough to allow surgical manipulation. Several polymers possess these suitable/ideal properties and many of them are Food and Drug Administration (FDA) approved for therapy. These polymers according to their origin include natural (e.g., collagen and silk) or synthetic (e.g., PLLA, poly(lactic-*co*-glycolic acid) (PLGA), PCL, and poly(glycerol-sebacate) (PGS)), which will be discussed below.

The very first step in this approach is to establish the biocompatibility of these biomaterials to RPC *in vitro* and in subretinal space. In earlier studies, researchers have utilized an established RPC line, D407, cultured on copolymers made of PLLA and PLGA. Although immortal cell line shows morphological similarities to *in vivo* tissues, stem cell-based approach more closely resembles RPCs. Later, hESCs were cultured on PLGA and parylene (a nonbiodegradable polymer), which supported in pigmentation and production of mature RPCs markers such as ZO-1, RPE65 and pigment epithelium-derived factor (PEDF), bestophin, and RDH5 (Liu et al., 2011). Similarly, some researchers focused on photoreceptor cell replacement using PLLA/PLGA copolymers. Although, these copolymers have helped in proliferation of RPCs, photoreceptor-specific expression was not observed (Lavik et al., 2005). Further, Ng et al. investigated PLGA composite graft with RPCs to generate immune-privilege site (Ng et al., 2007). Recently, one novel strategy in the field of ophthalmology using PLGA is the microencapsulation of glial cell line-derived neurotrophic factor with photoreceptors or retinal ganglion cells (RGCs) in glaucoma model (Checa-Casalengua et al., 2011). Later, Yao et al. showed that the incorporation of matrix metalloproteinase 2 in PLGA microsphere facilitated inhibitory barrier removal, retinal degeneration, and enhanced cell integration (Yao et al., 2011).

Further, Redenti et al. (2009) introduced microfabricated PGS scaffold (45 µm thick) using a replica molding technique, for the delivery of retinal stem–progenitor cells (RSPCs) to the subretinal space and reported similarity in mechanical properties of PGS with retinal tissue (Figure 8.2b). The superiority of PGS over PLA/PLGA on the basis of biodegradability and biocompatibility has seen ample documentation (Wang et al., 2002, 2003; Sundback et al., 2005) and also RSPCs showed enhanced attachment, proliferation, and migration on this scaffold. Further, the upregulation of glial fibrillary acidic protein and downregulation of immature markers (e.g., Pax6, Hes1, and Sox2) indicated a trend toward differentiation into RPCs (Neeley et al., 2008). In other study, one specially designed construct with PCL has been shown to support the RPC proliferation, migration, and integration to the host retina. This construct incorporated both short (2.5 µm) and long (25 µm) nanowires projecting from a thin base (5 µm), representing the thinnest polymer used in retinal transplantation (Redenti et al., 2008). Later, PCL combined with other biomaterials like chitosan was considered to produce chitosan-graft-poly(ε-caprolactone)/PCL (CS-PCL/PCL) by electrospinning (Chen et al., 2011). This hybrid scaffold system was further investigated for proliferation and differentiation of mice RPCs into retinal neuron cells. Therefore, characteristic features such as biocompatibility (VandeVord et al., 2002) and muco-adhesiveness of chitosan (He et al., 1998) make it an attractive delivery vehicle in the field of ophthalmology. Although, there are certain limitations on stability issues, researchers have developed methods like cross-linking with glutaraldehye or ginipin to overcome this problem (Lai and Li, 2010).

Intact sheet transplantation is another approach for subretinal cell delivery in addition to hydrogel or scaffold-based systems. It has been reported that retinal sheet transplantation overcomes the above-mentioned limitations of saline-based cell injection into subretinal space (Aramant and Seiler, 2002). However, a few drawbacks like improper development of outer segments or increased formation of rosettes are associated with this strategy. Scientists have later developed some procedures to overcome these problems. One of the examples includes use of modified gelatin membrane as delivery carriers for retinal sheets. Later, Lai et al. demonstrated that EDC cross-linked gelatin membrane showed better degradation profile and cytocompatibility in comparison with glutaraldehyde-treated membrane (Lai and Li, 2010). Similarly, biopolymer-coated polyimide membrane has been shown to support hESCs proliferation and its differentiation toward RPCs (Subrizi et al., 2012). In other study, Tao et al. designed the ultrathin (6 µm) micromachined poly(methyl methacrylate) or PMMA scaffolds that provided a suitable cyto-architectural environment for retinal tissue engineering and transplantation (Tao et al., 2007).

Collagen is another well-known biomaterial used in tissue engineering and drug delivery applications and is FDA approved. Lu et al. reported for the first time, the usage of collagen film (5 µm thick) as Bruch's membrane alternate for long-term sustainable growth of RPE cells (Lu et al., 2007). Similarly, *B. mori* silk fibroin films (3 µm thick) have also been used for targeted cell delivery in prosthesis of Bruch's membrane (Shadforth et al., 2012).

Hydrogel-based regenerative strategies for retinal degenerative diseases have overcome the barriers of cell survival and integration associated with subretinal delivery on solid scaffolds (Neeley et al., 2008; Redenti et al., 2008, 2009). The modulus of solid scaffolds does not match that of the retina and also lack the flexibility essential for subretinal delivery across the damaged retina (Tomita et al., 2005). Hydrogel-based approaches have advantages over saline-based cell delivery system, which leads to cell death or leakage and migration from the site of injection (Ballios et al., 2010). Further, evidences also suggest that this transient encapsulation of cells in hydrogels support their survival under adverse conditions within the diseased or damaged host target organs (Karoubi et al., 2009; Mayfield et al., 2014).

Further, Ballios et al. developed hyaluronan and methylcellulose (HAMC)-based cell delivery vehicle, which exhibited physical and biological properties ideal for delivery to the subretinal space. HAMC has been shown to support the retinal RPCs survival and proliferation *in vitro* and showed the biodegradability in the subretinal space over 7 days after *in vivo* transplantation. In addition, HAMC-based cell delivery system has also been reported to overcome the limitations (such as cellular aggregation and noncontiguous distribution) related to traditional saline-based cell delivery strategies (Ballios et al., 2010). A similar study showed that cell delivery with PLLA–PLGA polymer hydrogel increased the cell survival rate by 10 fold (Tomita et al., 2005). One of the recent works demonstrated the fabrication of PEG and poly(L-lysine (PLL)-based hydrogels with mechanical strength (elastic modulus, 3800–5700 kPa) similar to lamina of the retina. These hydrogel supported the survival, migration, and neurite outgrowth of RGCs and amacrine cells and provided insight for understanding neuronal integration and transplantation (Hertz et al., 2013). Recently, fibrin glue is introduced as an encapsulating material for subretinal delivery of RPCs and demonstrated enhanced adhesion, proliferation, and also differentiation of RPCs after encapsulation. Herein, the adhesion of RPCs to fibrin glue was mediated by RGD-independent mechanism (Ahmed et al., 2014).

8.3.7 Optic Nerve

The optic nerve is the second cranial nerve, which is a continuation of axons and ganglions of the retina. Each optic nerve comprises around 1 million nerve cells and connects the retina to the brain. The point from where the optic nerve begins in the retina is known as the optic disc or the optic nerve head. Glaucoma (optic neuropathy) is one of the leading causes of blindness in the world. It is well known that nerves do not regenerate once injured, therefore regenerating the damaged neuronal tissue is a tough task. The RGCs and nerve cells comprise the major part of the optic nerve and RGCs tend to direct their axons radially in the neuronal tissue (Kador et al., 2013).

Several implants have been generated to restore the functionality of the optic nerves. The idea is to maintain the functionality of the tissue by incorporating some kind of aligned material. Researchers compared the RGCs grown on electrospun scaffolds to RGCs just added to the tissue, and found that the RGCs on scaffolds maintained their axons in radial direction as the original tissue in comparison to mere addition of RGCs, which lead to the growth of axons in random directions (Kador et al., 2013) (Figure 8.2e). Further, protein-coated nanofibers or scaffolds (coated with growth factors as biological cues) and self-assembling proteins have demonstrated wider applications for axon regeneration (Chen and Rao, 2011). Incorporation of nanofibers with nanoparticles or nanospheres can help in the regeneration as well as redirection of the axon on application of magnetic field. A variety of biodegradable materials, which have been utilized to fabricate these electrospun fibers include poly(lactic-*co*-glycolic acid) (PLGA), PLLA (Yang et al., 2005), and poly(L-lactide-*co*-epsilon-caprolactone) (Bhang et al., 2007). However, the electrospun fibers alone do not provide complete solution to the problem. Therefore, polymers mixed with neurotropic proteins have also been recently generated in order to regenerate growth factor encapsulated fibers. In a recent research, the researchers implanted a nanofiber composite scaffold consisting of glial-derived growth factor *in vivo* into rat sciatic nerve (Chew et al., 2007). It was found that upon incorporation of the scaffold, not only the regeneration of nerve and myelinated axons increased but also the electro-physiologic functionality of the construct was maintained.

Several other scaffolds, which have been used for transplantation, include a polymer composed of polyglycolic acid (PGA, synthetic) and chitosan (a natural material derived from the exoskeleton of crustaceans). The polymer after fabrication was coated with a recombinant neuronal adhesion protein called L1 (Doherty et al., 1995). The incorporation of the adhesion protein onto the scaffold helped in development, elongation of axons, and regeneration of nerves (Roonprapunt et al., 2003).

In addition, nonprefabricated peptides, which are self-assembled *in vivo* in hamsters to form nanofiber scaffold have been successfully employed for optic nerve regeneration. On injecting the peptides, these peptides rapidly form scaffolds facilitating in bridging the tissue gap and exhibiting the return of functional orienting movement (Ellis-Behnke et al., 2006).

8.4 Recent Developments and Future Prospects of Ocular Tissue Engineering

There have been significant developments and advancement in ocular tissue engineering approaches in recent years. Moreover, progress in regenerative medicine for cornea and corneal stem cell research provides an optimistic prospect on their utilization to replace partial or full thickness damaged and or diseased corneas (Connon, 2015; Ghezzi et al., 2015).

A variety of natural biomaterials have been developed and modified to assist in these regenerative approaches, to regenerate the cornea to different degrees, starting from epithelial, stromal, endothelial layers, to full thickness corneal tissues. The utilization of natural biomaterials for ocular tissue engineering offers potential benefits over earlier used allogenic/synthetic biomaterials for corneal tissue regeneration (Lawrence et al., 2009; Wu et al., 2014). Natural origin biomaterials derived corneal substitutes hold great promise for long-term success and are being translated to human clinical trials due to its mimicking properties like native tissues. The traditional approach for ocular tissue engineering employs top–down approach, where cells are seeded on the surface of scaffolds for regeneration of tissues. However, in corneal regeneration, which is a highly organized tissue, this approach faces difficulty in recapitulating the necessary microstructural features. Therefore, researchers have focused on bottom–up approach for regenerating cornea, where main approach includes building of microtissues with repeated functional units (Connon, 2015). Recently, researchers have utilized RGD(S) peptide amphiphiles (PAs) for coating hydrophobic surfaces of striated polytetrafluoroethylene in order to obtain a highly organized tissue, with orientation of human cornea stromal fibroblasts and subsequent accumulation of ECM similar to *in vivo* conditions (Gouveia et al., 2013). Here, the PAs have been synthesized via self-assembly and form a supramolecular structure with geometrically defined nanoscale patterns, which is not possible to achieve with intact matrix macromolecules (Lutolf and Hubbell, 2005; Hamley, 2011).

However, with all the advancements in the field of biomaterials, corneal endothelial cell properties and current surgical procedures restricts the success of ocular tissue engineering strategies (Teichmann et al., 2013). Thus, regenerative medicine for cornea offers an attractive and promising approach for patients with corneal diseases. This approach has shown enormous promise in ocular tissue engineering and offers a paradigm shift from conventional corneal transplantation strategies to stem cell-based therapeutic reconstruction. Also, ophthalmology is the only field of medical science so far, which has gained maximum from regenerative medicine due to its accessibility, ease of follow-up, and immune-privileged nature. Apart from bone marrow transfusion, the other cell-based transplantation technique approved for patient care is LSC transplantation (Oie and Nishida, 2013; Dhamodaran et al., 2014). Novel approaches for delivery of LSCs on the corneal surface include use of contact lens as a substrate/carrier for expansion of cell. This delivery strategy has shown promising results, as stem cells maintained their phenotype and mitotic activity even after being transferred to the ocular surface (Brown et al., 2014; Gore et al., 2014).

Translational biomechanics in ophthalmology is a rapidly growing area, however, is still in its infancy. The ocular biomechanics greatly influences the refractive surgery and keratoconus and in turn remodeling of the targeted tissues. Therefore, research advancements, which include recognition of current clinical practices and how they are affected by ocular biomechanics, could make significant impact in diagnosis and treatment. In addition, an important challenge in ocular biomechanics research is measurement of biomechanical properties of all individual ocular tissues in *in vivo* conditions. With recent advancement in imaging technology and imaging processing techniques, this challenge would be realized in future and might benefit in the development of validated models for biomechanical testing (Girard et al., 2014). There are some emerging translational strategies that already exist, such as corneal stiffening and others are more likely to follow.

Future perspectives of ocular tissue engineering include the use of pluripotent stem cells or other stem cells and study of ocular biomechanics for regeneration of corneal tissues. Therefore, in order to translate ocular tissue engineering to clinics, attention is required to match current treatment options to human physiological requirements for *in vivo* remodeling/regeneration. In addition, the *in vitro* study of the corneal diseases would be useful as discovery tools for new treatment options (Ghezzi et al., 2015). However, a detailed and measured scientific approach would be very much required to ensure safety during transplantation and other treatment options.

References

Ahmad, I., Tang, L., Pham, H. 2000. Identification of neural progenitors in the adult mammalian eye. *Biochem Biophys Res Commun.* 270:517–521.

Ahmad, S., Fiqueiredo, F., Lako, M. 2006. Corneal epithelial stem cells: Characterization, culture and transplantation. *Regen Med.* 1:29–44.

Ahmed, T.A.E., Ringuette, R., Wallace, V.A., Griffith, M. 2014. Autologous fibrin glue as an encapsulating scaffold for delivery of retinal progenitor cells. *Front Bioeng Biotechnol.* 2:85.

Alqvere, P.V., Berglin, L., Gouras, P., Sheng, Y. 1996. Human fetal RPE transplants in age related macular degeneration (ARMD). *Invest Ophthalmol Vis Sci.* 37:S96.

Alqvere, P.V., Gouras, P., DafgårdKopp, E. 1999. Long-term outcome of RPE allografts in non-immunosuppressed patients with AMD. *Eur J Ophthalmol.* 9:217–230.

Altman, G.H., Diaz, F., Jakuba, C. et al. 2003. Silk-based biomaterials. *Biomaterials.* 24:401–416.

Ang, L.P.K., Tanioka, H., Kawasaki, S. et al. 2010. Cultivated human conjunctival epithelial transplantation for total limbal stem cell deficiency. *Invest Ophthalmol Vis Sci.* 51:758–764.

Aramant, R.B., Seiler, M.J. 2002. Retinal transplantation—Advantages of intact fetal sheets. *Prog Retin Eye Res.* 21:57–73.

Arfaj, A.K. 2015. Boston keratoprosthesis—Clinical outcomes with wider geographic use and expanding indications—A systematic review. *Saudi J Ophthalmol.* 29:212–221.

Arnhold, S., Klein, H., Semkova, I., Addicks, K., Schraermeyer, U. 2004. Neurally selected embryonic stem cells induce tumor formation after long-term survival following engraftment into the subretinal space. *Invest Ophthalmol Vis Sci.* 45:4251–4255.

Atala, A., Kasper, F.K., Mikos, A.G. 2012. Engineering complex tissues. *Sci Transl Med.* 4:160rv12.

Baino, F. 2011. Towards an ideal biomaterial for vitreous replacement: Historical overview and future trends. *Acta Biomater.* 7:921–935.

Ballios, B.G., Cooke, M.J., Kooy, D.V.D., Shoichet, M.S. 2010. A hydrogel-based stem cell delivery system to treat retinal degenerative diseases. *Biomaterials.* 31:2555–2564.

Barber, A.C., Hippert, C., Duran, Y. et al. 2013. Repair of the degenerate retina by photoreceptor transplantation. *Proc Natl Acad Sci USA.* 110:354–359.

Baum, B.J., Wang, S., Cukierman, E. et al. 1999. Re-engineering the functions of a terminally differentiated epithelial cell *in vivo. Ann N Y Acad Sci.* 875:294–300.

Beales, M.P., Funderburgh, J.L., Jester, J.V., Hassell, J.R. 1999. Proteoglycan synthesis by bovine keratocytes and corneal fibroblasts: Maintenance of the keratocyte phenotype in culture. *Invest Ophthalmol Vis Sci.* 40:1658–1663.

Berson, E.L., Rosner, B., Sandberg, M.A., Hayes, K.C., Nicholson, B.W., Weigel-DiFranco, C., Willett, W. 1993. A randomized trial of vitamin A and vitamin E supplementation for retinitis pigmentosa. *Arch Ophthalmol.* 111:761–772.

Berson, E.L., Rosner, B., Sandberg, M.A. et al. 2004. Further evaluation of docosahexaenoic acid in patients with retinitis pigmentosa receiving vitamin A treatment: Subgroup analyses. *Arch Ophthalmol.* 122:1306–1314.

Bhang, S.H., Lim, J.S., Choi, C.Y., Kwon, Y.K., Kim, B.S. 2007. The behavior of neural stem cells on biodegradable synthetic polymers. *J Biomater Sci Polym Ed.* 18:223–239.

Brown, K.D., Low, S., Mariappan, I. et al. 2014. Plasma polymer-coated contact lenses for the culture and transfer of corneal epithelial cells in the treatment of limbal stem cell deficiency. *Tissue Eng A.* 20:646–655.

Bullock, A.J., Higham, M.C., MacNeil, S. 2006. Use of human fibroblasts in the development of a xenobiotic-free culture and delivery system for human keratinocytes. *Tissue Eng.* 12:245–255.

Burk, R., Hey, H., Draeger, J., Armbrecht, U., Morszeck, M. 1986. Current status of PMMA intraocular lens sterilization. *Klin Monbl Augenheilkd.* 188:45–46.

BylsmaFranzco, G.W., Guymer, R.H. 2005. Treatment of age-related macular degeneration. *Clin Exp Optom.* 88:322–334.

Cavalieri, F., Miano, F., D'Antona, P., Paradossi, G. 2004. Study of gelling behavior of poly(vinyl alcohol)-methacrylate for potential utilizations in tissue replacement and drug delivery. *Biomacromolecules.* 5:2439–2446.

Cen, L., Liu, W., Cui, L., Zhang, W., Cao, Y. 2008. Collagen tissue engineering: Development of novel biomaterials and applications. *Pediatr Res.* 63:492–496.

Chan, I.M., Tolentino, F.I., Refojo, M.I., Fournier, G., Albert, D.M. 1984. Vitreous substitute: Experimental studies and review. *Retina.* 4:51–59.

Checa-Casalengua, P., Jiang, C., Bravo-Osuna, I. et al. 2011. Retinal ganglion cells survival in a glaucoma model by GDNF/Vit E PLGA microspheres prepared according to a novel microencapsulation procedure. *J Control Release.* 156:92–100.

Chen, D.F., Rao, R.C. 2011. Nanomedicine and optic nerve regeneration implications for ophthalmology. *US Ophtalmic Rev.* 4:108–111.

Chen, H., Fan, X., Xia, J., Chen, P., Zhou, X., Huang, J., Yu, J., Gu, P. 2011. Electrospun chitosan-graft-poly(ε-caprolactone)/poly(ε-caprolactone) nanofibrous scaffolds for retinal tissue engineering. *Int J Nanomed.* 6:453.

Chen, J., Altman, G.H., Karageorgiou, V., Horan, R., Collette, A., Volloch, V., Colabro, T., Kaplan, D.L. 2003a. Human bone marrow stromal cell and ligament fibroblast responses on RGD-modified silk fibers. *J Biomed Mater Res A.* 67:559–570.

Chen, J., Li, Q., Xu, J., Huang, Y., Ding, Y., Deng, H., Zhao, S., Chen, R. 2005. Study on biocompatibility of complexes of collagen–chitosan–sodium hyaluronate and cornea. *Artif Organs.* 29:104–113.

Chen, W., Ishikawa, M., Yamaki, K., Sakuragi, S. 2003b. Wistar rat palpebral conjunctiva contains more slow-cycling stem cells that have larger proliferative capacity: Implication for conjunctival epithelial homeostasis. *Jpn J Ophthalmol.* 47:119–128.

Chew, S.Y., Mi, R., Hoke, A., Leong, K.W. 2007. Aligned protein–polymer composite fibers enhance nerve regeneration: A potential tissue-engineering platform. *Adv Funct Mater.* 17:1288–1296.

Chirila, T.V., Barnard, Z., Zainuddin, Z., Harkin, D.G. 2007. Silk as substratum for cell attachment and proliferation. *Mater Sci Forum.* 561:1549–1552.

Chirila, T.V., Hong, Y. 1998. The vitreous humor. In *Handbook of Biomaterial Properties*, Black, J. and Hastings, G. (eds.), Springer, US, 125–131.

Cicero, S., Johnson, D., Reyntjens, S., Frase, S., Connell, S., Chow, L., Baker, S.J., Sorrentino, B.P., Dyer, M.A. 2009. Cells previously identified as retinal stem cells are pigmented ciliary epithelial cells. *Proc Natl Acad Sci.* 106:6685–6690.

Comer, G.M., Ciulla, T.A. 2005. Current and future pharmacological intervention for diabetic retinopathy. *Expert Opin Emerg Drugs.* 10:441–455.

Connon, C.J. 2015. Approaches to corneal tissue engineering: Top-down or bottom-up? *Procedia Eng.* 110:15–20.

Danysh, B.P., Duncan, M.K. 2009. The lens capsule. *Exp Eye Res.* 88:151–164.

Das, A.V., Mallya, K.B., Zhao, X., Ahmad, F., Bhattacharya, S., Thoreson, W.B., Hegde, G.V., Ahmad, I. 2006. Neural stem cell properties of Müller glia in the mammalian retina: Regulation by Notch and Wnt signaling. *Dev Biol.* 299:283–302.

Das, T., Cerro, M.D., Jalali, S. et al. 1999. The transplantation of human fetal neuroretinal cells in advanced retinitis pigmentosa patients: Results of a long-term safety study. *Exp Neurol.* 157:58–68.

Davidorf, F.H., Chambers, R.B., Kwon, O.W., Doyle, W., Gresak, P., Frank, S.G. 1990. Ocular toxicity of vitreal pluronic polyol F-127. *Retina.* 10:297–300.

de la Mata, A.D.L., Nieto-Miguel, T., López-Paniagua, M. et al. 2013. Chitosan–gelatin biopolymers as carrier substrata for limbal epithelial stem cells. *J Mater Sci Mater Med.* 24:2819–2829.

Del Rio-Tsonis, K.D., Tomarev, S.I., Tsonis, P.A. 1999. Regulation of Prox 1 during lens regeneration. *Invest Ophthalmol Vis Sci.* 40:2039–2045.

Deshpande, P., Notara, M., Bullett, N., Daniels, J., Haddow, D.B., MacNeil, S. 2009. Development of a surface-modified contact lens for the transfer of cultured limbal epithelial cells to the cornea for ocular surface diseases. *Tissue Eng A.* 15:2889–2902.

Dhamodaran, K., Subramani, M., Ponnalagu, M., Shetty, R., Das, D. 2014. Ocular stem cells: A status update! *Stem Cell Ther.* 5:1–12.

Doherty, P., Williams, E., Walsh, F.S. 1995. A soluble chimeric form of the L1 glycoprotein stimulates neurite outgrowth. *Neuron.* 14:57–66.

Doi, M., Refojo, M.F. 1994. Histopathology of rabbit eyes with intravitreous silicone–fluorosilicone copolymer oil. *Exp Eye Res.* 59:737–746.

Doillon, C.J., Watsky, M.A., Hakim, M., Wang, J., Munger, R., Laycock, N., Osborne, R., Griffith, M. 2003. A collagen-based scaffold for a tissue engineered human cornea: Physical and physiological properties. *Int J Artif Organs.* 26:764–773.

Du, Y., Funderburgh, M.L., Mann, M.M., SundarRaj, N., Funderburgh, J.L. 2005. Multipotent stem cells in human corneal stroma. *Stem Cells.* 23:1266–1275.

Duncan, T.J., Tanaka, Y., Shi, D., Kubota, A., Quantock, A.J., Nishida, K. 2010. Flow-manipulated, crosslinked collagen gels for use as corneal equivalents. *Biomaterials.* 31:8996–9005.

Ebrahimi, M., Taghi-Abadi, E., Baharvand, H. 2009. Limbal stem cells in review. *J Ophthalmic Vis Res.* 4:40.

Eguchi, G. 1993. Lens transdifferentiation in the vertebrate retinal pigmented epithelial cell. *Prog Retin Res.* 12:205–230.

Eguchi, G. 1998. Transdifferentiation as the basis of eye lens regeneration. In *Cellular and Molecular Basis of Regeneration: From Invertebrates to Humans*, Ferreti, P., Géraudie, J. (eds), 207–228. Wiley, Chichester.

Eiraku, M., Takata, N., Ishibashi, H., Kawada, M., Sakakura, E., Okuda, S., Sekiguchi, K., Adachi, T., Sasai, Y. 2011. Self-organizing optic-cup morphogenesis in three-dimensional culture. *Nature.* 472:51–56.

Ellis-Behnke, R.G., Liang, Y.X., You, S.W., Tay, D.K.C., Zhang, S., So, K.F., Schneider, G.E. 2006. Nano neuro knitting: Peptide nanofiber scaffold for brain repair and axon regeneration with functional return of vision. *Proc Natl Acad Sci USA.* 103:5054–5059.

Fan, T., Ma, X., Zhao, J., Wen, Q., Hu, X., Yu, H., Shi, W. 2013. Transplantation of tissue-engineered human corneal endothelium in cat models. *Mol Vis.* 19:400.

Feng, S., Chen, H., Liu, Y., Huang, Z., Sun, X., Zhou, L., Lu, X., Gao, Q. 2013. A novel vitreous substitute of using a foldable capsular vitreous body injected with polyvinylalcohol hydrogel. *Sci Rep.* 3:1838.

Fernandez-Vigo, J., Refojo, M.F., Verstraeten, T. 1990a. Evaluation of a viscoelastic solution of hydroxypropyl methylcellulose as a potential vitreous substitute. *Retina.* 10:148–152.

Fernandez-Vigo, J., Sabugal, J.F., Rey, A.D., Concheiro, A., Martinez, R. 1990b. Molecular weight dependence of the pharmacokinetic of hydroxypropyl methylcellulose in the vitreous. *J Ocul Pharmacol.* 6:137–142.

Ferrari, S., Iorio, E.D., Barbaro, V., Ponzin, D., Sorrentino, F.S., Parmeggiani, F. 2011. Retinitis pigmentosa: Genes and disease mechanisms. *Curr Genomics.* 12:238.

Foster, W.J. 2008. Vitreous substitutes. *Expert Rev Ophthalmol.* 3:211–218.

Francis, P.J., Berry, V., Moore, A.T., Bhattacharya, S. 1999. Lens biology: Development and human cataractogenesis. *Trends Genet.* 15:191–196.

Gao, Q., Mou, S., Ge, J., To, C.H., Hui, Y., Liu, A., Wang, Z., Long, C., Tan, J. 2008. A new strategy to replace the natural vitreous by a novel capsular artificial vitreous body with pressure-control valve. *Eye.* 22:461–468.

Geerling, G., Sieg, P., Bastian, G.O., Laqua, H. 1998. Transplantation of the autologous submandibular gland for most severe cases of keratoconjunctivitis sicca. *Ophthalmology.* 105:327–335.

George, A.J., Larkin, D.F. 2004. Corneal transplantation: The forgotten graft. *Am J Transplant.* 4:678–685.

Ghezzi, C.E., Jelena, R.K., David, L.K. 2015. Corneal tissue engineering: Recent advances and future perspectives. *Tissue Eng B: Rev.* 21:278–287.

Ghezzi, C.E., Muja, N., Marelli, B., Nazhat, S.N. 2011. Real time responses of fibroblasts to plastically compressed fibrillar collagen hydrogels. *Biomaterials.* 32:4761–4772.

Gil, E.S., Mandal, B.B., Park, S.H., Marchant, J.K., Omenetto, F.G., Kaplan, D.L. 2010. Helicoidal multi-lamellar features of RGD-functionalized silk biomaterials for corneal tissue engineering. *Biomaterials.* 31:8953–8963.

Girard, M.J.A., Dupps, W.J., Baskaran, M., Scarcelli, G., Yun, S.H., Quigley, H.A., Sigal, I.A., Strouthidis, N.G. 2014. Translating ocular biomechanics into clinical practice: Current state and future prospects. *Curr Eye Res.* 40:1–18.

Gore, A., Horwitz, V., Gutman, H., Tveria, L., Cohen, L., Cohen-Jacob, O., Turetz, J., McNutt, P., Dachir, S., Kadar, T. 2014. Cultivation and characterization of limbal epithelial stem cells on contact lenses with a feeder layer: Toward the treatment of limbal stem cell deficiency. *Cornea.* 33:65–71.

Gouveia, R.M., Castelletto, V., Alcock, S.G., Hamley, I.W., Connon, C.J. 2013. Bioactive films produced from self-assembling peptide amphiphiles as versatile substrates for tuning cell adhesion and tissue architecture in serum-free conditions. *J Mater Chem B.* 1:6157–6169.

Griffith, M., Osborne, R., Munger, R., Xiong, X., Doillon, C.J., Laycock, N.L., Hakim, M., Song, Y., Watsky, M.A. 1999. Functional human corneal equivalents constructed from cell lines. *Science.* 286:2169–2172.

Grolik, M., Szczubiałka, K., Wowra, B., Dobrowolski, D., Orzechowska-Wylęgała, B., Wylęgała, E., Nowakowska, M. 2012. Hydrogel membranes based on genipin-cross-linked chitosan blends for corneal epithelium tissue engineering. *J Mater Sci Mater Med.* 23:1991–2000.

Gualdoni, S., Baron, M., Lakowski, J., Decembrini, S., Smith, A.J., Pearson, R.A., Ali, R.R., Sowden, J.C. 2010. Adult ciliary epithelial cells, previously identified as retinal stem cells with potential for retinal repair, fail to differentiate into new rod photoreceptors. *Stem Cells.* 28:1048–1059.

Gupta, M.K., Khokhar, S.K., Phillips, D.M., Sowards, L.A., Drummy, L.F., Kadakia, M.P., Naik, R.R. 2007. Patterned silk films cast from ionic liquid solubilized fibroin as scaffolds for cell growth. *Langmuir.* 23:1315–1319.

Gwon, A., Gruber, L. 2010. Engineering the crystalline lens with a biodegradable or non-degradable scaffold. *Exp Eye Res.* 91:220–228.

Gwon, A., Gruber, L.J., Mantras, C. 1993. Restoring lens capsule integrity enhances lens regeneration in New Zealand albino rabbits and cats. *J Cataract Refract Surg.* 19:735–746.

Hamley, I.W. 2011. Self-assembly of amphiphilic peptides. *Soft Matter.* 7:4122–4138.

Han, B., Schwab, I.R., Madsen, T.K., Isseroff, R.R. 2002. A fibrin-based bioengineered ocular surface with human corneal epithelial stem cells. *Cornea.* 21:505–510.

Hanna, C., O'Brien, J.E. 1960. Cell production and migration in the epithelial layer of the cornea. *Arch Ophthalmol.* 64:536–539.

Hatfill, S.J., Margolis, L.B., Duray, P.H. 1996. *In vitro* maintenance of normal and pathological human salivary gland tissue in a NASA-designed rotating wall vessel bioreactor. *Cell Vis.* 3:397–401.

Hayashi, T., Mizuno, N., Owaribe, K., Kuroiwa, A., Okamoto, M. 2002. Regulated lens regeneration from isolated pigmented epithelial cells of newt iris in culture in response to FGF2/4. *Differentiation.* 70:101–108.

He, H., Yiu, S.C. 2014. Stem cell-based therapy for treating limbal stem cells deficiency: A review of different strategies. *Saudi J Ophthalmol.* 28:188–194.

He, P., Davis, S.S., Illum, L. 1998. *In vitro* evaluation of the mucoadhesive properties of chitosan microspheres. *Int J Pharm.* 166:75–88.

Hertz, J., Robinson, B., Valenzuela, D.A., Lavik, E.B., Goldberg, J.L. 2013. A tunable synthetic hydrogel system for culture of retinal ganglion cells and amacrine cells. *Acta Biomater.* 9:7622–7629.

Hirami, Y., Osakada, F., Takahashi, K., Okita, K., Yamanaka, S., Ikeda, H., Yoshimura, N., Takahashi, M. 2009. Generation of retinal cells from mouse and human induced pluripotent stem cells. *Neurosci Lett.* 458:126–131.

Hirayama, M., Ogawa, M., Oshima, M. et al. 2013. Functional lacrimal gland regeneration by transplantation of a bioengineered organ germ. *Nat Commun.* 4:2497.

Hoffmann, A., Nakamura, K., Tsonis, P.A. 2013. Intrinsic lens forming potential of mouse lens epithelial versus newt iris pigment epithelial cells in three-dimensional culture. *Tissue Eng C: Methods.* 20:91–103.

Hofmeister, F.M., Yalon, M.S., Iida, S., Goldberg, M.D. 1988. *In vitro* evaluation of iris chafe protection afforded by hydrophilic surface modification of polymethylmethacrylate intraocular lenses. *J Cataract Refract Surg.* 14:514–519.

Hogen-Esch, T.E., Shah, K.R., Fitzgerald, C.R. 1976. Development of injectable poly(glyceryl methacrylate) hydrogels for vitreous prosthesis. *J Biomed Mater Res.* 10:975–976.

Honda, N., Mimura, T., Usui, T., Amano, S. 2009. Descemet stripping automated endothelial keratoplasty using cultured corneal endothelial cells in a rabbit model. *Arch Ophthalmol.* 127:1321–1326.

Hong, Y., Chirila, T.V., Vijayasekaran, S., Shen, W., Lou, X., Dalton, P.D. 1998. Biodegradation *in vitro* and retention in the rabbit eye of crosslinked poly (1-vinyl-2-pyrrolidinone) hydrogel as a vitreous substitute. *J Biomed Mater Res.* 39:650–659.

Hsu, W.C., Spilker, M.H., Yannas, I.V., Rubin, P.A. 2000. Inhibition of conjunctival scarring and contraction by a porous collagen–glycosaminoglycan implant. *Invest Ophthalmol Vis Sci.* 41:2404–2411.

Ikeda, H.O., Sasaoka, N., Koike, M. et al. 2014. Novel VCP modulators mitigate major pathologies of rd10, a mouse model of retinitis pigmentosa. *Sci Rep.* 4:5970.

Inoue, T., Coles, K., Dorval, K. et al. 2010. Maximizing functional photoreceptor differentiation from adult human retinal stem cells. *Stem Cells.* 28:489–500.

Ishibashi, T., LEVEL-J Study Group. 2013. Maintenance therapy with pegaptanib sodium for neovascular age-related macular degeneration: An exploratory study in Japanese patients (LEVEL-J study). *Jpn J Ophthalmol.* 57:417–423.

Ito, M., Hayashi, T., Kuroiwa, A., Okamoto, M. 1999. Lens formation by pigmented epithelial cell reaggregate from dorsal iris implanted into limb blastema in the adult newt. *Dev Growth Differ.* 41:429–440.

Jhagta, H.S., Jain, P. 2015. Limbal stem cell deficiency: A review. *J Clin Ophthalmol Res.* 3:71.

Jung, J.C., Rio-tsonis, K.D., Tsonis, P.A. 1998. Regulation of homeobox-containing genes during lens regeneration. *Exp Eye Res.* 66:361–370.

Kador, K.E., Montero, R.B., Venugopalan, P. et al. 2013. Tissue engineering the retinal ganglion cell nerve fiber layer. *Biomaterials.* 34:4242–4250.

Karamichos, D. 2015. Ocular tissue engineering: Current and future directions. *J Funct Biomater.* 6:77–80.

Karl, M.O., Reh, T.A. 2010. Regenerative medicine for retinal diseases: Activating endogenous repair mechanisms. *Trends Mol Med.* 16:193–202.

Karoubi, G., Ormiston, M.L., Stewart, D.J., Courtman, D.W. 2009. Single-cell hydrogel encapsulation for enhanced survival of human marrow stromal cells. *Biomaterials.* 30:5445–5455.

Kawasaki, S., Tanioka, H., Yamasaki, K., Yokoi, N., Komuro, A., Kinoshita, S. 2006. Clusters of corneal epithelial cells reside ectopically in human conjunctival epithelium. *Invest Ophthalmol Vis Sci.* 47:1359–1367.

Kim, J.C., Tsenq, S.C. 1995. Transplantation of preserved human amniotic membrane for surface reconstruction in severely damaged rabbit corneas. *Cornea.* 14:473–484.

Kimura, Y., Madhavan, M., Call, M.K., Santiago, W., Tsonis, P.A., Lambris, J.D., Rio-Tsonis, K.D. 2003. Expression of complement 3 and complement 5 in newt limb and lens regeneration. *J Immunol.* 170:2331–2339.

Klassen, H., Warfvinge, K., Schwartz, P.H., Kiilgaard, J.F., Shamie, N., Jiang, C., Samuel, M., Scherfig, E., Prather, R.S., Young, M.J. 2008. Isolation of progenitor cells from GFP-transgenic pigs and transplantation to the retina of allorecipients. *Cloning Stem Cells.* 10:391–402.

Klassen, H.J., Ng, T.F., Kurimoto, Y., Kirov, I., Shatos, M., Coffey, P., Young, M.J. 2004. Multipotent retinal progenitors express developmental markers, differentiate into retinal neurons, and preserve light-mediated behavior. *Invest Ophthalmol Vis Sci.* 45:4167–4173.

Kleinberg, T.T., Tzekov, R.T., Stein, L., Ravi, N., Kaushal, S. 2011. Vitreous substitutes: A comprehensive review. *Surv Ophthalmol.* 56:300–323.

Kleinman, H.K., Martin, G.R. 2005. Matrigel: Basement membrane matrix with biological activity. *Semin Cancer Biol.* 15:378–386.

Knop, E., Knop, N. 2003. Eye-associated lymphoid tissue (EALT) is continuously spread throughout the ocular surface from the lacrimal gland to the lacrimal drainage system. *Ophthalmologe.* 100:929–942.

Kodama, R., Eguchi, G. 1995. From lens regeneration in the newt to in-vitro trans differentiation of vertebrate pigmented epithelial cells. *Semin Cell Biol.* 6:143–149.

Konomi, K., Zhu, C., Harris, D., Joyce, N.C. 2005. Comparison of the proliferative capacity of human corneal endothelial cells from the central and peripheral areas. *Invest Ophthalmol Vis Sci.* 46:4086.

Kruse, F.E. 1994. Stem cells and corneal epithelial regeneration. *Eye.* 8:170–183.

Kummer, M.P., Abbott, J.J., Dinser, S., Nelson, B.J. 2007. Artificial vitreous humor for in vitro experiments. In *Conferenc Proceedings of the IEEE Engineering in Medicine and Biology Society,* Lyon, France, 6407–6410.

Lace, R., Murray-Dunning, C., Williams, R. 2015. Biomaterials for ocular reconstruction. *J Mater Sci.* 50:1523–1534.

Lai, J.Y., Chen, K.H., Hsiue, G.H. 2007. Tissue-engineered human corneal endothelial cell sheet transplantation in a rabbit model using functional biomaterials. *Transplantation.* 84:1222–1232.

Lai, J.Y., Chen, K.H., Hsu, W.M., Hsiue, G.H., Lee, Y.H. 2006. Bioengineered human corneal endothelium for transplantation. *Arch Ophthalmol.* 124:1441–1448.

Lai, J.Y., Li, Y.T. 2010. Evaluation of cross-linked gelatin membranes as delivery carriers for retinal sheets. *Mat Sci Eng C.* 30:677–685.

Lai, J.Y., Li, Y.T., Cho, C.H., Yu, T.C. 2012. Nanoscale modification of porous gelatin scaffolds with chondroitin sulfate for corneal stromal tissue engineering. *Int J Nanomed.* 7:1101.

Lamba, D.A., Gust, J., Reh, T.A. 2009. Transplantation of human embryonic stem cell-derived photoreceptors restores some visual function in Crx-deficient mice. *Cell Stem Cell.* 4:73–79.

Lamba, D.A., Karl, M.O., Ware, C.B., Reh, T.A. 2006. Efficient generation of retinal progenitor cells from human embryonic stem cells. *Proc Natl Acad Sci USA.* 103:12769–12774.

Lamba, D.A., McUsic, A., Hirata, R.K., Wang, R., Russell, D., Reh, T.A. 2010. Generation, purification and transplantation of photoreceptors derived from human induced pluripotent stem cells. *PloS One.* 5:e8763.

Lang, R.A. 1999. Which factors stimulate lens fiber cell differentiation *in vivo*? *Invest Ophthalmol Vis Sci.* 40:3075–3078.

Lavik, E.B., Klassen, H., Warfvinge, K., Langer, R., Young, M.J. 2005. Fabrication of degradable polymer scaffolds to direct the integration and differentiation of retinal progenitors. *Biomaterials.* 26:3187–3196.

Lavker, R.M., Dong, G., Cheng, S.Z., Kudoh, K., Cotsarelis, G., Sun, T.T. 1991. Relative proliferative rates of limbal and corneal epithelia. Implications of corneal epithelial migration, circadian rhythm, and suprabasally located DNA-synthesizing keratinocytes. *Invest Ophthalmol Vis Sci.* 32:1864–1875.

Lavker, R.M., Sun, T.T. 2003. Epithelial stem cells: The eye provides a vision. *Eye.* 17:937–942.

Lawrence, B.D., Marchant, J.K., Pindrus, M.A., Omenetto, F.G., Kaplan, D.L. 2009. Silk film biomaterials for cornea tissue engineering. *Biomaterials.* 30:1299–1308.

Lawrence, B.D., Pan, Z., Liu, A., Kaplan, D.L., Rosenblatt, M.I. 2012a. Human corneal limbal epithelial cell response to varying silk film geometric topography *in vitro*. *Acta Biomater.* 8:3732–3743.

Lawrence, B.D., Pan, Z., Rosenblatt, M.I. 2012b. Silk film topography directs collective epithelial cell migration. *PLoS One* 7(11):e50190.

Lee, S.Y., Oh, J.H., Kim, J.C., Kim, Y.H., Kim, S.H., Choi, J.W. 2003. *In vivo* conjunctival reconstruction using modified PLGA grafts for decreased scar formation and contraction. *Biomaterials.* 24:5049–5059.

Liang, C., Peyman, G.A., Serracarbassa, P., Calixto, N., Chow, A.A., Rao, P. 1998. An evaluation of methylated collagen as a substitute for vitreous and aqueous humor. *Int Opthalmol.* 22:13–18.

Liang, Y., Liu, W., Han, B., Yang, C., Ma, Q., Zhao, W., Rong, M., Li, H. 2011. Fabrication and characters of a corneal endothelial cells scaffold based on chitosan. *J Mater Sci Mater Med.* 22:175–183.

Liu, L., Hu, Y., Zhu, D., Thomas, B., Ford, K., Ahuja, A.K., Thomas, B.B., Clegg, D.O., Hinton, D.R., Humayun, M.S. 2011. Human embryonic stem cell derived retinal pigment epithelial cells cultured on polymer substrates maintain a confluent monolayer structure in the subretinal space of implanted rats. *Invest Ophthalmol Vis Sci.* 52:3190–3190.

Lombaert, I.M., Brunsting, J.F., Wierenga, K., Faber, H., Stokman, M.A., Kok, T., Visser, W.H., Kampinga, H.H., de Haan, G., Coppes, R.P. 2008. Rescue of salivary gland function after stem cell transplantation in irradiated glands. *PloS One.* 3:e2063.

Long, C.J., Roth, M.R., Tasheva, E.S., Funderburgh, M., Smit, R., Conrad, G.W., Funderburgh, J.L. 2000. Fibroblast growth factor-2 promotes keratan sulfate proteoglycan expression by keratocytes *in vitro. J Biol Chem.* 275:13918–13923.

Los, L.I., van der Worp, R.J., Van Luyn, M.J., Hooymans, J.M. 2003. Age-related liquefaction of the human vitreous body: LM and TEM evaluation of the role of proteoglycans and collagen. *Invest Ophthalmol Vis Sci.* 44:2828–2833.

Lu, J.T., Lee, C.J., Bent, S.F., Fishman, H.A., Sabelman, E.E. 2007. Thin collagen film scaffolds for retinal epithelial cell culture. *Biomaterials.* 28:1486–1494.

Lutolf, M.P., Hubbell, J.A. 2005. Synthetic biomaterials as instructive extracellular microenvironments for morphogenesis in tissue engineering. *Nat Biotechnol.* 23:47–55.

Lynn, A.K., Yannas, I.V., Bonfield, W. 2004. Antigenicity and immunogenicity of collagen. *J Biomed Mater Res B.* 71:343–354.

Mantelli, F., Massaro-Giordano, M., Macchi, I., Lambiase, A., Bonini, S. 2013. The cellular mechanisms of dry eye: From pathogenesis to treatment. *J Cell Physiol.* 228:2253–2256.

Maruoka, S., Matsuura, T., Kawasaki, K., Okamoto, M., Yoshiaki, H., Kodama, M., Sugiyama, M., Annaka, M. 2006. Biocompatibility of polyvinyl alcohol gel as a vitreous substitute. *Curr Eye Res.* 31:599–606.

Maurice, D.M. 1957. The structure and transparency of the cornea. *J Physiol.* 136:263–286.

Mayfield, A.E., Tilokee, E.L., Latham, N., McNeill, B., Lam, B.K., Ruel, M., Suuronen, E.J., Courtman, D.W., Stewart, D.J., Davis, D.R. 2014. The effect of encapsulation of cardiac stem cells within matrix-enriched hydrogel capsules on cell survival, post-ischemic cell retention and cardiac function. *Biomaterials.* 35:133–142.

Messmer, E.M. 2015. The pathophysiology, diagnosis, and treatment of dry eye disease. *Dtsch Arztebl Int.* 112:71.

Mi, S., Chen, B., Wright, B., Connon, C.J. 2010. *Ex vivo* construction of an artificial ocular surface by combination of corneal limbal epithelial cells and a compressed collagen scaffold containing keratocytes. *Tissue Eng A.* 16:2091–2100.

Milliot, B. 1872. De la regeneration du cristallin chez quelques mammiferes (Regeneration lens in some mammals), Paris, France: Felix Alcan.

Mimura, T., Amano, S., Tabata, Y. 2011. Transplantation of corneal stroma reconstructed with gelatin and multipotent precursor cells from corneal stroma. In *Tissue Engineering for Tissue and Organ Regeneration*, Eberli, D. (ed.), INTECH Open Access Publisher, Croatia, European Union.

Mimura, T., Joyce, N.C. 2006. Replication competence and senescence in central and peripheral human corneal endothelium. *Invest Ophthalmol Vis Sci.* 47:1387.

Miura, K., Taki, C., Sunada, T., Nakatani, M., Nishimura, S. 2009. Ultrastructural study on lens regeneration around poly(vinylpyrrolidone) hydrogel implanted in rabbit eyes as an accommodative intraocular lens material. *Invest Ophthalmol Vis Sci.* 50:4381–4381.

Müller, L.J., Pels, L., Vrensen, G.F. 1995. Novel aspects of the ultrastructural organization of human corneal keratocytes. *Invest Ophthalmol Vis Sci.* 36:2557–2567.

Nakagawa, M., Tanaka, M., Miyata, T. 1997. Evaluation of collagen gel and hyaluronic acid as vitreous substitutes. *Ophthalmic Res.* 29:409–420.

Nakamura, K., Kurosaka, D., Bissen-Miyajima, H., Tsubota, K. 2001. Intact corneal epithelium is essential for the prevention of stromal haze after laser assisted *in situ* keratomileusis. *Br J Ophthalmol.* 85:209–213.

Nakamura, T., Inatomi, T., Sotozono, C., Koizumi, N., Kinoshita, S. 2015. Ocular surface reconstruction using stem cell and tissue engineering. *Prog Retin Eye Res.* pii: S1350-9462(15)00050-6.

Nakayasu, K., Tanaka, M., Konomi, H., Hayashi, T. 1986. Distribution of types I, II, III, IV and collagen in normal and keratoconus corneas. *Ophthalmic Res.* 18:1–10.

Neeley, W.L., Redenti, S., Klassen, H., Tao, S., Desai, T., Young, M.J., Langer, R. 2008. A microfabricated scaffold for retinal progenitor cell grafting. *Biomaterials.* 29:418–426.

Ng, T.F., Lavik, E., Keino, H., Taylor, A.W., Langer, R.S., Young, M.J. 2007. Creating an immune-privileged site using retinal progenitor cells and biodegradable polymers. *Stem Cells.* 25:1552–1559.

Nishida, K., Yamato, M., Hayashida, Y. et al. 2004a. Corneal reconstruction with tissue-engineered cell sheets composed of autologous oral mucosal epithelium. *New Engl J Med.* 351:1187–1196.

Nishida, K., Yamato, M., Hayashida, Y. et al. 2004b. Functional bioengineered corneal epithelial sheet grafts from corneal stem cells expanded *ex vivo* on a temperature-responsive cell culture surface. *Transplantation.* 77:379–385.

Nishitsuka, K., Kashiwagi, Y., Tojo, N., Kanno, C., Takahashi, Y., Yamamoto, T., Heldin, P., Yamashita, H. 2007. Hyaluronan production regulation from porcine hyalocyte cell line by cytokines. *Exp Eye Res.* 85:539–545.

Oie, Y., Nishida, K. 2013. Regenerative medicine for the cornea. *Biomed Res Int.* 2013:1–8 (Article ID 428247).

Orwin, E.J., Hubel, A. 2000. *In vitro* culture characteristics of corneal epithelial, endothelial, and keratocyte cells in a native collagen matrix. *Tissue Eng.* 6:307–319.

Osakada, F., Ikeda, H., Sasai, Y., Takahashi, M. 2009. Stepwise differentiation of pluripotent stem cells into retinal cells. *Nat Protoc.* 4:811–824.

Oshima, M., Mizuno, M., Imamura, A. et al. 2011. Functional tooth regeneration using a bioengineered tooth unit as a mature organ replacement regenerative therapy. *PloS One.* 6:e21531.

Ozcelik, B., Brown, K.D., Blencowe, A., Daniell, M., Stevens, G.W., Qiao, G.G. 2013. Ultrathin chitosan–poly(ethylene glycol) hydrogel films for corneal tissue engineering. *Acta Biomater.* 9:6594–6605.

Paulsen, F. 2008. Functional anatomy and immunological interactions of ocular surface and adnexa. *Dev Ophthalmol.* 41:21–35.

Pearson, R.A., Barber, A.C., West, E.L., MacLaren, R.E., Duran, Y., Bainbridge, J.W., Sowden, J.C., Ali, R.R. 2010. Targeted disruption of outer limiting membrane junctional proteins (Crb1 and ZO-1) increases integration of transplanted photoreceptor precursors into the adult wild-type and degenerating retina. *Cell Transplant.* 19:487.

Pe'er, J., Zajicek, G., Greifner, H., Kogan, M. 1996. Streaming conjunctiva. *Anat Rec.* 245:36–40.

Peh, G.S., Beuerman, R.W., Colman, A., Tan, D.T., Mehta, J.S. 2011. Human corneal endothelial cell expansion for corneal endothelium transplantation: An overview. *Transplantation.* 91:811–819.

Pellegrini, G., Golisano, O., Paterna, P., Lambiase, A., Bonini, S., Rama, P., De Luca, M. 1999. Location and clonal analysis of stem cells and their differentiated progeny in the human ocular surface. *J Cell Biol.* 145:769–782.

Pellegrini, G., Traverso, C.E., Franzi, A.T., Zingirian, M., Cancedda, R., De Luca, M. 1997. Long-term restoration of damaged corneal surfaces with autologous cultivated corneal epithelium. *Lancet.* 349:990–993.

Perry, H., Gopinath, A., Kaplan, D.L., Negro, L.D., Omenetto, F.G. 2008. Nano- and micropatterning of optically transparent, mechanically robust, biocompatible silk fibroin films. *Adv Mater.* 20:3070–3072.

Petrash, J.M. 2013. Aging and age-related diseases of the ocular lens and vitreous body. *Invest Ophthalmol Vis Sci.* 54:ORSF54.

Phu, D., Wray, L.S., Warren, R.V., Haskell, R.C., Orwin, E.J. 2010. Effect of substrate composition and alignment on corneal cell phenotype. *Tissue Eng A.* 17:799–807.

Purnell, B. 2008. New release: The complete guide to organ repair. *Science.* 322:1489–1489.

Rama, P., Bonini, S., Lambiase, A., Golisano, O., Paterna, De Luca, M., Pellegrini, G. 2001. Autologous fibrin-cultured limbal stem cells permanently restore the corneal surface of patients with total limbal stem cell deficiency. *Transplantation.* 72:1478–1485.

Ramachandran, R., Fausett, B.V., Goldman, D. 2010. Ascl1a regulates Müller glia dedifferentiation and retinal regeneration through a Lin-28-dependent, let-7 microRNA signalling pathway. *Nat Cell Biol.* 12:1101–1107.

Ramachandran, R., Zhao, X.F., Goldman, D. 2012. Insm1a-mediated gene repression is essential for the formation and differentiation of Müller glia-derived progenitors in the injured retina. *Nat Cell Biol.* 14:1013–1023.

Redenti, S., Neeley, W.L., Rompani, S., Saigal, S., Yang, J., Klassen, H., Langer, R., Young, M.J. 2009. Engineering retinal progenitor cell and scrollable poly(glycerol-sebacate) composites for expansion and subretinal transplantation. *Biomaterials.* 30:3405–3414.

Redenti, S., Tao, S., Yang, J., Gu, P., Klassen, H., Saigal, S., Desai, T., Young, M.J. 2008. Retinal tissue engineering using mouse retinal progenitor cells and a novel biodegradable, thin-film poly(e-caprolactone) nanowire scaffold. *J Ocul Biol Dis Infor.* 1:19–29.

Reichl, S., Borrelli, M., Geerling, G. 2011. Keratin films for ocular surface reconstruction. *Biomaterials.* 32:3375–3386.

Remington, S.G., Meyer, R.A. 2007. Lens stem cells may reside outside the lens capsule: An hypothesis. *Theor Biol Med Model.* 4:22.

Ren, R., Hutcheon, A.E.K., Guo, X.Q., Saeidi, N., Melotti, S.A., Ruberti, J.W., Zieske, J.D., Trinkaus-Randall, V. 2008. Human primary corneal fibroblasts synthesize and deposit proteoglycans in long-term 3-D cultures. *Dev Dynam.* 237:2705–2715.

Robert, Y., Gloor, B., Wachsmuth, E.D., Herbst, M. 1988. Evaluation of the tolerance of the intra-ocular injection of hydroxypropyl methylcellulose in animal experiments. *Klin Monarsbl Augenh.* 192:337–339.

Roonprapunt, C., Huang, W., Grill, R., Friedlander, D., Grumet, M., Chen, S., Schachner, M., Young, W. 2003. Soluble cell adhesion molecule L1-Fc promotes locomotor recovery in rats after spinal cord injury. *J Neurotrauma.* 20:871–882.

Schechter, B.A., Rand, W.J., Nagler, R.S., Estrin, I., Arnold, S.S., Villate, N., Velazquez, G.E. 2005. Corneal melt after amniotic membrane transplant. *Cornea.* 24:106–107.

Schermer, A., Galvin, S., Sun, T.T. 1986. Differentiation-related expression of a major 64 K corneal keratin *in vivo* and in culture suggests limbal location of corneal epithelial stem cells. *J Cell Biol.* 103:49–62.

Schrader, S., Kremling, C., Klinger, M., Laqua, H., Geerling, G. 2009a. Cultivation of lacrimal gland acinar cells in a microgravity environment. *Br J Ophthalmol.* 93:1121–1125.

Schrader, S., Notara, M., Beaconsfield, M., Tuft, S.J., Daniels, J.T., Geerling, G. 2009b. Tissue engineering for conjunctival reconstruction: Established methods and future outlooks. *Curr Eye Res.* 34:913–924.

Schrader, S., Wedel, T., Kremling, C., Laqua, H., Geerling, G. 2007. Amniotic membrane as a carrier for lacrimal gland acinar cells. *Graef Arch Clin Exp.* 245:1699–1704.

Scott, J.E. 2003. Elasticity in extracellular matrix "shape modules" of tendon, cartilage, etc.: A sliding proteoglycan-filament model. *J Physiol.* 553:335–343.

Selvam, S., Thomas, B., Trousdale, M.D., Stevenson, D., Schechter, J.E., Mircheff, A.K., Jacob, J.T., Smith, R.E., Yiu, S.C. 2007. Tissue-engineered tear secretory system: Functional lacrimal gland acinar cells cultured on matrix protein-coated substrata. *J Biomed Mater Res B.* 80:192–200.

Selvam, S., Thomas, B., Yiu, S.C. 2006. Tissue engineering: Current and future approaches to ocular surface reconstruction. *Ocul Surf.* 4:120–136.

Shackleton, M., Vaillant, F., Simpson, K.J., Stingl, J., Smyth, G.K., Asselin-Labat, M.L., Wu, L., Lindeman, G.J., Visvader, J.E. 2006. Generation of a functional mammary gland from a single stem cell. *Nature.* 439:84–88.

Shadforth, A.M., George, K.A., Kwan, A.S., Chirila, T.V., Harkin, D.G. 2012. The cultivation of human retinal pigment epithelial cells on *Bombyx mori* silk fibroin. *Biomaterials.* 33:4110–4117.

Sharma, K.K., Santhoshkumar, P. 2009. Lens aging: Effects of crystallins. *BBA Gen Subjects.* 1790:1095–1108.

Shimazaki, J., Yang, H.Y., Tsubota, K. 1997. Amniotic membrane transplantation for ocular surface reconstruction in patients with chemical and thermal burns. *Ophthalmology.* 104:2068–2076.

Shoval, A., Adams, C., David-Pur, M., Shein, M., Hanein, Y., Sernagor, E. 2009. Carbon nanotube electrodes for effective interfacing with retinal tissue. *Front. Neuroeng.* 2:4.

Sommer, F., Pollinger, K., Brandl, F., Weiser, B., Teßmar, J., Blunk, T., Göpferich, A. 2008. Hyalocyte proliferation and ECM accumulation modulated by bFGF and TGF-β1. *Graef Arch Clin Exp.* 246:1275–1284.

Subrizi, A., Hiidenmaa, H., Ilmarinen, T., Nymark, S., Dubruel, P., Uusitalo, H., Yliperttula, M., Urtti, A., Skottman, H. 2012. Generation of hESC-derived retinal pigment epithelium on biopolymer coated polyimide membranes. *Biomaterials.* 33:8047–8054.

Sumide, T., Nishida, K., Yamato, M. et al. 2006. Functional human corneal endothelial cell sheets harvested from temperature-responsive culture surfaces. *FASEB J.* 20:392–394.

Sundback, C.A., Shyu, J.Y., Wang, Y., Faquin, W.C., Langer, R.S., Vacanti, J.P., Hadlock, T.A. 2005. Biocompatibility analysis of poly(glycerol sebacate) as a nerve guide material. *Biomaterials.* 26:5454–5464.

Suzuki, S., Dawson, R.A., Chirila, T.V., Shadforth, A., Hogerheyde, T.A., Edwards, G.A., Harkin, D.G. 2015. Treatment of silk fibroin with poly(ethylene glycol) for the enhancement of corneal epithelial cell growth. *J Funct Biomater.* 6:345–366.

Sweeney, D.F., Millar, T.J., Raju, S.R. 2013. Tear film stability: A review. *Exp Eye Res.* 117:28–38.

Swindle, K.E., Hamilton, P.D., Ravi, N. 2006. Advancements in the development of artificial vitreous humor utilizing polyacrylamide copolymers with disulfide crosslinkers. *Polym Prepr.* 47:56–60.

Swindle-Reilly, K.E., Shah, M., Hamilton, D., Eskin, T.A., Kaushal, S., Ravi, N. 2009. Rabbit study of an in situ forming hydrogel vitreous substitute. *Invest Ophthalmol Vis Sci.* 50:4840–4846.

Talbot, M., Carrier, Giasson, C.J., Deschambeault, A., Guérin, S.L., Auger, F.A., Bazin, R., Germain, L. 2006. Autologous transplantation of rabbit limbal epithelia cultured on fibrin gels for ocular surface reconstruction. *Mol Vis.* 12:65–75.

Tan, D.T., Dart, J.K., Holland, E.J., Kinoshita, S. 2012. Corneal transplantation. *Lancet.* 379:1749–1761.

Tanioka, H., Kawasaki, S., Yamasaki, K., Ang, L.P., Koizumi, N., Nakamura, T., Yokoi, N., Komuro, A., Inatomi, T., Kinoshita, S. 2006. Establishment of a cultivated human conjunctival epithelium as an alternative tissue source for autologous corneal epithelial transplantation. *Invest Ophthalmol Vis Sci.* 47:3820.

Tao, S., Young, C., Redenti, S., Zhang, Y., Klassen, H., Desai, T., Young, M.J. 2007. Survival, migration and differentiation of retinal progenitor cells transplanted on micro-machined poly(methyl methacrylate) scaffolds to the subretinal space. *Lab Chip.* 7:695–701.

Taylor, L., Arnér, K., Engelsberg, K., Ghosh, F. 2013. Effects of glial cell line-derived neurotrophic factor on the cultured adult full-thickness porcine retina. *Curr Eye Res.* 38:503–515.

Teichmann, J., Valtink, M., Nitschke, M., Gramm, S., Funk, R.H., Engelmann, K., Werner, C. 2013. Tissue engineering of the corneal endothelium: A review of carrier materials. *J Funct Biomater.* 4:178–208.

Thorell, M.R., Nunes, R.P., Chen, G.W. et al. 2014. Response to aflibercept after frequent re-treatment with bevacizumab or ranibizumab in eyes with neovascular AMD. *Ophthal Surg Las IM.* 45:526–533.

Tiwari, S., Ali, M.J., Vemuganti, G.K. 2014. Human lacrimal gland regeneration: Perspectives and review of literature. *Saudi J Ophthalmol.* 28:12–18.

Tomita, M., Lavik, E., Klassen, H., Zahir, T., Langer, R., Young, M.J. 2005. Biodegradable polymer composite grafts promote the survival and differentiation of retinal progenitor cells. *Stem Cells.* 23:1579–1588.

Tosi, G.M., Massaro-Giordano, M., Caporossi, A., Toti, P. 2005. Amniotic membrane transplantation in ocular surface disorders. *J Cell Physiol.* 202:849–851.

Tsonis, P.A., Jang, W.O.N.H.E.E., Del Rio-Tsonis, K.A.T.I.A., Eguchi, G.O.R.O. 2001. A unique aged human retinal pigmented epithelial cell line useful for studying lens differentiation *in vitro*. *Int J Dev Biol.* 45:753–758.

Tsonis, P.A., Madhavan, M., Call, M.K., Gainer, S., Rice, A., Rio-Tsonis, D. 2004. Effects of a CDK inhibitor on lens regeneration. *Wound Repair Regen.* 12:24–29.

Tsonis, P.A., Trombley, M.T., Rowland, T., Chandraratna, R.A., Rio-Tsonis, D. 2000. Role of retinoic acid in lens regeneration. *Dev Dynam.* 219:588–593.

VandeVord, J., Matthew, H.W., DeSilva, S.P., Mayton, L., Wu, B., Wooley, H. 2002. Evaluation of the biocompatibility of a chitosan scaffold in mice. *J Biomed Mater Res*. 59:585–590.

Van Hoffelen, S.J., Young, M.J., Shatos, M.A., Sakaguchi, D.S. 2003. Incorporation of murine brain progenitor cells into the developing mammalian retina. *Invest Ophthalmol Vis Sci*. 44:426–434.

Vastine, D.W., Stewart, W.B., Schwab, I.R. 1982. Reconstruction of the periocular mucous membrane by autologous conjunctival transplantation. *Ophthalmology*. 89:1072–1081.

Vrana, N.E., Builles, N., Justin, V., Bednarz, J., Pellegrini, G., Ferrari, B., Damour, O., Hulmes, D.J., Hasirci, V. 2008. Development of a reconstructed cornea from collagen–chondroitin sulfate foams and human cell cultures. *Invest Ophthalmol Vis Sci*. 49:5325–5331.

Wang, S., Liu, W., Han, B., Yang, L. 2009. Study on a hydroxypropyl chitosan–gelatin based scaffold for corneal stroma tissue engineering. *Appl Surf Sci*. 255:8701–8705.

Wang, Y., Ameer, G.A., Sheppard, B.J., Langer, R. 2002. A tough biodegradable elastomer. *Nat Biotechnol*. 20:602–606.

Wang, Y., Kim, Y.M., Langer, R. 2003. *In vivo* degradation characteristics of poly(glycerol sebacate). *J Biomed Mater Res A*. 66:192–197.

Watanabe, R., Hayashi, R., Kimura, Y., Tanaka, Y., Kageyama, T., Hara, S., Tabata, Y., Nishida, K. 2011. A novel gelatin hydrogel carrier sheet for corneal endothelial transplantation. *Tissue Eng A*. 17:2213–2219.

Wei, Z.G., Cotsarelis, G., Sun, T.T., Lavker, R.M. 1995. Label-retaining cells are preferentially located in fornical epithelium: Implications on conjunctival epithelial homeostasis. *Invest Ophthalmol Vis Sci*. 36:236–246.

West, E.L., Pearson, R.A., Barker, S.E., Luhmann, U.F., Maclaren, R.E., Barber, A.C., Duran, Y., Smith, A.J., Sowden, J.C., Ali, R.R. 2010. Long-term survival of photoreceptors transplanted into the adult murine neural retina requires immune modulation. *Stem Cells*. 28:1997–2007.

Wilson, S.E., Netto, M., Ambrósio, R. 2003. Corneal cells: Chatty in development, homeostasis, wound healing, and disease. *Am J Ophthalmol*. 136:530–536.

Wirtschafter, J.D., Ketcham, J.M., Weinstock, R.J., Tabesh, T., McLoon, L.K. 1999. Mucocutaneous junction as the major source of replacement palpebral conjunctival epithelial cells. *Invest Ophthalmol Vis Sci*. 40:3138–3146.

Wong, W.L., Su, X., Li, X., Cheung, C.M.G., Klein, R., Cheng, C.Y., Wong, T.Y. 2014. Global prevalence of age-related macular degeneration and disease burden projection for 2020 and 2040: A systematic review and meta-analysis. *Lancet Glob Health*. 2:e106–e116.

World Health Organization. 2012. *Visual Impairment and Blindness*. Fact sheet 282.

Wu, J., Du, Y., Mann, M.M., Yang, E., Funderburgh, J.L., Wagner, W.R. 2013. Bioengineering organized, multilamellar human corneal stromal tissue by growth factor supplementation on highly aligned synthetic substrates. *Tissue Eng A*. 19:2063–2075.

Wu, J., Rnjak-Kovacina, J., Du, Y., Funderburgh, M.L., Kaplan, D.L., Funderburgh, J.L. 2014. Corneal stromal bioequivalents secreted on patterned silk substrates. *Biomaterials*. 35:3744–3755.

Xu, Y.G., Xu, Y.S., Huang, C., Feng, Y., Li, Y., Wang, W. 2008. Development of a rabbit corneal equivalent using an acellular corneal matrix of a porcine substrate. *Mol Vis*. 14:2180.

Yamada, T. 1977. Control mechanisms in cell-type conversion in newt lens regeneration. *Monogr Dev Biol*. 13:1.

Yamagami, S., Yokoo, S., Mimura, T., Takato, T., Araie, M., Amano, S. 2007. Distribution of precursors in human corneal stromal cells and endothelial cells. *Ophthalmology*. 114:433–439.

Yang, C., Yang, Y., Brennan, L., Bouhassira, E.E., Kantorow, M., Cvekl, A. 2010. Efficient generation of lens progenitor cells and lentoid bodies from human embryonic stem cells in chemically defined conditions. *FASEB J*. 24:3274–3283.

Yang, F., Murugan, R., Wang, S., Ramakrishna, S. 2005. Electrospinning of nano/micro scale poly(L-lactic acid) aligned fibers and their potential in neural tissue engineering. *Biomaterials*. 26:2603–2610.

Yang, J., Yamato, M., Nishida, K., Hayashida, Y., Shimizu, T., Kikuchi, A., Tano, Y., Okano, T. 2006. Corneal epithelial stem cell delivery using cell sheet engineering: Not lost in transplantation. *J Drug Target*. 14:471–482.

Yao, J., Tucker, B.A., Zhang, X., Checa-Casalengua, P., Herrero-Vanrell, R., Young, M.J. 2011. Robust cell integration from co-transplantation of biodegradable MMP2-PLGA microspheres with retinal progenitor cells. *Biomaterials*. 32:1041–1050.

Yoshino, K. 2000. Establishment of a human lacrimal gland epithelial culture system with *in vivo* mimicry and its substrate modulation. *Cornea*. 19: S26–S36.

Yoshino, K., Tseng, S.C., Pflugfelder, S.C. 1995. Substrate modulation of morphology, growth, and tear protein production by cultured human lacrimal gland epithelial cells. *Exp Cell Res*. 220:138–151.

Young, M.J. 2005. Stem cells in the mammalian eye: A tool for retinal repair. *APMIS*. 113:845–857.

Zeana, D., Becker, J., Kuckelkorn, R., Kirchhof, B. 1999. Perfluorohexyloctane as a long-term vitreous tamponade in the experimental animal. *Int Ophthalmol*. 23:17–24.

Zhou, H., Lu, Q., Guo, Q., Chae, J., Fan, X., Elisseeff, J.H., Grant, M.P. 2014. Vitrified collagen-based conjunctival equivalent for ocular surface reconstruction. *Biomaterials*. 35:7398–7406.

Zhou, Y., Wu, Z., Ge, J., Wan, P., Li, N., Xiang, P., Gao, Q., Wang, Z. 2011. Development and characterization of acellular porcine corneal matrix using sodium dodecylsulfate. *Cornea*. 30:73–82.

Zhu, X., Beuerman, R.W., Chan-Park, M.B., Cheng, Z., Ang, L.P., Tan, D.T. 2006. Enhancement of the mechanical and biological properties of a biomembrane for tissue engineering the ocular surface. *Ann Acad Med Singapore*. 35:210.

Zoukhri, D., Fix, A., Alroy, J., Kublin, C.L. 2008. Mechanisms of murine lacrimal gland repair after experimentally induced inflammation. *Invest Ophthalmol Vis Res*. 49:4399.

Zrenner, E. 2002. Will retinal implants restore vision? *Science*. 295:1022–1025.

Section IV

Tissue Engineering Strategies to Improve Transport, Metabolic, and Synthetic Functions

9

Tissue Engineering-Based Functional Restoration of Blood Vessels

Anuradha Subramanian

CONTENTS

9.1 Introduction

Regeneration of blood vessels has gained much focus for the treatment of cardiovascular disease, which is the primary cause of non-communicable disease death worldwide. American Heart Association reported an average of one death every 40 seconds, estimating the fatalities of more than 2150 Americans per day based on the 2011 death rate (Mozaffarian et al., 2015). Currently, autologous saphenous veins and internal mammary arteries are the major treatment options for the peripheral and cardiac bypass surgery, respectively (Catto et al., 2014). However, poor availability of the autologous vessels due to any vessels disease or trauma demands the use of available synthetic grafts such as expanded polytetrafluoroethylene (ePTFE) and Dacron (pethyethylene terephthalate). Conversely, use of synthetic grafts often causes the failure of graft especially small diameter (<6 mm) due to thrombosis, lack of growth potential with many long-term complications such as stenosis, thromboembolism, calcification, and infections (Hoenig et al., 2005; Bordenave et al., 2008; Peck et al., 2011; Rathore et al., 2012). Poor patency rate of synthetic materials is mainly due to the absence of endothelial monolayers as it lines the inner lumen of native blood vessel to provide selective permeability, thromboresistance, and structural integrity to the blood vessel (Vara et al., 2005). These limitations have urged the need for development of new blood vessel substitute resembling both the structure and function of native tissue. Tissue engineering is one of the promising approaches aiming to develop synthetic three-dimensional (3D) extracellular matrix (ECM) integrated with or without cells and growth factors to facilitate the functional tissue progression. As thorough understanding of blood vessel architecture and its components on the function aids the evolution of various tissue engineering strategies. This chapter outlines the hierarchical organization of vasculature, response of the tissues during injury, or specific diseases associated with the current clinical challenges. This chapter also highlights the updates of tissue engineering strategies and the existing limitations in an attempt to lead future accomplishments.

9.2 Hierarchical Organization of Vasculature

Blood vessels with varying sizes (large, medium, and small) extend to various parts of the body for transporting the nutrients, gasses, waste by-products, and also for mediating the immune defense. Blood vessels, except capillaries, consist of intricate tri-layered architecture with distinct cell and protein composition (Zhang et al., 2007). Inner lumen of blood vessels comprises longitudinally aligned monolayer of endothelium establishing the thromboresistant barrier between vessel walls and circulating blood with selective permeability, known as intimal layer. Apart from barrier function, endothelial cells regulate vessel tone, laminar blood flow, platelet aggregation, leukocyte attachment, migration, and proliferation of smooth muscle cells (SMCs) (Stegemann et al., 2007). A layer of basement membrane consisting of collagen IV and laminin with the layer of elastin (internal elastic lamina) is present beneath the intima. Multiple layers of circumferentially aligned muscle cells (SMCs) around the inner layer called media provide the contractile function to the blood vessels. This layer is rich in type I and III collagen with few proteins and proteoglycans due to the secretory characteristics of SMCs. The presence of fibrillar proteins and proteoglycans provides a mechanical strength against tension, shear, and compression, respectively. Layer rich in elastin named external elastic lamina separates media from adventia, the outer layer of vessel around the media. Advential layer comprises loose collagen matrix embedded with randomly distributed fibroblasts, which play a pivotal role in cell trafficking, immune response mediation, and vascular remodeling while providing a structural support (Nemeno-Guanzon et al., 2012).

9.3 Responses to Injury/Diseases

Though the platelets and monocytes circulate very close to walls of the blood vessels, they do not interact with endothelial cells as the endothelium integrity provides an anti-thrombogenic barrier. However, any injury, infection, or diseases may weaken the vascular wall due to loss of endothelial cells leading to aneurysm, dissection, and occlusion. As soon as the underlying subendothelial layer is exposed to blood, sequence of events are activated

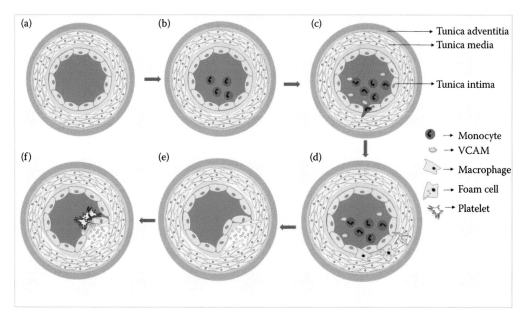

FIGURE 9.1
Response of blood vessels to injury/diseases. (a) Native blood vessels with intact endothelium; (b) monocytes circulation in native blood vessels; (c) endothelial dysfunction during injury; (d) migration of monocytes to medial layer and foam cell formation; (e) accumulation of fatty streaks with thin fibrin cap; and (f) platelet activation by fibrin cap rupture.

to bridge the defect (Figure 9.1). These include activation and adhesion of platelets on to the vessel wall; endothelial dysfunction leading to expression of various cell adhesion molecules facilitating the attachment of lymphocytes and monocytes to endothelial cells with the migration; and proliferation of SMCs (Mallat et al., 2000; Davignon and Ganz, 2004; Deanfield et al., 2007). Migration of monocytes into subendothelial layer becomes macrophage, which in turn differentiates to foam cells by the accumulation of oxidized low density lipoprotein (LDL). Apoptosis of foam cells stores the lipid rapidly, which are covered with thin fibrin cap in the intimal region. Rupturing of fibrin cap activates platelets to promote acute thrombosis as in Figure 9.1 (Ross, 1995; Bentzon et al., 2014). Thickening of intimal region occludes the blood flow to the adjacent tissues, which initiates the complex cellular changes transiently. However, severe or prolonged injury creates a hypoxic condition due to the lack of oxygen leading to the development of ischemia. Disturbance in the balance between the blood flow and metabolism of myocardium leads to the myocardial infarction.

9.4 Current Clinical Challenges in Restoration of Vasculature

Coronary artery bypass grafting is the gold standard clinical approach that involves the use of healthy blood vessels either taken from leg or chest to improve the blood flow. Arterial autografts are more preferable than venous grafts as it showed suitable mechanical strength and higher patency rate. However, donor site morbidity and donor availability are the major limitations (Piccone, 1987). Use of other biologic grafts such as allografts and xenografts (bovine) has also been limited due to aneurysm, disease transmission, and life-long immunosuppressive treatments. Synthetic grafts such as Dacron and ePTFE have been widely used as larger diameter grafts in high-flow and low-resistance conditions (Neff et al., 2011). Conversely, use of these grafts as for small diameter blood vessels provokes many complications such as thrombosis, calcification, aneurysm, poor compliance, and mismatch of mechanical properties with native blood vessels (Thomas et al., 2013). Failure of grafts may be due to acute thrombosis (<30 days), intimal hyperplasia (3 months to 2 years), or recurrence of atherosclerotic diseases (>2 years) (Conte et al., 2002; Thomas et al., 2013). These limitations of existing treatment strategies stipulate the requirement of vascular tissue engineering for small and large diameter blood vessel regeneration.

9.5 Tissue Engineering Strategies

Functional restoration of blood vessels based on tissue engineering involves the use of cells, biomaterials, and growth factors either singly or in combination to aid tissue progression. Biomaterial scaffolds exist as an ECM analog to establish cell–cell and cell–ECM communication by controlling the cell fate processes like adhesion, migration, proliferation, and functional gene expression (Bacakova et al., 2004; Bacakova, 2008). Generally, ideal scaffolds should be equivalent to or closely mimic the structural and porous architecture of ECM with the suitable biomechanical properties. In addition, scaffolds should be biocompatible, hemocompatible, biodegradable, nonimmunogenic, nontoxic, and nonthrombogenic. However, tissue engineering approaches for the development of blood vessels remain a challenge due to its intricate hierarchical organization of multilayer structure, distinctive mechanical strength to withstand the physiologic arterial pressure, disparity of ECM composition, and thickness from arteries and veins to capillaries. Many attempts either top-down or bottom-up approaches (Figure 9.2) have been made for the construction of tissue-engineered blood vessels, which includes the use of decellularized vasculature, biomaterial as scaffolds, cell sheet conduits, bioreactor-aided biofabrication, and bioprinting to address clinical challenges, which are discussed as follows.

9.5.1 Decellularized Strategies

Following the success of clinical translation of decellularized matrix-based trachea regeneration, investigations on the development of decellularized vessels have been growing due to its 3D microstructural and compositional similarities with native ECM (Piterina et al., 2009; Song and Ott, 2011). Decellularized matrix has other advantages such as biocompatibility, withholding native vessel's mechanical strength, augmentation of ECM via *de novo* synthesis, and abundance of allogenic and xenogenic sources (Badylak et al., 2009). Decellularization process involves the removal of all cellular components without altering chemical, mechanical, and biological integrity of the ECM by surfactant, mechanical, and enzymatic treatment (Rathore et al., 2012). These scaffolds have been stored like synthetic grafts either in hydrated or lyophilized form and would be used for scaffolding applications when required (Dahl et al., 2003; Quint et al., 2011). Hydrated form of native ECM possess adequate biomechanical properties and cellular in-growth potential, whereas dehydrated form of ECM holds extended shelf life and facilitates easy transportation (Badylak et al., 2009; Piterina et al., 2009). However, drawbacks such as lack of

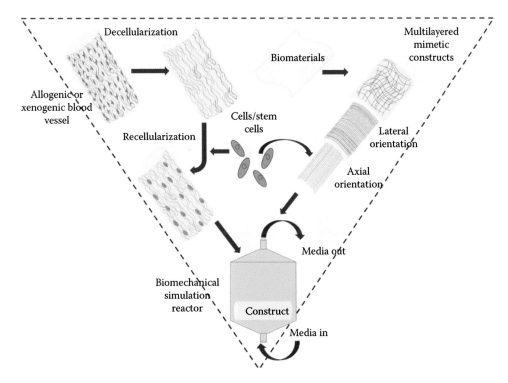

FIGURE 9.2
Top-down approaches for the fabrication of TEVGs.

anti-thrombogenic endothelium and threats of disease transmission limit its contributions in the tissue engineering field. Further, use of detergents and enzymes in decellularization process may promote shrinkage and affects the chemical, biomechanical, and biological properties of the ECM (L'Heureux et al., 1993; Gelse et al., 2003; Mano et al., 2007). Olausson et al. repopulated the allogenic decellularized ECM with autologous stem cells in order to achieve long-term immunosuppression (Olausson et al., 2012). Although seeding of patient's progenitor cells seems more promising, isolation and expansion of clinically meaningful number of cells either from bone marrow or whole blood are tricky. Olausson et al. have made an attempt to clinically transplant the tissue-engineered allogenic vein perfused with autologous peripheral whole blood into two pediatric patients suffering from hepatic portal vein thrombosis, thereby establishing re-endothelialization in decellularized vessel. However, one of the grafts was explanted after 7 months of implantation due to narrowing (Olausson et al., 2014). Instead of obtaining allogenic or xenogenic vessels for decellularization, allogenic aortic SMCs cultured on biodegradable polymeric scaffold under bioreactor conditions has been decellularized after maturation period (10 weeks) and used as arterial conduit (Quint et al., 2011). Hence, developing a vascular conduit with higher patency is indeed challenging due to the recurrence of lumen narrowing.

9.5.2 Biomaterial-Based Strategies

The basis of biomaterial strategy for tissue engineering comprises designing and fabrication of ideal vascular scaffolds for cell adhesion, migration, growth, and differentiation with appropriate choice of cells. These scaffolds provide a structural support to direct the new tissue formation. Multilayered blood vessel substitute was developed *in vitro* by Weinberg and Bell (1986) using bovine endothelial cells, SMCs, and adventitial fibroblast in collagen layers supported by Dacron mesh resembling mammalian muscular artery. Although this model exhibits maximal burst strength for 3–6 weeks, feasibility in the construction of tissue-engineered living vascular grafts has been well documented (Weinberg and Bell, 1986). Of various classes of biomaterials, polymers play a crucial role in tissue engineering technology due to its flexible physical, chemical, and biological properties. Choice of biomaterials in the development of scaffolds is based on the intended applications. Polymeric biomaterials are synthetic or natural with various merits and demerits. Status of various polymers explored in vascular reconstruction has been discussed in the following sections.

9.5.2.1 Synthetic Polymer-Based Approaches

Synthetic polymers such as ePTFE and polyethylene terephthalate (Dacron) have dominated the commercial market of vascular prostheses mainly for the larger diameter blood vessels (Whittemore et al., 1989; Greisler, 1990; Faries et al., 2000). Use of synthetic polymers offers more flexibility in the tailoring of elastic property of scaffolds. Although Teflon possesses electronegative luminal surface with porous architecture, poor patency rate (45%) was observed when used in femoropopliteal bypass surgery as compared to autologous vein grafts (60%–80%) (Johnson and Lee, 2000; Xue and Greisler, 2003). Similarly, Dacron has been widely used as aortic substitutes as it shows flexibility, elasticity, and kink-resistant properties (Ravi and Chaikof, 2010). However, Dacron showed lesser patency rate (56%) in femoral bypass surgery due to premature atherosclerosis (Thottappillil and Nair, 2015). Anti-thrombogenic property of ePTFE has been improved by developing shear stress resistant endothelium by fibrin glue precoating (Meinhart et al., 2001). Patency rate of the synthetic vascular substitutes was improved by functionalizing graft lumen by coatings, chemical, protein modifications, or endothelializations to improve nonthrombogenity and reduce inflammations (Walluscheck et al., 1996; Meinhart et al., 2001; Nishibe et al., 2001; Krijgsman et al., 2002; Li et al., 2005). Nondegradablility of these available grafts may promote long-term inflammations and demands the need of biodegradable synthetic grafts as it degrades with subsequent replacement of cell secreted native ECM in the void space. Degradable polymers such as polyglycolic acid (PGA), polylactic acid (PLA), poly-ε-caprolactone (PCL), polylactic-*co*-glycolic acid (PLGA), and polyglycerol sebacate (PGS) have been widely explored for potential vascular substitutes.

1. *PGA.* PGA is thermoplastic semicrystaline aliphatic polyesters that are degraded by hydrolytic breakdown of ester bonds (Gilding and Reed, 1979). Glycolic acid, a monomer unit of PGA is further metabolized into carbon dioxide and water (Dong et al., 2010). PGA loses its mechanical integrity in 4 weeks and is completely metabolized by 6 months (Ravi and Chaikof, 2010). This mechanical stability has been improved by the bovine SMC and endothelial cells seeded PGA scaffolds in bioreactors via the production of collagen from SMCs and its crosslinking (Niklason et al., 1999). Mechanical stiffness of PGA fails to confer elasticity of native arteries, which can be improved by the combination of copolymer of L-lactide and caprolactone. Ovine arterial cells seeded PGA scaffolds showed 73% of collagen content, presence of elastic fibers in media of tissue-engineered vessel walls with no sign of macroscopic calcification after 11 weeks of implantation in pulmonary arteries of lamb (Shinoka et al., 1998). Implantation of PGA submicron

fibers into rat model promoted fibrous encapsulation at implant interface by 7 days indicates the inflammatory characteristics and unsuitability of the use of PGA alone in long-term applications (Hajiali et al., 2011). Disadvantages such as poor mechanical property, acidic end products induced inflammatory responses, and poor long-term patency rate limits its potential applications in the tissue engineering field (Niklason et al., 1999, Higgins et al., 2003).

2. *PLA.* PLA is a biodegradable and biocompatible Food and Drug Administration (FDA)-approved thermoplastic aliphatic polyester. PLA is relatively more hydrophobic than PGA, which in turn lowers the degradation rate. Bettahalli et al. developed interconnected porous poly-L-lactic acid (PLLA) hollow fibers, which have been found to be permeating the bovine serum albumin at a permeance of 1963 L/m^2 h bar at 6 h (Bettahalli et al., 2011). Higher tensile strength and limited deformation are the major advantages of PLLA as it loses its mechanical integrity in several months to years. In addition, the implantation of PLA electrospun scaffolds showed less fibrotic zone, poor cell infiltration with the existence of fewer giant cells as compared to PGA fibers (Telemeco et al., 2005). Nanofiber/film composite made of PLGA resembling the morphology of natural ECM has supported the proliferation and extension of human umbilical vein endothelial cells in 6-day culture (Seo et al., 2008). PLGA scaffolds have also been designed for the spatial and temporal release of vascular endothelial growth factor to promote angiogenesis (Ennett et al., 2006). Bilayered tubular PLGA electrospun scaffolds has been cultured with canine bone marrow derived SMCs and endothelial cells. The cellular scaffold promoted neointimal layer formation with good patency by 3 weeks in artery of adult dog, whereas the acellular scaffold facilitated the thrombus formation and occlusion within a week (Kim et al., 2008).

3. *Polycaprolactone.* PCL is the semicrystalline hydrophobic polyester with low melting temperature of 54–60°C (Woodruff and Hutmacher, 2010). Advantages such as higher elasticity, slower degradation rate, and nontoxic metabolic end products with the ease of processing at low temperature have made them more promising substitutes for vascular tissue engineering (Nair and Laurencin, 2007; Thottappillil and Nair, 2015). Burst pressure of tubular PCL nanofibrous scaffolds (4000 mmHg) resemble the native vessels and also showed resistance to the physiological conditions of blood vessels (Drilling et al., 2009). Diban et al. developed hollow fiber PCL small diameter blood vessel substitute, which has been found to stimulate the attachment and proliferation of adipose stem cells (Diban et al., 2013). Further biomimicking multilayered arrangement of blood vessel fabricated by orienting PCL nanofibers of inner layer with longitudinal alignment and outer layer with circumferential alignment promoted endothelial cell attachment (Wu et al., 2010). PCL scaffolds implanted from rat arterial circulation exhibited homogenous neointimal formation and endothelialization with chondroid metaplasia after 6 months (de Valence et al., 2012). Copolymers such as poly(lactide-*co*-caprolactone) (PLCL) and poly(glycolide-*co*-caprolcatone) are also investigated for blood vessel regeneration due to their controllable degradation rate with low toxicity (Thottappillil and Nair, 2015). PLCL seeded with rabbit aortic SMCs under dynamic culture conditions has supported the SMC proliferation and collagen production (Jeong et al., 2005). Heparin-bonded poly(L-lactide-co-ϵ-caprolactone) demonstrated the biomechanical properties of canine femoral arteries and pre-endothelialized scaffolds showed 88.9% patency rate after 6 months in canine femoral artery replacement model (Wang et al., 2013).

4. *Polyglycerosorbate.* PGS is biodegradable polyester formed by the polycondesation of glycerol and sebasic acid. This elastomeric tough polymer exhibits high elongation with low modulus offering good biocompatibility and rapid degradation within 2 months *in vivo* (Wang et al., 2002). PGS-based biphasic tubular scaffolds have demonstrated nonthrombogenicity compared to synthetic grafts such as ePTFE and PLGA scaffolds (Motlagh et al., 2006). Porous PGS scaffolds cultured with adult primary baboon SMCs in bioreactor conditions for 3 weeks promoted mature elastin production and compliance equivalent to native arteries (Lee et al., 2011). Three months post-implanted PGS–PCL composite scaffolds in rat abdominal aorta did not provoke any stenosis (Wu et al., 2012).

5. *Polyurethane* is another choice of synthetic polymer for the fabrication of small diameter blood vessel substitute as it demonstrates higher elasticity and tensile strength along with biocompatibility (Grasl et al., 2010). Poly(ester urethane) urea nanofibrous scaffolds supported the proliferation and distribution of SMCs (Grasl et al., 2010). Polyurethane electrospun scaffolds implanted in rat abdominal aorta exhibited 95% patency rate by 6 months (Bergmeister et al., 2012). Hence, various nondegradable and degradable synthetic polymers have been widely explored for vascular tissue applications due to the lack of batch-to-batch variations with tailorable mechanical and biodegradable properties of scaffolds. However, none of the material is equivalent to endothelial non-thrombogenic barrier. Hence, the lack of biological recognition limits its potential applications as it is essential to promote endothelialization.

9.5.2.2 Natural Polymer-Based Approaches

Polymers derived from animal sources mimics the ECM components and in turn demonstrate biocompatibility and nontoxicity (Boccafoschi et al., 2007). Of many natural polymers, collagen, elastin, hyaluronan, fibrin, silk fibroin, gelatin, and chitosan have been extensively investigated for blood vessel regeneration.

1. *Collagen,* mainly type I collagen, is the most abundant component of ECM in blood vessel contributing mechanical support by limiting high strain deformation (Sankaran et al., 2015). Use of native structural proteins as biomaterials allows tissue progression as it has a specific cell-binding motifs. Collagen possesses integrin-binding motifs, which permit cell adhesion and other cell fate processes like migration, proliferation, and differentiation (Ravi and Chaikof, 2010). Further advantages such as low inflammatory, less antigenicity, biodegradability, and biocompatibility with cell adhering property make collagen a potential candidate for vascular applications (Couet et al., 2007; Marelli et al., 2012). Weinberg and Bell fabricated the first tissue-engineered vascular graft (TEVG) made of cell-seeded collagen gels resembling the intimal, medial, and adventitial layers of blood vessels. As these scaffolds ruptured at 10 mmHg, the burst strength of the scaffolds was improved to 40–70 mmHg by the incorporation of polyethylene terephthalate (PET) meshes. Vascular tissue mimetic architecture developed from cell-seeded multilayered collagen gels exhibited circularly aligned human SMCs, randomly dispersed fibroblast cells with the slightly extended parallel aligned endothelial cells to the tube axis (Weinberg and Bell, 1986). Reconstituted collagen films have been found to promote the adhesion and growth of endothelial and SMCs without altering the viscoelastic property of blood and did not support blood coagulation

(Boccafoschi et al., 2005). However, inferior mechanical stability under hemodynamic environment with physical stiffness and poor processability restricts the prospective applications (Zhang et al., 2007).

2. *Elastin.* Shortcomings of stiffer collagen provoked the search of elastic polymers for vascular applications. Elastin rich in arterial walls confers stretching, recoiling, and durability of the blood vessels (Rabaud et al., 1991). Tri-layered biomimetic vascular substitute has been developed by Boland et al. (2004) via electrospinning of collagen and elastin proteins. Insoluble nature of elastin showed difficulty in processing new biomaterials or mixing with other biomaterials (Thottappillil and Nair, 2015). Leach et al. synthesized water soluble α-elastin that are crosslinked with diepoxy resin to improve the stability of the elastin-based scaffolds (Leach et al., 2005). Dose-dependent effect of α-elastin in collagen gel has been observed on SMC and endothelial cell proliferation. At 5 mg/mL, α-elastin inhibits the SMC hyperplasia while stimulating the endothelial cell proliferation (Ito et al., 1997). Alternatively, polymers with repeats of pentapeptide sequences valine-proline-glycine-valine-glycine (VPGVG) demonstrated elastic properties, which are equivalent to native elastin (Ravi et al., 2009). Genetic engineering-based elastin mimetic diblock and triblock copolymers have been self-assembled into nano-textured hydrogel systems. Contents of collagen and elastin in collagen–elastin–glycosaminoglycan construct exhibited higher tensile strength and elasticity, respectively (Daamen et al., 2003). Mechanical strength of electrospun recombinant human tropoelastin was found to be equivalent to native elastin and supported the cobblestone morphology of endothelial cell after 48-h culture (McKenna et al., 2012). Coating of elastin onto the synthetic grafts such as ePTFE, Dacron, polycarbonate, and polyurethane improved hemocompatibility by reducing thrombogenicity, platelet adhesion, and activation (Woodhouse et al., 2004). Proliferation of SMCs results in arterial stenosis in the absence of extracellular elastin component (Gozna et al., 1974; Li et al., 1998; Ratcliffe, 2000; Kielty et al., 2002; Karnik et al., 2003; Long and Tranquillo, 2003). Hence, incorporation of elastin component is mandatory not alone to improve mechanical strength but also to prevent undesirable complications.

3. *Hyaluronan* is a nonsulfated linear glycosamino glycan comprising glucoronic acid and N-acetyl glucosamine. Hydrophilicity, biocompatibility, biodegradability, and nonadhesive property are the major advantages of hyaluronan (Catto et al., 2014). Further, Ramamurthi and Vesely (2005) reported that the use of hylan gels promotes the synthesis and organization of elastin matrix resembling native aortic valve. End-to-end implantation of HYAFF-11 tubes with 4 mm diameter in porcine model degraded completely after 5 months and replaced by neo-artery comprising organized collagen and elastin fibers, mature SMCs with the endothelial lining of lumen (Zavan et al., 2008).

4. *Fibrin* is insoluble protein matrix developed after tissue injury providing structural support for coordinating the cellular fate processes. Use of fibrin as scaffolding materials for many tissue engineering applications is growing due to the feasibility of isolating it from patient's whole blood and biodegradability in turn eliminating the immunological complications (Janmey et al., 2009). Unlike ECM, fibrin gels assembled quickly to form 3D network with high elastic modulus (Janmey et al., 2009). Firbin was used as coating material for many synthetic vascular grafts such as ePTFE to enhance the endothelialization and also prevent the loss of

endothelial cells due to the shear stress (Zilla et al., 1989; Deutsch et al., 2009). It has also been reported that the mature crosslinked fibrin matrix was reported to be fairly nonthrombogenic and reduce the thrombus formation. Composite vascular construct made by collagen and fibrin showed improved gel compaction, thereby contributing superior mechanical property compared to pure collagen and fibrin gels (Cummings et al., 2004). These fibrin gels have other desirable characteristics such as nontoxicity, nonimmunogenicity, cell-binding sites, biodegradability, self-assembling property, processability into any shape and size, and tunability of physical, chemical, and mechanical properties for tissue engineering applications (Shaikh et al., 2008).

5. *Silk fibroin* is a fibrillar protein produced from *Bombyx mori* silk worm consisting of mainly 43% glycine, 30% alanine, and 12% serine residues (Vepari and Kaplan, 2007). Excellent mechanical strength, toughness, biocompatibility, ease of processability, and functional modifications with minimal thrombogenicity are more attractive properties for the development of ideal vascular constructs (Lovett et al., 2007, 2008, 2010; Kundu et al., 2013). Silk biomaterial shows slow degradation behavior without eliciting immune response and absorbed very slowly *in vivo* (Cao and Wang, 2009). Silk fibroin protein electrospun into small diameter vascular grafts showed comparable tensile strength with native vessels and was also found to support both human endothelial and SMCs (Thottappillil and Nair, 2015). Silk-based vascular grafts demonstrated long-term patency with the intima and media like layer assembly by 12 months of post-implantation of rat abdominal aorta. Fibroin-based scaffolds showed higher patency rate; 85% as compared to ePTFE (30%) at 1 year implantation (Enomoto et al., 2010).

6. *Gelatin* is also one of the potential biomaterial for vascular tissue engineering applications due to its similarities with the collagen (Sell et al., 2009). Gelatin is derived from the collagen via denaturation consisting of amino acids such as glycine and proline as collagen. Type A gelatin possess more carboxylic groups facilitating functional modification as well as scaffold fabrication, whereas type B form of gelatin was found to enhance endothelial cell attachment (Thottappillil and Nair, 2015). Due to its upper critical solution temperature nature, gelatin becomes gel at below 37°C and transforms into sol at above the 37°C. Stability of gelatin has been improved by crosslinking, which in turn prolongs the degradation rate (Panzavolta et al., 2011). It was also reported that electrospun gelatin was found to possess higher tensile strength than collagen fibers (Sell et al., 2010).

9.5.2.3 Hybrid Biomaterials-Based Approaches

Limitations such as inferior mechanical strength and poor processability of natural polymers and lack of biorecognition motif in synthetic polymers demand the development of hybrid biomaterials (synthetic and natural), which in turn combine the advantages of the parent polymers while neutralizing the demerits of the two biomaterials (Catto et al., 2014). For example, gelatin was introduced at different weight ratios to PGA to alter the mechanical and biological properties of the vascular prosthesis (Hajiali et al., 2011). Similarly, PCL has been combined with natural proteins such as collagen or elastin to meet the desirable mechanical strength with adequate biological behavior in vascular regeneration (Tillman et al., 2009; McClure et al., 2010; Wise et al., 2011).

9.5.3 Scaffold-Free Strategies

Unlike traditional tissue engineering that requires the cells, signaling molecules, and scaffolds as ECM analog, scaffold-free tissue engineering demands the requirement of suitable cell source and stimulation to induce inherent capacity of the cells to synthesize tissue-specific ECM and matrix maturation for tissue organization (Kelm et al., 2010). Lack of exogenous biomaterial scaffold in these strategies insists the requirement of high cell density in order to establish cell–cell communication. Native tissue architecture with the functions has been developed using exogenous cues such as soluble growth factors, enzymes, and physical forces.

Ideal cell source should be nonimmunogenic, with ease of expansion in culture and functionally active (Zhang et al., 2007). Autologous vascular cells such as endothelial and SMCs do not stimulate the immune reaction (Niklason et al., 1999; Heydarkhan-Hagvall et al., 2006). However, expansion of adult autologous cells in culture is difficult due to limited proliferation of terminally differentiated cells. Length of the telomere at the ends of chromosomes is maintained by enzyme called telomerase, which consists of two subunits (RNA component and telomerase reverse transcriptase [TERT]). As most of the somatic cells do not express TERT, telomere shortening cannot be prevented leading to the cell senescence. Poh et al. have made an attempt to extend the life span of smooth muscle and endothelial cells harvested from elderly patients by transfecting with human TERT subunit (Poh et al., 2005). Use of allogenic source of cells poses the immune rejection problem. Although the pluripotent embryonic stem cells (ESCs) differentiate into SMCs, ethical concern, low induction efficiency, and tumorigenic potential

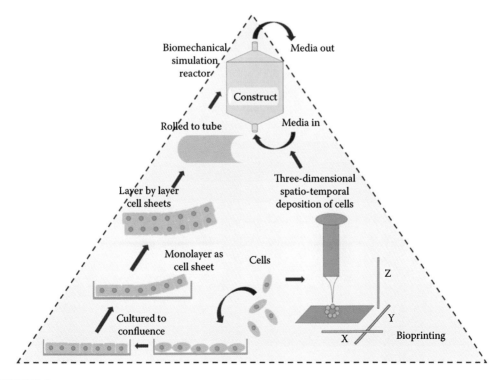

FIGURE 9.3
Bottom-up technology for the fabrication of TEVGs.

are the major limitations of ESCs (Levenberg et al., 2002; McCloskey et al., 2005; Zhang et al., 2007). Endothelial progenitor cells (EPCs) isolated from umbilical cord blood can be differentiated into mature endothelial cells as it has the *in vitro* expansion potential over 20 passages without losing the differentiation potential (Asahara et al., 1997). Further, EPCs play a vital role in angiogenesis, endothelium repair, and hemostasis (Nemeno-Guanzon et al., 2012). Another excellent choice of autologous cell source is bone marrow cells as it can be readily aspirated by semi-invasive technique and vascular differentiation potential.

Nevertheless high cell density and prolonged expansion process are required to fabricate tissue-engineered blood vessels; scaffold-free approaches such as cell sheet conduits, rapid prototyping/bioprinting, and bioreactor-based biofabrication have been exploited to circumvent problems like chronic inflammation, thrombosis, weak cell–cell communication, and rejections, which are associated with the scaffold-based strategies (L'Heureux et al., 2006). Figure 9.3 shows the bottom-up technology for the fabrication of vascular construct.

9.5.3.1 Cell Sheet Conduits

Cell sheet-based approach in regenerative medicine is "bottom-up" technology where functional units of tissue have been built to construct individual sections, which in turn combined together to generate tissue-engineered substitutes. Cell sheet transplantation receives much attention in tissue engineering applications as the artificial ECM promote inflammatory responses while degrading simultaneously (Shimizu, 2014). In addition, success of complete regeneration mainly depends on the establishment of strong cell–cell and cell–ECM communication. However, ECM analog failed to exhibit high cell density, in turn weakening the cell–cell interactions. Hence, cell sheets either two-dimensional monolayer or multilayer constructs has been used without any materials in cell sheet-based tissue engineering approach as it has the advantages of cell secreted native ECM. In addition, multiple cell types can also be micropatterned in these cell sheet construct (Guillotin and Guillemot, 2011). This cell sheet has also been rolled into tubular constructs for small diameter blood vessel grafts. Since the sheets consist of living cells with its own organized ECM, these conduits showed excellent mechanical strength. L' Heureux et al. developed tissue-engineered blood vessels-based cell sheets for adult arterial revascularization. Sheets of SMCs rolled around the mandrel to develop tunica media followed by the wrapping of fibroblast cells sheets to build tunica adventitia. Seeding of endothelial cells into the lumen surface of tubular construct has supported the development of tunica intimal layer as native vessels. This living tissue-engineered blood vessel has been cultured further under pulsatile bioreactor to enhance the rate of respective ECM production (L'Heureux et al., 1998). However, vulnerability to damage while handling and time-consuming process are the major limitations of sheet-based tissue engineering. Rayatpisheh et al. made an attempt to improve the stability of cell sheets and the rate of SMC maturation by integrating the cell sheet technology with electrospun scaffolding approach (Rayatpisheh et al., 2014).

9.5.3.2 Rapid Prototyping (Bioprinting)

Successful regeneration of vascular tissue is determined by the intricate architecture, cellularity, native ECM and desirable flexibility, and strength of functional vessels, while available cell sheet technology does not reproduce the structural organization despite having appropriate mechanical strength, and native ECM deposition. Further, time taken for the construction of sheet-based grafts is lengthy (several months). Hence, unmet need of existing technologies such as spatial and temporal precise patterning of cells and growth factors has been achieved by the emerging rapid prototypic technology, which involves the computer aided, automated 3D deposition of bioink using bioprinter. Bioprinting is the high throughput and easy scalable technology providing reproducible complex architectures of native tissue by positioning either cells or cell aggregates precisely.

In the case of building complex vasculature, bioprinting accomplishes the construction of hollow, branched, high aspect ratio tubular geometries by additive assembly. Small diameter, branched tubular constructs made of vascular tissue spheroids was printed using agarose rod-based templates of 300–500 μm diameters (Norotte et al., 2009). Faulkner-Jones et al. have developed viable spheroidal aggregates of human ESCs using valve-based bioprinter with reproducible controllable size and pluripotency. The spheroid formation has been initiated by printing an array with cell density gradient (Faulkner-Jones et al., 2013). Recently, co-axial printing of alginate loaded human umbilical vein SMCs and calcium crosslinker in sheath and core, respectively, demonstrated peripheral and luminal deposition of ECM by thick cell sheets for 6 weeks (Zhang et al., 2015). Bioprinting of agarose-based fibers as templates for microchannels fabrication, followed by the casting of photopolymerizable hydrogel precursor and crosslinking, aided in the hazzle-free removal of nonadhesive agarose forming perfusable vascular networks. Further, the gelatin methacrylated cell-laden hydrogel construct improved cellular viability, differentiation, and thereby functional endothelial monolayer formation (Bertassoni et al., 2014). The emergence of bioprinting warrants the integration of desired functions both biological and physicochemical of constructs, in addition to the rheology of printable bioink for the building of 3D complex functional branched blood vessels (Hoch et al., 2014).

9.5.3.3 Bioreactors

Blood vessels are one of the complex dynamic tissues, constantly subjected to physical forces. Bioreactors are another scaffold-free strategy for the *ex vivo* engineering of 3D blood vessels as it can provide physical and biological signals under controlled environmental conditions. Treating aged patients with autologous grafts for revascularization still remains a challenge due to telomeric erosion and senescence of cells. Poh et al. have made an attempt to fabricate autologous blood vessels against atheroscelorsis using adult human telomerase reverse transcriptase (hTERT)—SMCs under pulsatile flow bioreactor system at 165 beats per minute. After 7 weeks of culture, endothelial cells at the density of 2.7×10^6 cells/mL were injected into the vessel lumen to establish the endothelium (Poh et al., 2005). When the endothelial cells are exposed to cyclic strain in dynamic conditions, the mechanical strength of the scaffolds was found to be increased due to the overexpression of matrix remodeling protein MMP2, whereas the exposure to shear stress alters the orientation of cells and increases the endothelial cell adhesion (Seliktar et al., 2001; Braddon et al., 2002; Lee et al., 2002; Nerem, 2003; Seliktar et al., 2003). SMCs have transdifferentiated from its contractile phenotype into synthetic phenotype after injury or atherosclerotic diseases in arteries due to the injury-induced phenotypic plasticity (Speer et al., 2009). Transdifferentiation of SMCs and calcification has been controlled while exposing the SMC to cyclic strain (Nikolovski et al., 2003). Thus, bioreactors play a vital role in the ECM production, phenotypic stability of vascular cells by the simulation of tissue dynamics.

9.6 Tissue-Engineered Blood Vessels: A Clinical Success

The ultimate goal of regenerative medicine is to develop TEVGs with potential to be translated from bench-to-bed side. In an effort to translate the TEVGs to the clinics, grafts investigated in preclinical animal models have been implanted in patients. In 2001, Shinoka et al. accomplished the first TEVG transplantation for high-flow low-pressure pulmonary venous system in a 4-year-old patient and 24 other pediatric, young patients. The graft comprised PGA or PLLA fiber meshes coated with L-lactide and ε-caprolactone (50:50) copolymer, enriched *in vitro* with autologous vascular cells sourced from peripheral vein biopsies. The follow up recorded no sign of calcification, obstruction, stenosis, thrombosis, or aneurysm after 2 years and no mortality with 16% stenosis in smaller diameter (<18 mm) grafts after 7 years (long term) (Catto et al., 2014). Later, in 2005, autologous bone marrow-derived mononuclear cells from iliac crest was preferred for faster culturing (2 days) to overcome the delay caused in culturing autologous vascular cells (10 days). The graft exhibited good patency in all the 42 patients for 32 months (Shin'oka et al., 2005).

Completely autologous TEVGs developed by cell sheet engineering were implanted in 10 patients for hemodialysis by McAllister et al. (2009). Patients with end-stage renal disease and hemodialysis failure were implanted with TEVGs as arteriovenous shunts in the upper arm. The TEVGs consisted of homogenous tissue generated by wounding autologous fibroblasts sheet with autologous endothelial cells seeded onto the inner layer few days prior to surgical implantation. This autologous TEVGs showed poor compliance during implantation and only 50% patency after 3–6 months, although the TEVGs was subjected to constraints like frequent rupture and hemodynamic load (McAllister et al., 2009).

9.7 Summary and Future Prospective

This chapter mainly focused on top-down and bottom-up strategies for the development of TEVGs. Immunogenicity of decellularization based scaffolds has been reduced with the recellularization by autologous cells. As the decellularized matrix requires extreme processing conditions, various biomaterials from natural and synthetic sources have been explored for vascular regeneration. Commercially available synthetic grafts such as Dacron, ePTFE shows good patency in larger arteries but cannot be an ideal substitute for smaller arteries. Many attempts to improve endothelialization in the lumen of synthetic grafts have increased the patency. However, nondegradable nature of polymers restricts its utility due to chronic inflammations. Hence, designing biodegradable vascular scaffolds with ideal characteristics such as biomechanical, physicochemical, and biological properties similar to native ECM has evidenced biomaterial combinations with complementary features. Further clinical trials of autologous cells seeded biomaterial substrate exhibited patency in patients for several years. However, limitations such as presence of residual biomaterials with the inflammatory responses, poor long-term patency, and inferior cell–cell interaction stipulate the exploitation of bottom-up approaches in vasculature regeneration. Unlike ECM analogous scaffold-based approaches, cell sheet engineering stimulates the self-generation of native ECM by autologous cells with mechanical properties identical to native. Lengthy processing for the expansion of cell sheets with poor structural organization has been overcome by the rapid prototyping (bioprinting) technology, which achieves spatio-temporal deposition of cells. Simulation of biomechanics to enhance the tissue-specific ECM production *in vitro* and *ex vivo* engineering of the developed constructs has emerged as promising. Therefore, fabrication of wholesome vasculature with intricate architecture, dynamic functions with biomechanical properties necessitates overcoming the lacuna in the existing strategies by superimposing top-down and bottom-up approaches to act in unison.

References

Asahara, T., Murohara, T., Sullivan, A. et al. 1997. Isolation of putative progenitor endothelial cells for angiogenesis. *Science*. 275:964–967.

Bacakova, L. 2008. Cell colonization control by physical and chemical modification of materials. In: Kimura, D. (ed.), *Cell Growth Processes: New Research*. Nova Science, Huntington, New York, pp. 5–56.

Bacakova, L., Filova, E., Rypacek, F., Svorcik, V., Stary, V. 2004. Cell adhesion on artificial materials for tissue engineering. *Physiol Res*. 53:S35–S45.

Badylak, S. F., Freytes, D. O., Gilbert, T. W. 2009. Extracellular matrix as a biological scaffold material: Structure and function. *Acta Biomater*. 5:1–13.

Bentzon, J. F., Otsuka, F., Virmani, R., Falk, E. 2014. Mechanisms of plaque formation and rupture. *Circ Res*. 114:1852–1866.

Bergmeister, H., Grasl, C., Walter, I. et al. 2012. Electrospun small diameter polyurethane vascular grafts: Ingrowth and differentiation of vascular specific host cells. *Artif Organs*. 36:54–61.

Bertassoni, L. E., Cecconi, M., Manoharan, V. et al. 2014. Hydrogel bioprinted microchannel networks for vascularization of tissue engineering constructs. *Lab Chip*. 14:2202–2211.

Bettahalli, N. M. S., Steg, H., Wessling, M., Stamatialis, D. 2011. Development of poly (L-lactic acid) hollow fiber membranes for artificial vasculature in tissue engineering scaffolds. *J. Membr. Sci*. 371:117–126.

Boccafoschi, F., Habermehl, J., Vesentini, S., Mantovani, D. 2005. Biological performances of collagen-based scaffolds for vascular tissue engineering. *Biomaterials*. 26:7410–7417.

Boccafoschi, F., Rajan, N., Habermehl, J., Mantovani, D. 2007. Preparation and characterization of a scaffold for vascular tissue engineering by direct-assembling of collagen and cells in a cylindrical geometry. *Macromol Biosci*. 7:719–726.

Boland, E. D., Matthews, J. A., Pawlowski, K. J., Simpson, D. G., Wnek, G. E., Bowlin, G. L. 2004. Electrospinning collagen and elastin: Preliminary vascular tissue engineering. *Front Biosci*. 9:1422–1432.

Bordenave, L., Menu, P., Baquey, C. 2008. Developments towards tissue-engineered, small-diameter arterial substitutes. *Expert Rev Med Devices*. 5:337–347.

Braddon, L. G., Karoyli, D., Harrison, D. G., Nerem, R. M. 2002. Maintenance of a functional endothelial cell monolayer on a fibroblast/polymer substrate under physiologically relevant shear stress conditions. *Tissue Eng*. 8:695–708.

Cao, Y., Wang, B. 2009. Biodegradation of silk biomaterials. *Int. J. Mol. Sci*. 10:1514–1524.

Catto, V., Farè, S., Freddi, G., Tanzi, C. M. 2014. Vascular tissue engineering: Recent advances in small diameter blood vessel regeneration. *ISRN Vasc. Med*. 2014: 1–27 (Article ID 923030).

Conte, M. S., Mann, M. J., Simosa, H. F., Rhynhart, K. K., Mulligan, R. C. 2002. Genetic interventions for vein bypass graft disease: A review. *J Vasc Surg*. 36:1040–1052.

Couet, F., Rajan, N., Mantovani, D. 2007. Macromolecular biomaterials for scaffold-based vascular tissue engineering. *Macromol Biosci*. 7:701–718.

Cummings, C. L., Gawlitta, D., Nerem, R. M., Stegemann, J. P. 2004. Properties of engineered vascular constructs made from collagen, fibrin, and collagen–fibrin mixtures. *Biomaterials*. 25:3699–3706.

Daamen, W. F., van Moerkerk, H. T., Hafmans, T. et al. 2003. Preparation and evaluation of molecularly-defined collagen–elastin–glycosaminoglycan scaffolds for tissue engineering. *Biomaterials.* 24:4001–4009.

Dahl, S. L., Koh, J., Prabhakar, V., Niklason, L. E. 2003. Decellularized native and engineered arterial scaffolds for transplantation. *Cell Transplant.* 12:659–666.

Davignon, J., Ganz, P. 2004. Role of endothelial dysfunction in atherosclerosis. *Circulation.* 109(suppl III):III-27–III-32.

Deanfield, J. E., Halcox, J. P., Rabelink, T. J. 2007. Endothelial function and dysfunction: Testing and clinical relevance. *Circulation.* 115:1285–1295.

Deutsch, M., Meinhart, J., Zilla, P. et al. 2009. Long-term experience in autologous *in vitro* endothelialization of infrainguinal ePTFE grafts. *J Vasc Surg.* 49:352–362.

de Valence, S., Tille, J. C., Mugnai, D. et al. 2012. Long term performance of polycaprolactone vascular grafts in a rat abdominal aorta replacement model. *Biomaterials.* 33:38–47.

Diban, N., Haimi, S., Bolhuis-Versteeg, L. et al. 2013. Development and characterization of poly(ε-caprolactone) hollow fiber membranes for vascular tissue engineering. *J Membr. Sci.* 438:29–37.

Dong, Y., Yong, T., Liao, S., Chan, C. K., Stevens, M. M., Ramakrishna, S. 2010. Distinctive degradation behaviors of electrospun polyglycolide, poly(dl-lactide-co-glycolide), and poly(l-lactide-co-ε-caprolactone) nanofibers cultured with/without porcine smooth muscle cells. *Tissue Eng A.* 16:283–298.

Drilling, S., Gaumer, J., Lannutti, J. 2009. Fabrication of burst pressure competent vascular grafts via electrospinning: Effects of microstructure. *J Biomed Mater Res A.* 88:923–934.

Ennett, A. B., Kaigler, D., Mooney, D. J. 2006. Temporally regulated delivery of VEGF *in vitro* and *in vivo*. *J Biomed Mater Res A.* 79:176–184.

Enomoto, S., Sumi, M., Kajimoto, K. et al. 2010. Long-term patency of small-diameter vascular graft made from fibroin, a silk-based biodegradable material. *J Vasc Surg.* 51:155–164.

Faries, P. L., Logerfo, F. W., Arora, S., Hook, S., Pulling, M. C., Akbari, C. M., Campbell, D. R., Pomposelli, F. B. Jr. 2000. A comparative study of alternative conduits for lower extremity revascularization: All-autogenous conduit versus prosthetic grafts. *J Vasc Surg.* 32:1080–1090.

Faulkner-Jones, A., Greenhough, S., King, J. A., Gardner, J., Courtney, A., Shu, W. 2013. Development of a valve-based cell printer for the formation of human embryonic stem cell spheroid aggregates. *Biofabrication.* 5:015013.

Gelse, K., Pöschl, E., Aigner, T. 2003. Collagens—Structure, function, and biosynthesis. *Adv Drug Deliv Rev.* 55:1531–1546.

Gilding, D. K., Reed, A. M. 1979. Biodegradable polymers for use in surgery—Polyglycolic/poly(lactic acid) homo- and copolymers: 1. *Polymer.* 20:1459–1464.

Gozna, E. R., Mason, W. F., Marble, A. E., Winter, D. A., Dolan, F. G. 1974. Necessity for elastic properties in synthetic arterial grafts. *Can J Surg.* 17:176–179 passim.

Grasl, C., Bergmeister, H., Stoiber, M., Schima, H., Weigel, G. 2010. Electrospun polyurethane vascular grafts: *In vitro* mechanical behavior and endothelial adhesion molecule expression. *J Biomed Mater Res A.* 93:716–723.

Greisler, H. P. 1990. Interactions at the blood/material interface. *Ann Vasc Surg.* 4:98–103.

Guillotin, B., Guillemot, F. 2011. Cell patterning technologies for organotypic tissue fabrication. *Trends Biotechnol.* 29:183–190.

Hajiali, H., Shahgasempour, S., Naimi-Jamal, M. R., Peirovi, H. 2011. Electrospun PGA/gelatin nanofibrous scaffolds and their potential application in vascular tissue engineering. *Int J Nanomed.* 6:2133–2141.

Heydarkhan-Hagvall, S., Esguerra, M., Helenius, G., Soderberg, R., Johansson, B. R, Risberg, B. 2006. Production of extracellular matrix components in tissue engineered blood vessels. *Tissue Eng.* 12:831–842.

Higgins, S. P., Solan, A. K., Niklason, L. E. 2003. Effects of polyglycolic acid on porcine smooth muscle cell growth and differentiation. *J Biomed Mater Res A.* 67:295–302.

Hoch, E., Tovar, G. E. M., Borchers, K. 2014. Bioprinting of artificial blood vessels: Current approaches towards a demanding goal. *Eur J Cardiothorac Surg.* 46:767–778.

Hoenig, M. R., Campbell, G. R., Rolfe, B. E., Campbell, J. H. 2005. Tissue-engineered blood vessels alternative to autologous grafts? *Arterioscler Thromb Vasc Biol.* 25:1128–1134.

Ito, S., Ishimaru, S., Wilson, S. E. 1997. Inhibitory effect of type 1 collagen gel containing alpha-elastin on proliferation and migration of vascular smooth muscle and endothelial cells. *Cardiovasc Surg.* 5:176–183.

Janmey, P. A., Winer, J. P., Weisel, J. W. 2009. Fibrin gels and their clinical and bioengineering applications. *J. R. Soc. Interface.* 6:1–10.

Jeong, S. I., Kwon, J. H., Lim, J. I. et al. 2005. Mechano-active tissue engineering of vascular smooth muscle using pulsatile perfusion bioreactors and elastic PLCL scaffolds. *Biomaterials.* 26:1405–1411.

Johnson, W. C., Lee, K. K. 2000. A comparative evaluation of polytetrafluoroethylene, umbilical vein, and saphenous vein bypass grafts for femoral-popliteal above-knee revascularization: A prospective randomized Department of Veterans Affairs cooperative study. *J Vasc Surg.* 32:268–277.

Karnik, S. K., Brooke, B. S., Antonio, B. G., Sorensen, L., Wythe, J. D., Schwartz, R. S. 2003. A critical role for elastin signaling in vascular morphogenesis and disease. *Development.* 130:411–423.

Kelm, J. M., Lorber, V., Snedeker, J. G. et al. 2010. A novel concept for scaffold-free vessel tissue engineering: Self-assembly of microtissue building blocks. *J Biotechnol.* 148:46–55.

Kielty, C. M., Sherratt, M. J., Shuttleworth, C. A. 2002. Elastic fibres. *J. Cell Sci.* 115:2817–2828.

Kim, M. J., Kim, J., Yi, G., Lim, S., Hong, Y. S., Chung, D. J. 2008. *In vitro* and *in vivo* application of PLGA nanofiber for artificial blood vessel. *Macromol Res.* 16:345–352.

Krijgsman, B., Seifalian, A. M., Salacinski, H. J., Tai, N. R., Punshon, G., Fuller, B. J., Hamilton, G. 2002. An assessment of covalent grafting of RGD peptides to the surface of a compliant poly(carbonate-urea) urethane vascular conduit versus conventional biological coatings: Its role in enhancing cellular retention. *Tissue Eng.* 8:673–680.

Kundu, B., Rajkhowa, R., Kundu, S. C., Wang, X. 2013. Silk fibroin biomaterials for tissue regenerations. *Adv Drug Deliv Rev.* 65:457–470.

L'Heureux, N., Dusserre, N., Konig, G. et al. 2006. Human tissue engineered blood vessels for adult arterial revascularization. *Nat Med.* 12:361–365.

L'Heureux, N., Germain, L., Labbé, R., Auger, F. A. 1993. *In vitro* construction of a human blood vessel from cultured vascular cells: A morphologic study. *J Vasc Surg.* 17:499–509.

L'Heureux, N., Pâquet, S., Labbé, R., Germain, L., Auger, F. A. 1998. A completely biological tissue-engineered human blood vessel. *FASEB J.* 12:47–56.

Leach, J. B., Wolinsky, J. B., Stone, P. J., Wong, J. Y. 2005. Crosslinked alpha-elastin biomaterials: Towards a processable elastin mimetic scaffold. *Acta Biomater.* 1:155–164.

Lee, A. A., Graham, D. A., Dela Cruz, S., Ratcliffe, A., Karlon, W. J. 2002. Fluid shear stress-induced alignment of cultured vascular smooth muscle cells. *J Biomech Eng.* 124:37–43.

Lee, K., Stolz, D. B., Wang, Y. 2011. Substantial expression of mature elastin in arterial constructs. *Proc Natl Acad Sci USA.* 108:2705–2710.

Levenberg, S., Golub, J. S., Amit, M., Itskovitz-Eldor, J., Langer, R. 2002. Endothelial cells derived from human embryonic stem cells. *Proc Natl Acad Sci USA.* 99:4391–4396.

Li, C., Hill, A., Imran, M. 2005. *In vitro* and *in vivo* studies of ePTFE vascular grafts treated with P15 peptide. *J Biomater Sci Polym Ed.* 16:875–891.

Li, D. Y., Brooke, B., Davis, E. C., Mecham, R. P., Sorensenk, L. K., Boakk, B. B. 1998. Elastin is an essential determinant of arterial morphogenesis. *Nature.* 393:276–280.

Long, J. L., Tranquillo, R. T. 2003. Elastic fiber production in cardiovascular tissue-equivalents. *Matrix Biol.* 22:339–350.

Lovett, M., Cannizzaro, C., Daheron, L., Messmer, B., Vunjak-Novakovic, G., Kaplan, D. L. 2007. Silk fibroin microtubes for blood vessel engineering. *Biomaterials.* 28:5271–5279.

Lovett, M., Eng, G., Kluge, J. A., Cannizzaro, C., Vunjak-Novakovic, G., Kaplan, D. L. 2010. Tubular silk scaffolds for small diameter vascular grafts. *Organogenesis.* 6:217–224.

Lovett, M. L., Cannizzaro, C. M., Vunjak-Novakovic, G., Kaplan, D. L. 2008. Gel spinning of silk tubes for tissue engineering. *Biomaterials.* 29:4650–4657.

Mallat, Z., Benamer, H., Hugel, B., Benessiano, J., Steg, P. G., Freyssinet, J. M., Tedgui, A. 2000. Elevated levels of shed membrane microparticles with procoagulant potential in the peripheral circulating blood of patients with acute coronary syndromes. *Circulation*. 101:841–843.

Mano, J. F., Silva, G. A., Azevedo, H. S. et al. 2007. Natural origin biodegradable systems in tissue engineering and regenerative medicine: Present status and some moving trends. *J R Soc Interface*. 4:999–1030.

Marelli, B., Achilli, M., Alessandrino, A. et al. 2012. Collagen reinforced electrospun silk fibroin tubular construct as small calibre vascular graft. *Macromol Biosci*. 12:1566–1574.

McAllister, T. N., Maruszewski, M., Garrido, S. A. et al. 2009. Effectiveness of haemodialysis access with an autologous tissue-engineered vascular graft: A multicentre cohort study. *Lancet*. 373:1440–1446.

McCloskey, K. E., Gilroy, M. E., Nerem, R. M. 2005. Use of embryonic stem cell-derived endothelial cells as a cell source to generate vessel structures *in vitro*. *Tissue Eng*. 11:497–505.

McClure, M. J., Sell, S. A., Simpson, D. G., Walpoth, B. H., Bowlin, G. L. 2010. A three-layered electrospun matrix to mimic native arterial architecture using polycaprolactone, elastin, and collagen: A preliminary study. *Acta Biomater*. 6:2422–2433.

McKenna, K. A., Hinds, M. T., Sarao, R. C. et al. 2012. Mechanical property characterization of electrospun recombinant human tropoelastin for vascular graft biomaterials. *Acta Biomater*, 8:225–233.

Meinhart, J. G., Deutsch, M., Fischlein, T., Howanietz, N., Fröschl, A., Zilla, P. 2001. Clinical autologous *in vitro* endothelialization of 153 infrainguinal ePTFE grafts. *Ann Thorac Surg*. 71:S327–S331.

Motlagh, D., Yang, J., Lui, K. Y., Webb, A. R., Ameer, G. A. 2006. Hemocompatibility evaluation of poly(glycerol-sebacate) *in vitro* for vascular tissue engineering. *Biomaterials*. 27:4315–4324.

Mozaffarian, D., Benjamin, E. J., Go, A. S. et al. 2015. Heart disease and stroke statistics—2015 update: A report from the American Heart Association. *Circulation*. 131:e29–e322.

Nair, L. S., Laurencin, C. T. 2007. Biodegradable polymers as biomaterials. *Prog Polym Sci*. 32:762–798.

Neff, L. P., Tillman, B. W., Yazdani, S. K. et al. 2011. Vascular smooth muscle enhances functionality of tissue-engineered blood vessels *in vivo*. *J Vasc Surg*. 53:426–434.

Nemeno-Guanzon, J. G., Lee, S., Berg, J. R. et al. 2012. Trends in tissue engineering for blood vessels. *J Biomed Biotechnol*. 2012:1–14.

Nerem, R. M. 2003. Role of mechanics in vascular tissue engineering. *Biorheology*. 40:281–287.

Niklason, L. E., Gao, J., Abbott, W. M., Hirschi, K. K., Houser, S., Marini, R., Langer, R. 1999. Functional arteries grown *in vitro*. *Science*. 284:489–493.

Nikolovski, J., Kim, B. S., Mooney, D. J. 2003. Cyclic strain inhibits switching of smooth muscle cells to an osteoblast-like phenotype. *FASEB J*. 17:455–457.

Nishibe, T., O'Donnel, S., Pikoulis, E., Rich, N., Okuda, Y., Kumada, T., Kudo, F., Tanabe, T., Yasuda, K. 2001. Effects of fibronectin bonding on healing of high porosity expanded polytetrafluoroethylene grafts in pigs. *J Cardiovasc Surg (Torino)*. 42:667–673.

Norotte, C., Marga, F., Niklason, L., Forgacs, G. 2009. Scaffold-free vascular tissue engineering using bioprinting. *Biomaterials*. 30:5910–5917.

Olausson, M., Kuna, V. K., Travnikova, G. et al. 2014. *In vivo* application of tissue-engineered veins using autologous peripheral whole blood: A proof of concept study. *EBioMedicine*. 1:72–79.

Olausson, M., Patil, P. B., Kuna, V. K. et al. 2012. Transplantation of an allogeneic vein bioengineered with autologous stem cells: A proof-of-concept study. *Lancet*. 380:230–237.

Panzavolta, S., Gioffrè, M., Focarete, M. L., Gualandi, C., Foroni, L., Bigi, A. 2011. Electrospun gelatin nanofibers: Optimization of genipin cross-linking to preserve fiber morphology after exposure to water. *Acta Biomater*. 7:1702–1709.

Peck, M., Gebhart, D., Dusserre, N., McAllister, T. N., L'Heureux, N. 2011. The evolution of vascular tissue engineering and current state of the art. *Cells Tissues Organs*. 195:144–158.

Piccone, V. 1987. Alternative techniques in coronary artery reconstruction. In: Sawyer, P. N. (ed.), *Modern Vascular Grafts*. McGraw-Hill, New York, pp. 253–260.

Piterina, A. V., Cloonan, A. J., Meaney, C. L. et al. 2009. ECM-based materials in cardiovascular applications: Inherent healing potential and augmentation of native regenerative processes. *Int J Mol Sci*. 10:4375–4417.

Poh, M., Boyer, M., Solan, A., Dahl, S. L., Pedrotty, D., Banik, S. S., McKee, J. A., Klinger, R. Y., Counter, C. M., Niklason, L. E. 2005. Blood vessels engineered from human cells. *Lancet.* 365:2122–2124.

Quint, C., Kondo, Y., Manson, R. J., Lawson, J. H., Dardik, A., Niklason, L. E. 2011. Decellularized tissue-engineered blood vessel as an arterial conduit. *PNAS.* 108:9214–9219.

Rabaud, M., Lefebvre, F., Ducassou, D. 1991. *In vitro* association of type III collagen with elastin and with its solubilized peptides. *Biomaterials.* 12:313–319.

Ramamurthi, A., Vesely, I. 2005. Evaluation of the matrix-synthesis potential of crosslinked hyaluronan gels for tissue engineering of aortic heart valves. *Biomaterials.* 26:999–1010.

Ratcliffe, A. 2000. Tissue engineering of vascular grafts. *Matrix Biol.* 19:353–357.

Rathore, A., Cleary, M., Naito, Y., Rocco, K., Breuer, C. 2012. Development of tissue engineered vascular grafts and application of nanomedicine. *Wiley Interdiscip Rev Nanomed Nanobiotechnol.* 4:257–272.

Ravi, S., Chaikof, E. L. 2010. Biomaterials for vascular tissue engineering. *Regen Med.* 5:107.

Ravi, S., Qu, Z., Chaikof, E. L. 2009. Polymeric materials for tissue engineering of arterial substitutes. *Vascular.* 17:S45–S54.

Rayatpisheh, S., Heath, D. E., Shakouri, A., Rujitanaroj, P., Chewa, S. Y., Chan-Park, M. B. 2014. Combining cell sheet technology and electrospun scaffolding for engineered tubular, aligned, and contractile blood vessels. *Biomaterials.* 35:2713–2719.

Ross, R. 1995. Cell biology of atherosclerosis. *Annu Rev Physiol.* 57:791–804.

Sankaran, K. K., Subramanian, A., Krishnan, U. M., Sethuraman, S. 2015. Nanoarchitecture of scaffolds and endothelial cells in engineering small diameter vascular grafts. *Biotechnol J.* 10:96–108.

Seliktar, D., Nerem, R. M., Galis, Z. S. 2001. The role of matrix metalloproteinase-2 in the remodeling of cell-seeded vascular constructs subjected to cyclic strain. *Ann Biomed Eng.* 29:923–934.

Seliktar, D., Nerem, R. M., Galis, Z. S. 2003. Mechanical strain-stimulated remodeling of tissue-engineered blood vessel constructs. *Tissue Eng.* 9:657–666.

Sell, S. A., McClure, M. J., Garg, K., Wolfe, P. S., Bowlin, G. L. 2009. Electrospinning of collagen/biopolymers for regenerative medicine and cardiovascular tissue engineering. *Adv Drug Deliv Rev.* 61:1007–1019.

Sell, S. A., Wolfe, P. S., Garg, K., McCool, J. M., Rodriguez, I. A., Bowlin, G. L. 2010. The use of natural polymers in tissue engineering: A focus on electrospun extracellular matrix analogues. *Polymers.* 2:522–553.

Seo, H. J., Yu, S. M., Lee, S. H., Choi, J. B., Park, J.-C., Kim, J. K. 2008. Effect of PLGA nano-fiber/film composite on HUVECs for vascular graft scaffold. In: Lim C., Goh, J. H. (eds), *13th International Conference on Biomedical Engineering*, Singapore, 23, pp. 2147–2150.

Shaikh, F. M., Callanan, A., Kavanagh, E. G., Burke, P. E., Grace, P. A., McGloughlin, T. M. 2008. Fibrin: A natural biodegradable scaffold in vascular tissue engineering. *Cells Tissues Organs.* 188:333–346.

Shimizu, T. 2014. Cell sheet-based tissue engineering for fabricating 3-dimensional heat tissues. *Circ J.* 78:2594–2603.

Shin'oka, T., Matsumura, G., Hibino, N. et al. 2005. Midterm clinical result of tissue-engineered vascular autografts seeded with autologous bone marrow cells. *J Thorac Cardiovasc Surg.* 129:1330–1338.

Shinoka, T., Shum-Tim, D., Ma, P. X. et al. 1998. Creation of viable pulmonary artery autografts through tissue engineering. *J Thorac Cardiovasc Surg.* 115:536–545.

Song, J. J., Ott, H. C. 2011. Organ engineering based on decellularized matrix scaffolds. *Trends Mol Med.* 17:424–432.

Speer, M. Y., Yang, H. Y., Brabb, T. et al. 2009. Smooth muscle cells give rise to osteochondrogenic precursors and chondrocytes in calcifying arteries. *Circ Res.* 104:733–741.

Stegemann, J. P., Kaszuba, S. N., Rowe, S. L. 2007. Review: Advances in vascular tissue engineering using protein-based biomaterials. *Tissue Eng.* 13:2601–2613.

Telemeco, T. A., Ayres, C., Bowlin, G. L. et al. 2005. Regulation of cellular infiltration into tissue engineering scaffolds composed of submicron diameter fibrils produced by electrospinning. *Acta Biomater* 1:377–385.

Thomas, A. C., Campbell, G. R., Campbell, J. H. 2003. Advances in vascular tissue engineering. *Cardiovasc Pathol*. 12:271–276.

Thomas, L. V., Lekshmi, V., Nair, P. D. 2013. Tissue engineered vascular grafts-preclinical aspects. *Int J Cardiol*. 167:1091–1100.

Thottappillil, N., Nair, P. D. 2015. Scaffolds in vascular regeneration: Current status. *Vasc Health Risk Manag*. 11:79–91.

Tillman, B. W., Yazdani, S. K., Lee, S. J., Geary, R. L., Atala, A., Yoo, J. J. 2009. The *in vivo* stability of electrospun polycaprolactonecollagen scaffolds in vascular reconstruction. *Biomaterials*. 30:583–588.

Vara, D. S., Salacinski, H. J., Kannan, R. Y., Bordenave, L., Hamilton, G., Seifalian, A. M. 2005. Cardiovascular tissue engineering: State of the art. *Pathol Biol (Paris)*. 53:599–612.

Vepari, C., Kaplan, D. L. 2007. Silk as a biomaterial. *Prog. Polym. Sci*. 32:991–1007.

Walluscheck, K. P., Steinhoff, G., Kelm, S., Haverich, A. 1996. Improved endothelial cell attachment on ePTFE vascular grafts pretreated with synthetic RGD-containing peptides. *Eur J Vasc Endovasc Surg*. 12:321–330.

Wang, S., Mo, X. M., Jiang, B. J., Gao, C. J., Wang, H. S., Zhuang, Y. G., Qiu, L. J. 2013. Fabrication of small-diameter vascular scaffolds by heparin-bonded P(LLA-CL) composite nanofibers to improve graft patency. *Int J Nanomed*. 8:2131–2139.

Wang, Y., Ameer, G. A., Sheppard, B. J., Langer, R. 2002. A tough biodegradable elastomer. *Nat. Biotechnol*. 20:602–606.

Weinberg, C. B., Bell, E. 1986. A blood vessel model constructed from collagen and cultured vascular cells. *Science*. 231:397–400.

Whittemore, A. D., Kent, K. C., Donaldson, M. C., Couch, N. P., Mannick, J. A. 1989. What is the proper role of polytetrafluoroethylene grafts in infrainguinal reconstruction? *J Vasc Surg*. 10:299–305.

Wise, S. G., Byrom, M. J., Waterhouse, A., Bannon, P. G., Ng, M. K. C., Weiss, A. S. 2011. A multilayered synthetic human elastin/polycaprolactone hybrid vascular graft with tailored mechanical properties. *Acta Biomater*. 7:295–303.

Woodhouse, K. A., Klement, P., Chen, V. et al. 2004. Investigation of recombinant human elastin polypeptides as non-thrombogenic coatings. *Biomaterials*. 25:4543–4553.

Woodruff, M. A., Hutmacher, D. W. 2010. The return of a forgotten polymer—Polycaprolactone in the 21st century. *Prog Polym Sci*. 35:1217–1256.

Wu, H., Fan, J., Chu, C. C., Wu, J. 2010. Electrospinning of small diameter 3-D nanofibrous tubular scaffolds with controllable nanofiber orientations for vascular grafts. *J Mater Sci Mater Med*. 21:3207–3215.

Wu, W., Allen, R. A., Wang, Y. 2012. Fast degrading elastomer enables rapid remodeling of a cell-free synthetic graft into a neo-artery. *Nat Med*. 18:1148–1153.

Xue, L., Greisler, H. P. 2003. Biomaterials in the development and future of vascular grafts. *J Vasc Surg*. 37:472–480.

Zavan, B., Vindigni, V., Lepidi, S. et al. 2008. Neoarteries grown *in vivo* using a tissue-engineered hyaluronan-based scaffold. *FASEB J*. 22:2853–2861.

Zhang, W. J., Liu, W., Cui, L., Cao, Y. 2007. Tissue engineering of blood vessel. *J Cell Mol Med*. 11:945–957.

Zhang, Y., Yu, Y., Akkouch, A., Dababneh, A., Dolatia, F., Ozbolat, I. T. 2015. *In vitro* study of directly bioprinted perfusable vasculature conduits. *Biomater. Sci*. 3:134–143.

Zilla, P., Fasol, R., Preiss, P. et al. 1989. Use of fibrin glue as a substrate for *in vitro* endothelialization of PTFE vascular grafts. *Surgery*. 105:51522.

10

Bioartificial Pancreas

Clancy J. Clark and Emmanuel C. Opara

CONTENTS

10.1 Introduction

The pancreas is an endocrine and exocrine organ located centrally posterior to the stomach. It is vital in maintaining glucose control and facilitates the digestion and intestinal absorption of carbohydrates, proteins, and lipids. The ductal network and acinar cells involved in the exocrine function of the pancreas comprise 95% of the pancreatic mass. Clusters of cells called islets of Langerhans represent the endocrine component of the pancreas. Islets consist of four main cell types: alpha cells secrete glucagon, increasing blood glucose; beta cells secrete insulin, decreasing blood glucose; delta cells secrete somatostatin, which helps regulate alpha and beta cells; and gamma cells secrete pancreatic polypeptide. The interplay between these cells within islets of Langerhans helps regulate glucose metabolism and homeostasis.

Destruction of islets of Langerhans or cellular resistance to insulin causes diabetes mellitus. In type 1 diabetes, β cells are destroyed through an immune-mediated mechanism with onset of disease occurring mainly in childhood. Type 2 diabetes develops in the setting of obesity, sedentary lifestyle, and poor diet. In type 2 diabetes, cells throughout the body fail to respond to insulin. Type 3 diabetes is a newly recognized category of diabetes arising from pancreatic disease, including trauma/injury, chronic pancreatitis, malignancy, or drug toxicity (Ewald and Bretzel, 2013).

Diseases of the pancreas, including pancreatitis, pancreatic cancer, and diabetes, have a significant impact on a patient's quality of life and result in substantial financial burden for society. As of 2012, 86 million Americans aged 20 and older have prediabetes and 9.3% suffer from diabetes (29.1 million) (American Diabetes Association, 2015). Globally, more than 1.5 million people died secondary to diabetes in 2012, and by 2030, diabetes will be the seventh leading cause of death (WHO, 2015). Diabetes results in significant long-term morbidity and mortality. Cardiovascular and cerebrovascular effects of diabetes lead to hypertension, myocardial infarction, stroke, kidney dysfunction, vision impairment, sensory loss, limb loss, and wound infection. In the United States, diabetes cost $245 billion in 2012 (American Diabetes Association, 2015).

Management of diabetes focuses on glycemic control through pharmacological therapy. Patients with type 2 diabetes can be managed with a variety of medicines, including metformin, short- and long-acting insulin, sulfonylureas, meglitinides, thiazolidinedione, alpha-glucosidase, GLP-1 receptor agonists, DPP-4 inhibitors, and SGLT-2 inhibitors (Nathan, 2015). For patients with insulin deficiency, standard treatment is daily injections of exogenous insulin. Thirty years ago, the Diabetes Control and Complications Trial demonstrated that well-controlled glycemia can prevent the development of secondary complications of diabetes (Gubitosi-Klug, 2014). Follow-up studies have confirmed the benefit of tight glucose control (Aiello and Sun, 2015). However, good glycemic control does not prevent or reverse diabetic retinopathy, nephropathy, and neuropathy (The Diabetes Control and Complications Trial Research Group, 1993). Potential complications linked with intensive insulin therapy include weight gain and hypoglycemia (The Diabetes Control and Complications Trial Research Group, 1988, 1993; Lebovitz, 2011).

Given the challenges patients face with current treatment options and socioeconomic burden of diabetes worldwide, alternative treatment options have been explored, including transplantation of beta cells using whole pancreas or individual islets. Previous studies indicate that pancreas transplant may prevent secondary diabetic complications in type 1 and type 2 diabetics (Ciancio and Burke, 2014). In contrast to exogenous insulin administration, transplantation can achieve normoglycemia along with prevention and even reversal of certain secondary diabetic complications, such as nephropathy and coronary artery disease (Ciancio and Burke, 2014). While there are clear advantages of pancreas transplant, immunosuppressive drugs have significant short- and long-term risks, such as infection or secondary malignancy (White et al., 2009).

In 1966, the first combined kidney–pancreas transplantation was performed at the University of Minnesota by Kelly and Lillehei (Kelly et al., 1967). From 1966 to 2008, over 30,000 pancreas transplants (22,000 in the United States) have been performed (Gruessner and Sutherland, 2008). Unfortunately, given the complexity of whole pancreas transplant, patients are at risk of procedure-related complications, including bleeding, infection, pancreatic fistula, and anastomotic leak. Transplantation of isolated islet cells has demonstrated some promise (Kendall and Robertson, 1997; Weir and Bonner-Weir, 1997; Kenyon et al., 1998; Harlan et al., 2009). Following the initial report of isolating islets from the rat pancreas, this approach has resulted in significant investigation (Lacy and Kostianovsky, 1967). In 2000, the Edmonton group introduced a method of islet transplantation using glucocorticoid-free immunosuppressive regimen (Shapiro et al., 2000).

Despite the initial promising results of islet cell transplantation, it has been difficult to generalize. From a total of 1 million islets in the normal human pancreas, only 50% are successfully isolated on a consistent basis (Hatziavramidis et al., 2013). Allogenic cells used in islet cell transplant induce an immune response, and to avoid rejection, patients require chronic immunosuppression. Most importantly, the severe shortage of human donors is a significant barrier to clinical islet transplantation (Lacy and Kostianovsky, 1967; Kendall and Robertson, 1997; Weir and Bonner-Weir, 1997; Kenyon et al., 1998; Robertson, 2000; Shapiro et al., 2000; Ryan et al., 2001; Rother and Harlan, 2004; Ryan et al., 2005; Harlan et al., 2009).

Bioartificial pancreas is a promising device to replace β-cells and may address issues associated with shortages in donor islets and need for long-term immunosuppression. A well-designed bioartificial pancreas should be capable of producing adequate insulin to treat all forms of diabetes and perform as a pancreas replacement.

10.1.1 Defining the Bioartificial Pancreas

The bioartificial pancreas is a bioengineered device that is implanted, secretes insulin in response to blood glucose, and helps regulate glucose homeostasis. Simple islet cell transplant without immunosuppression is not possible given allogenic immune response. For type 1 diabetes, preexisting antibodies and immune cells against β-cell surface epitopes and insulin will also destroy transplanted islets (Jansson and Hellerström, 1983). Therefore, the bioengineered pancreas must immune-isolate islets to avoid rejection. One strategy for immune isolation is biocoating or encapsulation of allogenic or xenogeneic islet cells before implantation. The bioengineered pancreas could address issues of limited human islet cell availability, enable prolonged euglycemia, and avoid risks associated with immunosuppression.

The two functions of a successful bioartificial pancreas are (1) improved glycemic control by minimizing blood glucose fluctuations and (2) reproduction of normal stimulation of the liver by the pancreas, helping to normalize carbohydrate and lipid metabolism.

10.2 Approaches to Fabricating a Bioartifical Pancreas

A couple of approaches to engineering a bioartificial pancreas have been proposed. One approach involves using gene therapy technology in which a genetically engineered virus that may transform host cells into insulin-producing cells is introduced into a patient. Another approach is to bioengineer an islet cell delivery system that protects islets and increases their short- and long-term viability using an encapsulation technique. In this chapter, we will focus on microencapsulation as a method of engineering bioartificial pancreas.

Microencapsulation is the process of enclosing micron-sized particles or droplets in an inert shell. The encapsulation process both protects and isolates the contents from the external environment. The products obtained by this process are called microparticles, microcapsules, and microspheres (Ghosh, 2006). Particles typically range from 200 to 1000 microns in diameter (Pareta et al., 2012b). Microencapsulation has mostly been applied to large-scale industrial processes of emulsification, coacervation, spray drying, fluidized bed coating, etc., mainly for applications in the chemicals (detergents, cosmetics, printing ink, etc.), textiles, food, and paper industry (Tewes et al., 2006). With recent technological advancements, microencapsulation has gained significant interest among bioengineers and researchers. Microencapsulation of pancreatic islet cells is one of many applications of this exciting technology.

10.2.1 Isolation of Pancreatic Islets

Isolation of functional and intact pancreatic islets is technically challenging and the key first step in constructing a bioengineered pancreas. Various isolation techniques have been proposed and involve preservation, dissociation, and purification (Kin, 2010). The process of islet isolation has significant impact on clinical outcomes (Lakey et al., 2002). Using collagenase and proteases, islets are separated from the intercellular collagen matrix. Following dissociation, the islets need to be washed and purified. Bacterial cultures are obtained to avoid infection at the time of transplant. The length of exposure to collagenase and proteases determines to an extent the intra-islet cell–cell adhesion disruption and separation for the extra-islet cell matrix. Shorter exposure time can result in low islet yields but longer exposure can lead to loss of islet cell integrity and viability.

10.2.2 Methods of Encapsulation

A variety of encapsulation methods have been investigated. Industrial bulk microencapsulation processes include spray drying, hot melt, coacervation and phase separation, atomization, pan coating, solvent evaporation, and fluidized bed/air suspension coating. High-quality microcapsules, however, are not required in the food and cosmetic industry. For the creation of encapsulated islets, one requires monodispersed, highly controllable microencapsulation. The commonly employed devices for microencapsulation of cells and biological materials are coaxial airflow droplet generator, electrostatic generator, vibration method, jet cutter, and shear flow-driven methods (Figure 10.1).

10.2.3 Biomaterials

Islets are encapsulated in a protective coating for immunoisolation (Opara et al., 2010) (Figure 10.2). Therefore, the biomaterials used must be biocompatible and semipermeable. The protective coating should be able to exchange hormones, nutrients, and oxygen. Biocompatibility of encapsulated pancreatic islets is measured by the extent of fibrosis at the implantation site. The most common materials used for microencapsulation are agarose, alginate, chitosan, cellulose, copolymers of acrylonitrile, poly(hydroxyethylmethacrylate–methyl methacrylate) (HEMA–MMA), and polyethylene glycol (PEG) (Lim and Sun, 1980; Dawson et al., 1987; Iwata et al., 1989; Kessler et al., 1991; Zielinski and Aebischer, 1994;

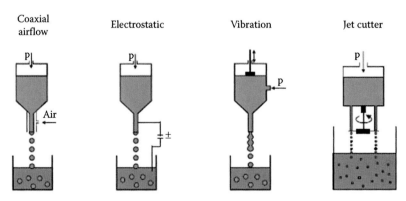

FIGURE 10.1
Schematic representation of the various microencapsulation methods. (From Prusse, U. et al. 2008. *Chem Pap.* 62: 364–74. With permission.)

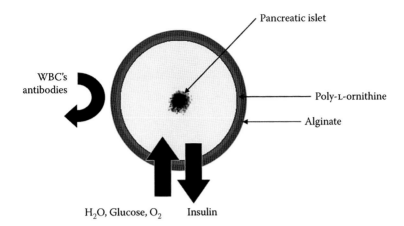

FIGURE 10.2
Illustration of the principle of microencapsulation technology. (From Opara, E. C. et al. 2010. *J Investig Med.* 58: 831–7. With permission.)

Cruise et al., 1999; Risbud and Bhonde, 2001). Hydrogels, such as alginate, are structurally soft and pliable, resulting in less irritation to the neighboring tissues after implantation. Alginate hydrogels also are permeable to low-molecular-weight molecules. This makes hydrogels a favorable method of encapsulation (Pareta et al., 2012b).

10.2.3.1 Alginate

Alginate is the most studied hydrogel for pancreatic islet encapsulation. Alginate molecules are linear block copolymers of β-ᴅ-mannuronic (M) and α-ʟ-guluronic acids (G), which form a gel in the presence of divalent ions such as calcium or barium (Pareta et al., 2012b). Barium is toxic to humans; therefore, gelling of alginate is performed with calcium. Alginate gelling can be performed in multiple environmental and physiological conditions, making it very suitable for islet encapsulation. Importantly, alginate can encapsulate pancreatic islets at normal physiological conditions. Islet encapsulation with alginate has improved islet viability and does not interfere with cellular function (Fritschy et al., 1991; Sandler et al., 1997; De Haan et al., 2003). In animal and human studies of implanted alginate-based capsules, they have remained stable for years (Soon-Shiong et al., 1994; Sun et al., 1996). Also, since alginates are negatively charged, the attachment of immune cells to the microcapsule is decreased (Pareta et al., 2012b).

10.2.3.2 Poly-ʟ-Lysine

One challenge of working with alginate is its stability. Coating alginate beads with poly-ʟ-lysine (PLL) can increase membrane stability but maintain a permeable membrane (Pareta et al., 2012b). PLL, therefore, is a commonly used polycation solution for stabilizing alginate in the encapsulation process. This stable PLL–alginate construct enables long-term xenograft transplantation.

Numerous studies have demonstrated that the alginate–PLL–alginate construct is effective in small animal, large animal, and human studies (Lim and Sun, 1980; O'Shea et al., 1984; Sun et al., 1984; O'Shea and Sun, 1986; Fan et al., 1990; Fritschy et al., 1991; Lum et al., 1992; Soon-Shiong et al., 1992; Elliott et al., 2000; Kendall et al., 2001; Calafiore et al., 2006).

However, free, unbound PLL stimulates an inflammatory response and fibrosis of microcapsules after implantation (Thu et al., 1996; Strand et al., 2001). Recent studies reported that PLL does not form a simple membrane layer separate from alginate (King et al., 1987; Clayton et al., 1991; Strand et al., 2001). Even in encapsulation systems where an outer alginate layer is used, PLL is still present (Pareta et al., 2012b). This likely increases the chance of an inflammatory response and fibrotic overgrowth (King et al., 1987; Clayton et al., 1991; Strand et al., 2001). Scar and fibrosis around implanted microcapsules will alter capsule permeability, leading to islet cell dysfunction and decreased islet cell viability (De Vos et al., 2006). The surface roughness of the PLL layer, as demonstrated by atomic force microscopy may also induce significant fibrotic overgrowth. However, properly bound PLL microcapsules can be safely implanted with minimal inflammatory response.

10.2.3.3 Poly-L-Ornithine

Poly-L-ornithine (PLO) is an alternative to PLL. PLO is a widely used positively charged biomaterial that can be used for forming a permselective coating (Darrabie et al., 2005). This permselectivity decreases pore size and capsule swelling, creating more stable capsule able to provide immune isolation for islet cells without impairing oxygen and nutrient diffusion (Opara et al., 2010). We have demonstrated that PLO has improved mechanical properties compared with PLL (Darrabie et al., 2005). Also, the immune response to PLO is less than PLL (Basta et al., 1991; Calafiore et al., 1997; Kizilel et al., 2005). When compared to alginate–PLL microcapsules, alginate–PLO microcapsules have decreased swelling and bursting under osmotic stress (Darrabie et al., 2005). Bead swelling can lead to increased pore size and membrane permeability. Disrupted pores will lead to inappropriate diffusion of cytokines and thus decreases islet cell viability (Thu et al., 1996). Our prior work indicates that the improved mechanical properties of the alginate–PLO construct versus alginate–PLL may be due to the shorter monomer structure of PLO (Darrabie et al., 2005). Long-term studies in rodents, dogs, and pigs investigating intraperitoneal injection employing alginate–PLO microcapsules demonstrated long-term stability of microcapsules up to 1 year postimplant without significant fibrosis (De Vos et al., 2006).

10.2.4 Islet Encapsulation

Islet encapsulation is done in aqueous dispersion with low agitation, in the presence of iso-osmotic salt, glucose, and oxygen in the media under normal physiological pH (Pareta et al., 2013). Alginate beads are coated with a cationic poly(amino acid), such as PLL or PLO, to improve structure durability while maintaining permeability (Chaikof, 1999; Opara et al., 2013). Then, an outer layer of alginate is applied. This layering of an alginate–PLL/PLO–alginate construct is known as alginate-PLL/PLO-alginate (APA) microcapsules (Pareta et al., 2013). Figure 10.3 shows encapsulated islets in APA microcapsules.

Capsule size is important for maintaining islet cell viability. In most tissues, the maximum diffusion distance for effective oxygen and nutrient diffusion from blood capillary to cells is about 200 μm (Pareta et al., 2013). A diffusion gradient is also found within the microcapsule, as well as, within the pancreatic islet. Larger capsules result in decreased exchange of oxygen, hormones, and nutrients. Therefore, microcapsules are preferred over macrocapsules (Pareta et al., 2013). Forming of microcapsules require interfacial precipitation of alginate using a divalent cation, such as calcium or barium. This alginate solution is combined with pancreatic islets to form encapsulated islets. The formation of individual capsules is based on suspension of this solution and using a variety of techniques, including air jet

Bioartificial Pancreas 237

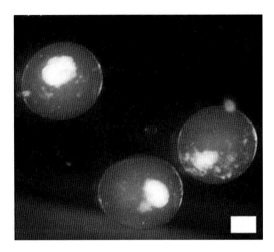

FIGURE 10.3
Encapsulated islets in an alginate microcapsule. Scale = 100 μm.

spray method, electrostatic generators, submerged oscillating coaxial extrusion nozzles, conformal coatings, and spinning disk atomization (Dawson et al., 1987; Wolters et al., 1991; Hallé et al., 1994; Hsu et al., 1994; Senuma et al., 2000; Desmangles et al., 2001; Prüsse et al. 2008). In our lab, the most commonly used method is air jet spray using a two-channel air droplet microencapsulator (Pareta et al., 2013). The alginate–islet cell suspension is allowed to drip through an inner channel and the droplet is formed using shear forces from an outer channel of air. The microcapsule size can be adjusted by changing the diameter of the inner and outer channels. Pancreatic islet cell microencapsulation is performed rapidly at controlled temperatures (around 4°C) to decrease hypoxic damage and improve islet viability.

Unfortunately, our current microencapsulation process is slow and is not able to efficiently form large numbers of encapsulated pancreatic islets. Given the capsulation process is performed in room air, it induces hypoxic stress and will result in increased islet cell loss if performed over an extended period (De Vos et al., 1997; Opara et al., 2010). A multichannel air jacket microfluidic device may be able to overcome barriers to scaling up islet cell microencapsulation. Multichannel devices can increase the speed of encapsulation eight times faster than conventional methods (Pareta et al., 2014b). Initial results indicate no negative impact on pancreatic islet function (Pareta et al., 2014b). Additionally, using rapid prototyping technology, scale-up of this microfluidic approach can also be cost-efficient (Tendulkar et al., 2011).

Decreased capsule size improves pancreatic islet viability and function and will also decrease total transplant volume. Recent investigations have, therefore, focused on reducing bead diameter from larger 800-μm bead to much smaller 185-μm bead. This new bead size is four times smaller than conventional beads (Pareta et al., 2012a). The diffusion of oxygen and nutrients is improved with the smaller-diameter beads. Smaller capsule size also appears to have improved stability *in vivo* over larger capsules (Omer et al., 2005; Pareta et al., 2013). Unfortunately, reduced microcapsule size can result in an increased percent of exposed islets, thus inducing an inflammatory or rejection response. To adjust for protruding islets, the pancreatic islet density in the alginate microbead is decreased, but then this may lead to increased number of empty capsules. Therefore, an optimal islet density must be determined during the scaling-up process to produce microcapsules with a low percent of exposed islets, few empty capsules, and minimal irregularities or imperfections.

10.2.5 Microcapsules as an Immune Barrier

Uncoated non-permselective alginate microbeads are very permeable (>600 kD) and permit uptake of IgG (150 kD) and thyroglobulin (669 kD) (Pareta et al., 2013). For example, uncoated alginate capsules contain IgG and C3 component after 1 week of transplant (Lanza et al., 1995). With uncoated microcapsules, small molecules produced by macrophages and T-cells, such as IL-1β, TNF-α, and IFN-γ, can easily enter capsules and destroy the encapsulated islets (Van Schilfgaarde and de Vos, 1999). As discussed above, coating alginate microcapsules with a barrier of PLO or PLL can help create an immune barrier. The positively charged polyamino acid molecules create an alginate–PLL or alginate–PLO construct (Thu et al., 1996). The construct reduces the pore size of the microcapsule, resulting in a decrease in the exchange of small molecules between the host and the microcapsule (King et al., 1987; Hallé et al., 1994; Kulseng et al., 1997). The addition of an outer layer of alginate, creating an alginate–PLL/PLO–alginate construct, can help decrease the fibrous reaction, resulting in exposed polyamino acid (Pareta et al., 2014b). The first permselective biomaterial developed was PLL. More recent studies indicated that PLO significantly reduces the immune response compared with PLL and has been shown to strengthen microcapsules (Lim and Sun, 1980; Darrabie et al., 2001; Pareta et al., 2013).

10.2.6 Transplantation Site

Survival of transplanted pancreatic islets is dependent on rapid engraftment by minimizing the interval of islet hypoxia. Therefore, proximity to the bloodstream is a major predictor of graft viability. The optimal site for transplantation of pancreatic islets is not clear. For example, the portal vein is frequently used for human islet cell transplant but is limited by small graft volume. For animals, pancreatic islet cells are typically implanted into the peritoneal cavity (Pareta et al., 2013). It is technically easier to implant islets into the peritoneum and as it has a large capacity (Elliott et al., 2000; Calafiore et al., 2006). However, there are several disadvantages to using the peritoneum. First, transplanted pancreatic islet cells are vulnerable to intraperitoneal T-cells and macrophages (Van Schilfgaarde and de Vos, 1999; De Vos et al., 2003; De Groot et al., 2004; Safley et al., 2005). Second, islets have less access to the vasculature (Van Schilfgaarde and de Vos, 1999; De Vos et al., 2002). Given the pitfalls of peritoneal implantation, multiple alternative sites have been investigated, including the liver, portal vein, kidney capsule, subcutaneously, and into an omental pouch (Kin et al., 2003; Toso et al., 2005; Dufrane et al., 2006a,b; Kobayashi et al., 2006; Moya et al., 2010a,b; Opara et al., 2010). As noted before, the portal vein has limited transplant volume and is prone to thrombosis. Implantations under the skin and in the kidney capsule also have not demonstrated improved results. Both are limited by transplant volume and less cellular overgrowth compared with pancreatic islets transplanted into the peritoneum.

Within the peritoneum, an omental pouch may be the optimal target transplantation site. It is well vascularized and does not have a limited volume (Kin et al., 2003). The omentum is easily accessible and a small pouch can be created with suture (Pareta et al., 2013). Pancreatic islets are then placed in the center of this pouch (Kin et al., 2003). In recent studies, encapsulated islets implanted into an omental pouch appear to function better than encapsulated islets implanted free in the peritoneum (Kobayashi et al., 2006). Long-term survival of encapsulated islets in an omental pouch has also been demonstrated (Pareta et al., 2014a).

10.2.7 Islet Graft Vascularization and Angiogenesis

While we have improved the microencapsulation process and have identified suitable target transplant sites, long-term survival of implanted pancreatic islets is still limited by graft vascularization. After implantation, pancreatic islet viability is dependent on the levels of oxygen, hormones, and nutrients. The pancreas is a highly vascular organ and islets receive a significant percent of the pancreas blood volume (Lifson et al., 1980; Jansson and Hellerström, 1983). From the point of pancreas resection through the processing of pancreatic islet isolation, individual islets have no vascular supply (Brissova et al., 2004). Prolonged lack of blood supply results in ischemia of pancreatic islets and can result in poor engraftment of the islets and poor islet function. Islet cells are most susceptible to damage in the first 3 days (Davalli et al., 1996).

Microvasculature forms in 10–14 days after transplant in successful pancreatic islet grafts (Menger et al., 1994; Merchant et al., 1997; Vajkoczy et al., 1995; Beger et al., 1998; Furuya et al., 2003). For encapsulated islets, islet cells depend on the diffusion of oxygen and nutrients. A hypoxic environment will lead to cell death (Vasir et al., 1998). Addition of angiogenic stimulating proteins, such as growth factor, fibroblast growth factor 1 (FGF-1), within encapsulated islets may improve survival of transplanted islets (Lai et al., 2005, Miao et al., 2005, Rivas-Carrillo et al., 2006; Opara et al., 2010). Durability of neovasculature resulting from growth factors, however, has not been well investigated and may be abnormal and unsustainable vasculature formation (Pareta et al., 2013). Controlled, sustained release of FGF-1 allows for normal vessel growth limited to the site of implantation (Moya et al., 2009). Additionally, methods for generating alginate–PLO–alginate constructs for sustained release of FGF-1 have been investigated and have been shown to cause significant angiogenesis over controls when implanted into the omental pouches of rats for 2 weeks (Khanna et al., 2010; Opara et al., 2010).

10.2.8 Antioxidants and Islet Transplantation

Hypoxia during the isolation process results in the release of oxygen-free radicals (superoxide oxygen, hydrogen peroxide, hydroxyl radicals, and peroxynitrite), leading to oxidative stress (Pareta et al., 2012). After implantation, pancreatic islets are then exposed to free radicals, which further injure pancreatic islets (Wiegand et al., 1993; Pareta et al., 2012). Normally, tissues can clear free radicals but when the free radicals cannot be cleared, it results in oxidative stress (Opara, 2006). This persistent oxidative stress can impact survival of transplanted islets. For example, transplanted beta cells have been shown to be damaged as a result of oxidative stress (Rabinovitch and Suarez-Pinzon, 1998). Potentially, the addition of free radical scavengers may improve the viability of transplanted islets (Monfared, 2009). In one study, the addition of Trolox, a water-soluble derivative of vitamin E, improved islet function following isolation and during encapsulation (Stiegler et al., 2010).

10.3 Clinical Trials in Microencapsulation of Islet Cells

Transplantation of encapsulated pancreatic islet cells has been investigated in animal trials and small human clinical trials (Table 10.1). Studies have demonstrated successful and

TABLE 10.1

Summary of Large Animal and Human Studies

Study	Model	Type of Graft	Islet Equivalents (IEQ/kg Body Weight)	Duration of Insulin Independence
Soon-Shiong et al. (1992)	Canine	Allograft		63–107 days
Sun et al. (1996)	Primate	Xenograft (porcine)	7500–17,500	120–803 days
Dufrane et al. (2006a)	Primate	Xenograft (porcine)	15,000	
Wang et al. (2008)	Canine	Allograft	55,270–87,031	50–214 days
Kendall et al. (2001)	Primate	Xenograft (porcine)	15,000	Up to 9 months
Soon-Shiong et al. (1994)	Human	Allograft	15,000	9 months
Calafiore et al. (1997)	Human	Allograft	400,000–600,000 total IEQ	
Elliott et al. (2007)	Human	Xenograft (porcine)	15,000	

Note: With the exception of Dufrane et al. (2006a), where encapsulated islets were implanted within the kidney capsule, all studies implanted encapsulated islets intraperitoneally with either PLL or PLO barriers.

sustained insulin production in mouse, rat, canine, pig, and primates. Results obtained in allo- and xenotransplantation approaches are encouraging (Soon-Shiong et al., 1992; Kendall et al., 2001; Calafiore, 2004; Dufrane et al., 2006a,b; Wang et al., 2008). Phase I and II human clinical trials are currently underway by Living Cell Technologies (Clinical Trials. gov., 2014; Diabecell: Development to Date, 2015).

Several pilot clinical studies have been conducted to evaluate transplantation of micro-encapsulated pancreatic islet cells in humans. These studies have demonstrated stabilization of blood glucose levels and decrease in insulin requirements but have not enabled long-term insulin independence (Calafiore et al., 2006; Elliott et al., 2007). In a case report by Soon-Shiong et al. (1994), encapsulated islets were transplanted by injection into the peritoneal cavity. This type 1 diabetic patient observed stabilization of blood glucose over the 9-month observation period (Soon-Shiong et al., 1994).

In 2009, Living Cell Technologies (LCT Global) began Phase I/IIa clinical trials with its encapsulated neonatal islet xenotransplant program in Russia. According to the information available from the LCT website, eight patients received the microencapsulated pig islet implants (DIABECELL) of varying strengths and number of doses (Diabecell: Development to Date, 2015). LCT further outlined that the trial successfully met its endpoints of demonstrating safety and tolerability (Diabecell: Development to Date, 2015). Preliminary unpublished data by LCT indicates that patients had improved blood glucose with decrease in insulin requirements and better blood glucose control (Diabecell: Development to Date, 2015). Phase IIa clinical trials are now underway in New Zealand and Argentina. Patients are receiving various doses of microencapsulated porcine islets ranging from 5000 to 20,000 IEQ/kg. Initial findings reported by LCT indicate improvements in HbA1c, improvements in hypoglycemia unawareness, and a positive impact on quality of life. Implanted microencapsulated xenotransplants appear to be safe and well tolerated.

10.3.1 Current Challenges in Clinical Application

Since the introduction of microencapsulation technology by Bisceglie in the 1930s, we have made significant progress toward engineering a bioartificial pancreas (Bisceglie, 1933). Clinic trials are demonstrating promising results. However, there are certain challenges that still prevent this versatile technology from wide-scale use, including (1) scale-up devices for microencapsulation, (2) improved internal oxygen and nutrients transfer to promote cell viability, (3) reducing the total transplant volume, (4) determining an optimal implantation site, (5) reduction of inflammatory response after transplant of the encapsulated islet cells, (6) complete encapsulation of all the cells, (7) efficient islet isolation, and (8) improved purification and storage techniques (Pareta et al., 2012). Table 10.2 summarizes several of these barriers and strategies to overcome them.

The biggest challenge facing the field of islet cell microencapsulation is scaling up of the manufacturing process. There is currently no commercially available microencapsulation device that satisfactorily meets the optimum requirements for islet microencapsulation (Pareta et al., 2014b). The two most commonly used devices for microencapsulation are the electrostatic bead generator and the air-syringe pump droplet generator (Wolters et al., 1991; Hsu et al., 1994; Park et al., 2011). Current devices are unable to produce high numbers of numerous capsules in a short interval of time. Processing times need to decrease to prevent loss of islets and the total number of islets encapsulated during this process need to increase. For treatment of the diabetic patient, 1 million islets are required. We estimated that 100 hours would be required to complete the encapsulation of 1 million islets (Pareta et al., 2014b). However, in practice, the process may in fact be two times longer (De Vos et al., 1997).

Importantly, islet cells do not expand in culture and are difficult to maintain in culture. Therefore, methods to improve cell viability are highly desirable in islet cell transplantation. Microcapsules can limit the supply of nutrients and oxygen and directly impact islet cell viability. This is further exasperated by the hypoxic environment encountered during islet transplantation (Opara et al., 2010; Opara and Harrison, 2013). Different polymeric materials, such as agarose and alginate, used for encapsulation have different permeabilities to oxygen (Li et al., 1996). To overcome oxygen diffusion limitation and enhance cell viability, oxygen delivery systems such as micro- and nanoparticulate oxygen generators and perfluorocarbon (PFC) may be included in an encapsulation matrix (Chin et al., 2008).

The optimal site for bioartificial pancreas implantation is a matter of intense research (Merani et al., 2008). The peritoneal cavity has been used in numerous studies because of

TABLE 10.2

Current Barriers to Success of Encapsulated Islet Cell Transplantation

Barriers to Microcapsule Transplantation	Strategies for Clinical Success
Loss of viability during islet isolation and encapsulation	Improved enzymatic blends and process control to maximize pure islet yield
	Culture media for long-term *in vitro* culture and encapsulation
	Scalable microfluidic encapsulation devices
Failure to revascularize on transplantation	Better vascularized implant site
	Co-encapsulation with angiogenic factors to promote revascularization
	Co-encapsulation with antioxidants to counter oxidative stress
Inflammatory reaction	Good hydrogel coating
	Immunoisolation barriers with no surface exposure
Inadequate islet mass	Xenotransplants
	Stem cell and gene therapy-based approaches

Source: Reproduced from Pareta, R. A. et al. 2012b. Bioartificial pancreas: Evaluation of crucial barriers to clinical application. In *Organ Donation and Transplantation—Public Policy and Clinical Perspectives*, ed. G. Randhawa, 239–266, Intech Open Science. With permission.

technical ease of accessibility and its huge capacity to accommodate a large islet cell volume. Alternative sites have included the subcutaneous space, the kidney capsule, and the omentum. Our group has recently proposed that transplantation of microencapsulated islets in the omentum via an omentum pouch should be adequate to meet the oxygen needs of islets and easy retrieval of the encapsulated islets for posttransplant analyses (Opara et al., 2010; Pareta et al., 2014a).

Reducing the total volume of transplanted cells and complete cell encapsulation are major concerns for implementation of microencapsulated islet technology. Large-diameter capsules limit the transfer of oxygen and nutrients to the pancreatic islets within the microcapsule (Pareta et al., 2013). However, small capsules result in high ratio of empty capsules and incomplete encapsulation. Sorting encapsulated islets from empty and incomplete encapsulated islets can decrease overall transplant and decrease the immune response at the time of transplantation, albeit, it increases the laboriousness of the encapsulation process. In recent years, new techniques, such as conformal coating and islet enclosure, molecular entrapment, and nanoencapsulation of islets have been developed, but their impacts are yet to be determined (Tendulkar et al., 2013).

10.4 Conclusions

Engineering of a bioartificial pancreas through the microencapsulation of islet cells is a promising treatment option for endocrine diseases of the pancreas. Despite the apparent simplicity of islet cell encapsulation, few clinical trials exist. We are just beginning to understand the critical requirements for optimal encapsulation of islets in a microcapsule structure. Failures of successful islet cell encapsulation have been due to unpurified alginate, surface exposure of PLL, rough external surface, and low surface-to-volume ratio (Pareta et al., 2012b). High-throughput devices for making encapsulated islets are emerging and the encapsulation time will need to decrease, making microencapsulation a viable method for constructing a bioartificial pancreas.

Shortage of human pancreatic islets will limit the generalization of these techniques. However, regeneration therapy and xenotransplantation techniques may negate this issue of islet shortage. Various strategies are being explored to improve islet graft viability and longevity. These strategies will need to be combined to ensure optimal creation of encapsulated pancreatic islets for transplantation. Advances in micro-manufacturing, pharmacology, biomaterials, genetic engineering, micro-coating, and biological processing will undoubtedly lead to improvements in designing of the optimal bioartificial pancreas that would act as an effective alternative treatment for diabetes.

References

Aiello, L. P., Sun, W. 2015. Intensive diabetes therapy and ocular surgery in type 1 diabetes. *N Engl J Med*. 372: 1722–33.

American Diabetes Association. 2015. *Statistics about Diabetes*. http://www.diabetes.org/diabetes-basics/statistics/ (accessed January 1, 2015).

Basta, B. P. G., Faloerni, A., Calcinaro, F., Pietropaolo, M., Calafiore, R. 1991. Immunoprotection of pancreatic islet grafts within artificial microcapsules. *Int J Artif Organs*. 14: 789–91.

Beger, C., Cirulli, V., Vajkoczy, P., Halban, P. A., Menger, M. D. 1998. Vascularization of purified pancreatic islet-like cell aggregates (pseudoislets) after syngeneic transplantation. *Diabetes*. 47: 559–65.

Bisceglie, V. 1933. Über die antineoplastische immunität; heterologe Einpflanzung von Tumoren in Hühner-embryonen (About antineoplastic immunity: Heterologous implantation of tumors in chicken embryos). *Ztschr Krebsforsch*. 40: 122–40.

Brissova, M., Fowler, M., Wiebe, P. et al. 2004. Intraislet endothelial cells contribute to revascularization of transplanted pancreatic islets. *Diabetes*. 53: 1318–25.

Calafiore, R., Basta, G., Boselli, C. et al. 1997. Effects of alginate/polyaminoacidic coherent microcapsule transplantation in adult pigs. *Transplant Proc*. 29: 2126–7.

Calafiore, R., Basta, G., Luca, G. et al. 2004. Grafts of microencapsulated pancreatic islet cells for the therapy of diabetes mellitus in non-immunosuppressed animals. *Biotechnol Appl Biochem*. 39: 159–64.

Calafiore, R., Basta, G., Luca, G. et al. 2006. Microencapsulated pancreatic islet allografts into nonimmunosuppressed patients with type 1 diabetes. *Diab Care*. 29: 137–8.

Chaikof, E. L. 1999. Engineering and material considerations in islet cell transplantation. *Annu Rev Biomed Eng*. 1: 103–27.

Chin, K., Khattak, S. F., Bhatia, S. R., Roberts, S. C. 2008. Hydrogel-perfluorocarbon composite scaffold promotes oxygen transport to immobilized cells. *Biotechnol Prog*. 24: 358–66.

Ciancio, G., Burke, G. W. 2014. Type 2 diabetes: Is pancreas transplantation an option? *Curr Diab Rep*. 14: 542.

Clayton, H. A., London, N. J., Colloby, P. S., Bell, P. R., James, R. F. 1991. The effect of capsule composition on the biocompatibility of alginate-poly-L-lysine capsules. *J Microencapsul*. 8: 221–33.

Clinical Trials.gov. 2014. Open-Label Investigation of the Safety and Effectiveness of DIABECELL(R) in Patients with Type I Diabetes Mellitus. http://www.otsuka.com/en/hd_release/release/pdf.php?news=1011 (accessed October 6, 2015).

Cruise, G. M., Hegre, O. D., Lamberti, F. V. et al. 1999. *In vitro* and *in vivo* performance of porcine islets encapsulated in interfacially photopolymerized poly(ethylene glycol) diacrylate membranes. *Cell Transplant*. 8: 293–306.

Darrabie, M., Freeman, B. K., Kendall, W. F., Hobbs, H. A., Opara, E. C. 2001. Durability of sodium sulfate-treated polylysine-alginate microcapsules. *J Biomed Mater Res*. 54: 396–9.

Darrabie, M. D., Kendall, W. F., Opara, E. C. 2005. Characteristics of poly-L-ornithine-coated alginate microcapsules. *Biomaterials*. 26: 6846–52.

Davalli, A. M., Scaglia, L., Zangen, D. H., Hollister, J., Bonner-Weir, S., Weir, G. C. 1996. Vulnerability of islets in the immediate posttransplantation period: Dynamic changes in structure and function. *Diabetes*. 45: 1161–7.

Dawson, R. M., Broughton, R. L., Stevenson, W. T., Sefton, M. V. 1987. Microencapsulation of CHO cells in a hydroxyethyl methacrylate-methyl methacrylate copolymer. *Biomaterials*. 8: 360–6.

De Groot, M., Schuurs, T. A., Van Schilfgaarde, R. 2004. Causes of limited survival of microencapsulated pancreatic islet grafts. *J Surg Res*. 121: 141–50.

De Haan, B. J., Faas, M. M., De Vos, P. 2003. Factors influencing insulin secretion from encapsulated islets. *Cell Transplant*. 12: 617–25.

Desmangles, A. I., Jordan, O., Marquis-Weible, F. 2001. Interfacial photopolymerization of β cell clusters: Approaches to reduce coating thickness using ionic and lipophilic dyes. *Biotechnol Bioeng*. 72: 634–41.

De Vos, P., De Haan, B. J., Van Schilfgaarde, R. 1997. Upscaling the production of microencapsulated pancreatic islets. *Biomaterials*. 18: 1085–90.

De Vos, P., Faas, M. M., Strand, B., Calafiore, R. 2006. Alginate-based microcapsules for immunoisolation of pancreatic islets. *Biomaterials*. 27: 5603–17.

De Vos, P., Hamel, A. F., Tatarkiewicz, K. 2002. Considerations for successful transplantation of encapsulated pancreatic islets. *Diabetologia*. 45: 159–73.

De Vos, P., Smedema, I., van Goor, H. et al. 2003. Association between macrophage activation and function of micro-encapsulated rat islets. *Diabetologia.* 46: 666–73.

Diabetes Control and Complications Trial Research Group. 1988. Weight gain associated with intensive therapy in the diabetes control and complications trial. The DCCT Research Group. *Diab Care.* 11: 567–73.

Diabetes Control and Complications Trial Research Group. 1993. The effect of intensive treatment of diabetes on the development and progression of long-term complications in insulin-dependent diabetes mellitus. *N Engl J Med.* 329: 977–86.

Dufrane, D., Goebbels, R. M., Saliez, A., Guiot, Y., Gianello, P. 2006a. Six-month survival of microencapsulated pig islets and alginate biocompatibility in primates: Proof of concept. *Transplantation.* 81: 1345–53.

Dufrane, D., Steenberghe, M. V., Goebbels, R. M., Saliez, A., Guiot, Y., Gianello, P. 2006b. The influence of implantation site on the biocompatibility and survival of alginate encapsulated pig islets in rats. *Biomaterials.* 27: 3201–8.

Elliott, R. B., Escobar, L., Garkavenko, O. et al. 2000. No evidence of infection with porcine endogenous retrovirus in recipients of encapsulated porcine islet xenografts. *Cell Transplant.* 9: 895–901.

Elliott, R. B., Escobar, L., Tan, P. L. J., Muzina, M., Zwain, S., Buchanan, C. 2007. Live encapsulated porcine islets from a type 1 diabetic patient 9.5 yr after xenotransplantation. *Xenotransplantation.* 14: 157–61.

Ewald, N., Bretzel, R. G. 2013. Diabetes mellitus secondary to pancreatic diseases (type 3c)—Are we neglecting an important disease? *Eur J Intern Med.* 24: 203–6.

Fan, M. Y., Lum, Z. P., Fu, X. W., Levesque, L., Tai, I. T., Sun, A. M. 1990. Reversal of diabetes in BB rats by transplantation of encapsulated pancreatic islets. *Diabetes.* 39: 519–22.

Fritschy, W. M., Strubbe, J. H., Wolters, G. H., van Schilfgaarde, R. 1991. Glucose tolerance and plasma insulin response to intravenous glucose infusion and test meal in rats with microencapsulated islet allografts. *Diabetologia.* 34: 542–7.

Furuya, H., Kimura, T., Murakami, M., Katayama, K., Hirose, K., Yamaguchi, A. 2003. Revascularization and function of pancreatic islet isografts in diabetic rats following transplantation. *Cell Transplant.* 12: 537–44.

Ghosh, S. K. 2006. Functional coatings and microencapsulation: A general perspective, In *Functional Coatings: By Polymer Microencapsulation,* ed. S. K. Ghosh, 1–28, Wiley-VCH Verlag GmbH & Co. KGaA, Weinheim, FRG.

Gruessner, A. C., Sutherland, D. E. R. 2008. Pancreas transplant outcomes for United States (US) cases as reported to the United Network for Organ Sharing (UNOS) and the International Pancreas Transplant Registry (IPTR). *Clin Transpl.* 2008: 45–56.

Gubitosi-Klug, R. A. 2014. The diabetes control and complications trial/epidemiology of diabetes interventions and complications study at 30 years: Summary and future directions. *Diab Care.* 37: 44–9.

Hallé, J. P., Leblond, F. A., Pariseau, J. F., Jutras, P., Brabant, M. J., Lepage, Y. 1994. Studies on small (<300 microns) microcapsules: II—Parameters governing the production of alginate beads by high voltage electrostatic pulses. *Cell Transplant.* 3: 365–72.

Harlan, D. M., Kenyon, N. S., Korsgren, O., Roep, B. O. 2009. Current advances and travails in islet transplantation. *Diabetes.* 58: 2175–84.

Hatziavramidis, D. T., Karatzas, T. M., Chrousos, G. P. 2013. Pancreatic islet cell transplantation: An update. *Ann Biomed Eng.* 41: 469–76.

Hsu, B. R., Chen, H. C., Fu, S. H., Huang, Y. Y., Huang, H. S. 1994. The use of field effects to generate calcium alginate microspheres and its application in cell transplantation. *J Formos Med Assoc.* 93: 240–5.

Iwata, H., Amemiya, H., Matsuda, T., Takano, H., Hayashi, R., Akutsu, T. 1989. Evaluation of microencapsulated islets in agarose gel as bioartificial pancreas by studies of hormone secretion in culture and by xenotransplantation. *Diabetes.* 38: 224–5.

Jansson, L., Hellerström, C. 1983. Stimulation by glucose of the blood flow to the pancreatic islets of the rat. *Diabetologia.* 25: 45–50.

Kelly, W. D., Lillehei, R. C., Merkel, F. K., Idezuki, Y., Goetz, F. C. 1967. Allotransplantation of the pancreas and duodenum along with the kidney in diabetic nephropathy. *Surgery*. 61: 827–37.

Kendall, D. M., Robertson, R. P. 1997. Pancreas and islet transplantation: Challenges for the twenty-first century. *Endocrinol Metab Clin North Am*. 26: 611–30.

Kendall, W. F., Collins, B. H., Opara, E. C. 2001. Islet cell transplantation for the treatment of diabetes mellitus. *Expert Opin Biol Ther*. 1: 109–19.

Kenyon, N. S., Ranuncoli, A., Masetti, M., Chatzipetrou, M., Ricordi, C. 1998. Islet transplantation: Present and future perspectives. *Diabetes Metab Rev*. 14: 303–13.

Kessler, L., Pinget, M., Aprahamian, M., Dejardin, P., Damgé, C. 1991. *In vitro* and *in vivo* studies of the properties of an artificial membrane for pancreatic islet encapsulation. *Horm Metab Res*. 23: 312–7.

Khanna, O., Moya, M. L., Opara, E. C., Brey, E. M. 2010. Synthesis of multilayered alginate microcapsules for the sustained release of fibroblast growth factor-1. *J Biomed Mater Res— Part A*. 95: 632–40.

Kin, T. 2010. Islet isolation for clinical transplantation. *Adv Exp Med Biol*. 654: 683–710.

Kin, T., Korbutt, G. S., Rajotte, R. V. 2003. Survival and metabolic function of syngeneic rat islet grafts transplanted in the omental pouch. *Am J Transplant*. 3: 281–5.

King, G., Daugulis, J., Faulkner, P., Goosen, M. F. 1987. Alginate-polylysine microcapsules of controlled membrane molecular weight cutoff for mammalian cell culture engineering. *Biotechnol Prog*. 3: 231–40.

Kizilel, S., Garfinkel, M., Opara, E. 2005. The bioartificial pancreas: Progress and challenges. *Diabetes Technol Ther*. 7: 968–85.

Kobayashi, T., Aomatsu, Y., Iwata, H. et al. 2006. Survival of microencapsulated islets at 400 days posttransplantation in the omental pouch of NOD mice. *Cell Transplant*. 15: 359–65.

Kulseng, B., Thu, B., Espevik, T., Skjåk-Bræk, G. 1997. Alginate polylysine microcapsules as immune barrier: Permeability of cytokines and immunoglobulins over the capsule membrane. *Cell Transplant*. 6: 387–94.

Lacy, P. E., Kostianovsky, M. 1967. Method for the isolation of intact islets of Langerhans from the rat pancreas. *Diabetes*. 16: 35–9.

Lai, Y., Schneider, D., Kidszun, A. et al. 2005. Vascular endothelial growth factor increases functional beta-cell mass by improvement of angiogenesis of isolated human and murine pancreatic islets. *Transplantation*. 79: 1530–6.

Lakey, J. R. T., Tsujimura, T., Shapiro, A. M. J., Kuroda, Y. 2002. Preservation of the human pancreas before islet isolation using a two-layer (UW solution-perfluorochemical) cold storage method. *Transplantation*. 74: 1809–11.

Lanza, R. P., Kühtreiber, W. M., Ecker, D., Staruk, J. E., Chick, W. L. 1995. Xenotransplantation of porcine and bovine islets without immunosuppression using uncoated alginate microspheres. *Transplantation*. 59: 1377–84.

Lebovitz, H. E. 2011. Insulin: Potential negative consequences of early routine use in patients with type 2 diabetes. *Diab Care*. 34: S225–30.

Li, R. H., Altreuter, D. H., Gentile, F. T. 1996. Transport characterization of hydrogel matrices for cell encapsulation. *Biotechnol Bioeng*. 50: 365–73.

Life Cell Technologies. 2015. Diabecell: Development to Date. http://www.otsuka.com/en/hd_release/release/pdf.php?news=1011 (accessed October 6, 2015).

Lifson, N., Kramlinger, K. G., Mayrand, R. R., Lender, E. J. 1980. Blood flow to the rabbit pancreas with special reference to the islets of Langerhans. *Gastroenterology*. 79: 466–73.

Lim, F., Sun, A. M. 1980. Microencapsulated islets as bioartificial endocrine pancreas. *Science*. 210: 908–10.

Lum, Z. P., Krestow, M., Tai, I. T., Vacek, I., Sun, A. M. 1992. Xenografts of rat islets into diabetic mice. An evaluation of new smaller capsules. *Transplantation*. 53: 1180–3.

Menger, M. D., Vajkoczy, P., Beger, C., Messmer, K. 1994. Orientation of microvascular blood flow in pancreatic islet isografts. *J Clin Invest*. 93: 2280–5.

Merani, S., Toso, C., Emamaullee, J., Shapiro, M. J. 2008. Optimal implantation site for pancreatic islet transplantation. *Br J Surg*. 95: 1449–61.

Merchant, F. A., Diller, K. R., Aggarwal, S. J., Bovik, A. C. 1997. Angiogenesis in cultured and cryo-preserved pancreatic islet grafts. *Transplantation*. 63: 1652–60.

Miao, G., Mace, J., Kirby, M. et al. 2005. Beneficial effects of nerve growth factor on islet transplantation. *Transplant Proc*. 37: 3490–2.

Monfared, M. S. S. 2009. Islet transplantation and antioxidant management: A comprehensive review. *World J Gastroenterol*. 15: 1153.

Moya, M. L., Cheng, M. H., Huang, J. J. et al. 2010a. The effect of FGF-1 loaded alginate microbeads on neovascularization and adipogenesis in a vascular pedicle model of adipose tissue engineering. *Biomaterials*. 31: 2816–26.

Moya, M. L., Garfinkel, M. R., Liu, X. et al. 2010b. Fibroblast growth factor-1 (FGF-1) loaded microbeads enhance local capillary neovascularization. *J Surg Res*. 160: 208–12.

Moya, M. L., Lucas, S., Francis-Sedlak, M. et al. 2009. Sustained delivery of FGF-1 increases vascular density in comparison to bolus administration. *Microvasc Res*. 78: 142–7.

Nathan, D. M. 2015. Diabetes: Advances in diagnosis and treatment. *JAMA*. 314: 1052–62.

Omer, A., Duvivier-Kali, V., Fernandes, J. et al. 2005. Long-term normoglycemia in rats receiving transplants with encapsulated islets. *Transplantation*. 79: 52–8.

Opara, E. C. 2006. Oxidative stress. *Dis Mon*. 52: 183–98.

Opara, E. C., Harrison, B. S. 2013. The bioartificial pancreas: How should we address the issue of oxygen delivery? *JSM Regen Med Bio Eng*. 1: 1001.

Opara, E. C., McQuilling, J. P., Farney, A. C. 2013. Microencapsulation of pancreatic islets for use in a bioartificial pancreas. *Methods Mol Biol*. 1001: 261–6.

Opara, E. C., Mirmalek-Sani, S. H., Khanna, O., Moya, M. L. B. E. 2010. Design of a bioartificial pancreas. *J Investig Med*. 58: 831–7.

O'Shea, G. M., Goosen, M. F., Sun, A. M. 1984. Prolonged survival of transplanted islets of Langerhans encapsulated in a biocompatible membrane. *Biochim Biophys Acta*. 804: 133–6.

O'Shea, G. M., Sun, A. M. 1986. Encapsulation of rat islets of Langerhans prolongs xenograft survival in diabetic mice. *Diabetes*. 35: 943–6.

Pareta, R., McQuilling, J. P., Sittadjody, S. et al. 2014a. Long-term function of islets encapsulated in a redesigned alginate microcapsule construct in omentum pouches of immune-competent diabetic rats. *Pancreas*. 43: 605–13.

Pareta, R., Sanders, B., Babbar, P. et al. 2012a. Immunoisolation: Where regenerative medicine meets solid organ transplantation. *Expert Rev Clin Immunol*. 8: 685–92.

Pareta, R., Farney, A. C., Opara, E. C. 2013. Design of a bioartificial pancreas. *Pathobiology*. 80: 194–202.

Pareta, R., McQuilling, J. P., Farney, A. C., Opara, E. C. 2012b. Bioartificial pancreas: Evaluation of crucial barriers to clinical application. In *Organ Donation and Transplantation—Public Policy and Clinical Perspectives*, ed. G. Randhawa, 239–266, Intech Open Science. http://www.intechopen.com/books/organ-donation-and-transplantation-public-policy-and-clinical-perspectives

Pareta, R., McQuilling, J. P., Farney, A. C., Opara, E. C. 2014b. Microencapsulation technology. In *Regenerative Medicine Applications in Organ Transplantation*, ed. G. Orlando, 627–635, Elsevier, Amsterdam.

Park, C. H., Chung, N., Lee, J. 2011. Monodisperse red blood cell-like particles via consolidation of charged droplets. *J Colloid Interface Sci*. 361: 423–8.

Prüsse, U., Bilancetti, L., Bučko, M. et al. 2008. Comparison of different technologies for alginate beads production. *Chem Pap*. 62: 364–74.

Rabinovitch, A., Suarez-Pinzon, W. L. 1998. Cytokines and their roles in pancreatic islet beta-cell destruction and insulin-dependent diabetes mellitus. *Biochem Pharmacol*. 55: 1139–49.

Risbud, M. V., Bhonde, R. R. 2001. Suitability of cellulose molecular dialysis membrane for bioartificial pancreas: *In vitro* biocompatibility studies. *J Biomed Mater Res*. 54: 436–44.

Rivas-Carrillo, J. D., Navarro-Alvarez, N., Soto-Gutierrez, A. et al. 2006. Amelioration of diabetes in mice after single-donor islet transplantation using the controlled release of gelatinized FGF-2. *Cell Transplant*. 15: 939–44.

Robertson, R. P. 2000. Successful islet transplantation for patients with diabetes—Fact or fantasy? *N Engl J Med*. 343: 289–90.

Rother, K. I., Harlan, D. M. 2004. Challenges facing islet transplantation for the treatment of type 1 diabetes mellitus. *J Clin Invest*. 114: 877–83.

Ryan, E. A., Lakey, J. R. T., Rajotte, R. V. 2001. Clinical outcomes and insulin secretion after islet transplantation with the edmonton protocol. *Diabetes*. 50: 710–9.

Ryan, E. A., Paty, B. W., Senior, P. A. et al. 2005. Five-year follow-up after clinical islet transplantation. *Diabetes*. 54: 2060–9.

Safley, S. A., Kapp, L. M., Tucker-Burden, C., Hering, B., Kapp, J. A., Weber, C. J. 2005. Inhibition of cellular immune responses to encapsulated porcine islet xenografts by simultaneous blockade of two different costimulatory pathways. *Transplantation*. 79: 409–18.

Sandler, S., Andersson, A., Eizirik, D. L. et al. 1997. Assessment of insulin secretion *in vitro* from microencapsulated fetal porcine islet-like cell clusters and rat, mouse, and human pancreatic islets. *Transplantation*. 63: 1712–8.

Senuma, Y., Lowe, C., Zweifel, Y., Hilborn, J. G., Marison, I. 2000. Alginate hydrogel microspheres and microcapsules prepared by spinning disk atomization. *Biotechnol Bioeng*. 67: 616–22.

Shapiro, A. M., Lakey, J. R., Ryan, E. A. et al. 2000. Islet transplantation in seven patients with type 1 diabetes mellitus using a glucocorticoid-free immunosuppressive regimen. *N Engl J Med*. 343: 230–8.

Soon-Shiong, P., Feldman, E., Nelson, R. et al. 1992. Successful reversal of spontaneous diabetes in dogs by intraperitoneal microencapsulated islets. *Transplantation*. 54: 769–74.

Soon-Shiong, P., Heintz, R. E., Merideth, N. et al. 1994. Insulin independence in a type 1 diabetic patient after encapsulated islet transplantation. *Lancet*. 343: 950–1.

Stiegler, P., Stadlbauer, V., Hackl, F. et al. 2010. Prevention of oxidative stress in porcine islet isolation. *J Artif Organs*. 13: 38–47.

Strand, B. L., Ryan, L., In't Veld, P. et al. 2001. Poly-L-lysine induces fibrosis on alginate microcapsules via the induction of cytokines. *Cell Transplant*. 10: 263–75.

Sun, A. M., O'Shea, G. M., Goosen, M. F. 1984. Injectable microencapsulated islet cells as a bioartificial pancreas. *Appl Biochem Biotechnol*. 10: 87–99.

Sun, Y., Ma, X., Zhou, D., Vacek, I., Sun, A. M. 1996. Normalization of diabetes in spontaneously diabetic cynomologus monkeys by xenografts of microencapsulated porcine islets without immunosuppression. *J Clin Invest*. 98: 1417–22.

Tendulkar, S., McQuilling, J. P., Childers, C., Pareta, R., Opara, E. C., Ramasubramanian, M. K. 2011. A scalable microfluidic device for the mass production of microencapsulated islets. *Transpl Proc*. 43: 3184–7.

Tendulkar, S., Ramasubramanian, M. K., Opara, E. C. 2013. Microencapsulation: The emerging role of microfluidics. *Micro Nanosyst*. 5: 194–208.

Tewes, F., Boury, F., Benoit, A. 2006. Biodegradable microspheres: Advances in production technology. In *Microencapsulation: Methods and Industrial Applications*, ed. S. Benita, 1–54, CRC Press, New York.

Thu, B., Bruheim, P., Espevik, T., Smidsro, O., Soon-Shiong, P., Skjak-Braek, G. 1996. Alginate polycation microcapsules. I. Interaction between alginate and polycation. *Biomaterials*. 17: 1031–40.

Toso, C., Mathe, Z., Morel, P. et al. 2005. Effect of microcapsule composition and short-term immunosuppression on intraportal biocompatibility. *Cell Transplant*. 14: 159–67.

Vajkoczy, P., Menger, M. D., Simpson. E., Messmer, K. 1995. Angiogenesis and vascularization of murine pancreatic islet isografts. *Transplantation*. 60: 123–7.

Van Schilfgaarde, R., de Vos, P. 1999. Factors influencing the properties and performance of microcapsules for immunoprotection of pancreatic islets. *J Mol Med (Berl)*. 77: 199–205.

Vasir, B., Aiello, L. P., Yoon, K. H., Quickel, R. R., Bonner-Weir, S., Weir, G. C. 1998. Hypoxia induces vascular endothelial growth factor gene and protein expression in cultured rat islet cells. *Diabetes*. 47: 1894–903.

Wang, T., Adcock, J., Kühtreiber, W. et al. 2008. Successful allotransplantation of encapsulated islets in pancreatectomized canines for diabetic management without the use of immunosuppression. *Transplantation*. 85: 331–7.

Weir, G. C., Bonner-Weir, S. 1997. Scientific and political impediments to successful islet transplantation. *Diabetes.* 46: 1247–56.

White, S. A., Shaw, J. A., Sutherland, D. E. R. 2009. Pancreas transplantation. *Lancet.* 373: 1808–17.

WHO Diabetes Fact Sheet. 2015. *WHO.* http://www.who.int/mediacentre/factsheets/fs312/en/ (accessed January 1, 2015).

Wiegand, F., Kröncke, K. D., Kolb-Bachofen, V. 1993. Macrophage-generated nitric oxide as cytotoxic factor in destruction of alginate-encapsulated islets. Protection by arginine analogs and/or coencapsulated erythrocytes. *Transplantation.* 56: 1206–12.

Wolters, G. H., Fritschy, W. M., Gerrits, D., van Schilfgaarde, R. 1991. A versatile alginate droplet generator applicable for microencapsulation of pancreatic islets. *J Appl Biomater.* 3: 281–6.

Zielinski, B. A., Aebischer, P. 1994. Chitosan as a matrix for mammalian cell encapsulation. *Biomaterials.* 15: 1049–56.

11

Progress in Tissue Engineering Approaches toward Hepatic Diseases Therapeutics

Janani Radhakrishnan and Swaminathan Sethuraman

CONTENTS

11.1 Introduction

Liver failures at end stage necessitate transplantation of whole organ or tissue as gold standard treatment for potential functional substitution of diseased hepatic tissue (Zheng et al., 2015). From the time of inception, orthotopic liver transplantation procedures have been progressively refined with appreciable success rates around 86% and 72% of 1- and

5-year survival rates, respectively (Vacanti and Kulig, 2014). However, the clinical shortage of organ availability causes over 1500 deaths of 17,000 patients in waitlist every year in the United States alone (Vacanti and Kulig, 2014). Various extracorporeal liver assist devices both nonbiological and bioartificial are being adopted temporarily for the survival of patients with impaired functioning of liver (Du et al., 2014). Apart from limited availability of donor organs, management of patient condition during the delay, immunosuppression regime, long-term hospitalization, trained expertise requirement, and high costs are other constraints that complicates the clinical scenario of liver diseases (Chistiakov, 2012; Vacanti and Kulig, 2014). Therefore, these limitations warrant the application of tissue engineering strategies for the repair and regeneration of liver tissue. Conceptually, tissue engineering embodies the application of biomaterials alone or in combination with cells and biomolecules to facilitate the progression of functional tissue (Ananthanarayanan et al., 2011; Cassidy, 2014). Tissue regeneration established by extracellular matrix (ECM) analogs, biochemical milieu, and mechanical properties determines the fate of cellular and biological processes. Liver tissue-engineered matrices should essentially be three-dimensional (3D) and provide growth permissive environment for hepatocytes adhesion, cell–matrix interactions, phenotype and function retention, desired porosity for nutrients, and gas diffusion with neovascularization (Vasanthan et al., 2012). Although various biomaterials, both natural and synthetic-based 3D biomimetic scaffolds, have been fabricated and investigated for liver tissue engineering, restoration of long-term multiple functions of the complex hepatic tissue remains challenging. The advancement in strategies has evidenced stem cell-based organogenesis and the emergence of rapid prototyping by spatiotemporal positioning of multiple cells that potentially prints 3D complex hepatic tissue.

11.2 Liver Diseases: Pathology, Responses, and Therapeutic Interventions

Liver is the largest internal organ with complex architecture and variety of cells, majorly hepatocytes (60%), organized precisely (Kulig and Vacanti, 2004; Vasanthan et al., 2012). The parenchymal hepatocytes, precursor hepatic cells (ito and oval), Kuppfer cells, stellate cells, epithelial cells, biliary epithelial cells, sinusoidal epithelial cells, and fibroblasts constitute the bulk of the tissue in addition to the complex array of endothelial cells and vasculature (Kulig and Vacanti, 2004). Liver consistently performs significant metabolic activities such as glycogen storage, cytochrome P-450 activity, urea production, synthesis of carbohydrates, lipids, proteins, and hormones, detoxification, excretion, and biotransformation (Kulig and Vacanti, 2004; Vacanti and Kulig, 2014; Zhang et al., 2010). The unique superior self-intrinsic regenerative potential of liver cells effectively restores function and mass of native organ after injuries or partial hepatectomy upto 70% (Vacanti and Kulig, 2014; Zhang et al., 2010). The signaling molecules from prostaglandins initiate liver regeneration after hepatectomy. In fibrotic liver, elevated levels of anti-mitogenic growth factors such as transforming growth factor beta-1 causes apoptosis in hepatocytes, pro-fibrotic and antimitotic effects terminating regeneration (Zhang et al., 2010). In addition, mitogen hepatocyte growth factor, angiogenic factors like vascular endothelial growth factor, activation of hepatic stellate cells, and Kupffer cells, inflammatory cytokines play positive and negative regulators of regeneration, respectively (Hu and Li, 2015; Vasanthan et al., 2012; Zhang et al., 2010). In spite of the high regenerative potential, liver is frequently vulnerable to extensive damage caused by drugs, toxins, and viral infections; excessive and prolonged inflammation antagonizes regeneration (Palakkan et al., 2013; Zhang et al., 2010). The etiology of acute liver diseases that does not affect liver architecture includes direct injury, hepatocytes loss due to drug overdose, ingestion of poisonous substances, Wilson's disease, and Reye syndrome (Bhatia et al., 2014; Zhang et al., 2010), while hepatitis infections and alcohol abuse caused fibrosis contributes to chronic liver failure (Zhang et al., 2010). On the other hand, genetic defects in hepatocytes impairs metabolism and causes fatal deficiencies in hepatic functions (Zhang et al., 2010). Culmination of the causation for liver failure by treating infections, halting alcohol consumptions is followed to manage the condition in patients with failure at different stages. However, the treatment for life-threatening end stages of chronic liver diseases is liver transplantation (Zhang et al., 2010). Transplantation strategies apart from whole organ transplantation include reduced size liver transplantation and split-liver transplantation from living donor for substituting a diseased failed liver (Kulig and Vacanti, 2004). The limitation in donor availability and immunological complications are unfavorable, seeking the utilization of cell-based, orthotopic, matrix-based strategies, or transient extracorporeal devices for the treatment of liver diseases at different stages.

11.3 Cell-Based Therapeutics

Earliest source of cells for hepatic regeneration are both fresh and cryopreserved hepatocytes as it has efficient proliferative potential for transplantation. However, sparse availability of hepatocytes demands the requirement of other cell sources such as progenitors/stem cells with proliferative, prolonged survival, and hepatogenic differentiation and functions (Zhang et al., 2010). In addition to direct cell transplantation therapy, artificial liver support systems and tissue engineering strategies require hepatogenic cells to restore the multiple functions of liver. Various sources such as primary hepatocytes, human and porcine, stem cells (adult, embryonic, induced pluripotent cells), fetal and oval cells have been widely explored for hepatic regeneration that are discussed in the following section (Lee et al., 2015).

11.3.1 Choice of Cell Source

11.3.1.1 *Primary Hepatocytes*

11.3.1.1.1 *Human Hepatocytes*

Hepatocytes are the functional unit of liver and used for the restoration of hepatic tissue as it has the potential to replicate and repopulate the liver mass (Vasanthan et al., 2012). The infusion of isolated hepatocytes is less invasive, cost effective, reproducible, and expandable for the treatment of multiple patients compared to whole organ transplantation in metabolic liver diseases, acute and chronic failures clinically, and in preclinical trials (Bhatia et al., 2014; Lee et al., 2015; Ohashi et al., 2012). Eventually, in clinical trials, patients were treated with orthotopic liver transplantation as the efficiency reduced over time, thus restricting the potential of hepatocytes toward temporary treatment, which bridge the gap during the wait for donor organ (Bhatia et al., 2014). Other constraints include clinically relevant cell number for restoration of hepatic function, time scale for acute condition, and severely damaged unfavorable parenchymal structure in chronic liver failure hinders effective engraftment of required cell number. The minimal potential of adult hepatocytes to divide *in vitro* and transdifferentiation has led to exploration of xenogenic sources, *in vitro* sandwich and spheroid cultures for retention of functionality (Lee et al., 2015).

11.3.1.1.2 Porcine Hepatocytes

Porcine hepatocytes are metabolically similar to humans and are frequently opted source for extracorporeal bioartificial liver system (BAL) and implantable systems (Lee et al., 2015; Struecker et al., 2014). These xenogeneic cells exhibit potential under specific pathogen-free conditions and immunosuppression regime (Lee et al., 2015). Although available in plenty and less immunogenic, possibility of zoonotic disease transmission, protein–protein incompatibility, and physiologic disparity between humans and pigs restricts utility of porcine hepatocytes (Lee et al., 2015; Vacanti and Kulig, 2014).

11.3.1.2 Human Hepatocyte Cell Lines

The spontaneous proliferative hepatocyte cell lines established from human hepatomas have been examined as alternatives for the less proliferative primary hepatocytes (Kulig and Vacanti, 2004). This source provides unlimited expansion but is inferior in performing essential liver functions (Bhatia et al., 2014). C3A cell line derived from HepG2 hepatoma sourced cell line used in extracorporeal liver assist device exhibited enhanced synthesis of albumin and alpha-fetoprotein with nitrogen-metabolizing ability and no tumorigenicity (Lee et al., 2015; Vasanthan et al., 2015). However, inferior drug metabolism, ammonia elimination, amino acid metabolism, and cytochrome P450s function were caused by lack of complete urea-enzyme complex and less number of mitochondria (Lee et al., 2015). In view of attaining better functioning of cell lines over HepG2, primary hepatocytes were immortalized by Simian Virus 40 T antigen (SV40 T antigen) transfection, co-transfection of albumin-promoter-regulated antisense constructs and transcription factor E2F, and D1 cyclin genes (Palakkan et al., 2013; Zhang et al., 2010). In addition to inferior functioning, the uncertainty of tumorigenicity restricts its utility in implantable strategies (Lee et al., 2015; Palakkan et al., 2013). However, strategies such as reversible immortalization, incorporation of suicide gene sensitive to antiviral drugs have been explored to combat tumorigenicity of oncogenes. Thus, extensive examination for the safe long-term application should be ensured (Lee et al., 2015).

11.3.1.3 Human Fetal Hepatocytes

Fetal liver cells and fetal liver transplantation have exhibited improvement clinically in some acute liver failure patient studies (Lee et al., 2015). Human fetal hepatocytes (Hfh) have advantages such as higher proliferation and less tumorigenic risk than adult hepatocytes and immortalized cells, respectively (Barakat et al., 2012). However, the functions of ammonia removal and urea synthesis did not match the efficiency of primary adult hepatocytes and hence were not suitable for use in BALs. Concerns such as tumorigenicity, availability, and incomplete differentiation remain to be resolved prior to potential application (Lee et al., 2015).

11.3.1.4 Oval Cells

Oval cells are facultative stem cells anatomically located at the terminal branches of biliary trees called the canals of Hering, and secrete molecular markers of adult hepatocytes, cholangiocytes, and fetal hepatoblasts (Chistiakov, 2012; Lee et al., 2015). These hepatic stem/progenitor cells are activated after injury to repair, and repopulate the liver tissue by differentiating to hepatocytes, bile duct cells and expressing specific markers of hepatocytes and cholangiocytes. However, the self-renewal, differentiation, and functions require thorough analysis before it reaches the clinic (Chistiakov, 2012; Lee et al., 2015).

11.3.1.5 Stem Cells

Stem cells isolated from adults, embryo, extraembryonal, and induced pluripotent stem cells (iPSCs) have been explored for their availability, high proliferation, low immune rejection, and hepatic differentiation potential (Hu and Li, 2015).

11.3.1.5.1 Embryonic and iPSCs

The pluripotency, availability, and unlimited proliferation have brought forth embryonic stem cells for alternate source to derive hepatocyte-like cells (Lee et al., 2015; Palakkan et al., 2013). Although examined for utilization in BALs, the ethical concerns, immune compatibility, and teratoma induction from the remnant nondifferentiated cells in the cell mass restricts application as transplantable source (Palakkan et al., 2013). However, the development of iPSCs by reprogramming differentiated adult cells to possess stemness has overcome the ethical and immune concerns, while the teratoma issue remains to be addressed (Bhatia et al., 2014; Palakkan et al., 2013). The efficient differentiation of embryonic and iPSCs to hepatocytes *in vitro* has been investigated for application in BAL, short-term drug and toxicity evaluation, and other hepatic tissue engineering strategies (Du et al., 2014; Palakkan et al., 2013; Zhang et al., 2014). These sources require deeper assessment of the remaining concerns prior to be used in cell-based therapeutics (Palakkan et al., 2013).

11.3.1.5.2 Adult Stem Cells

Teratoma risk-free adult stem cells avoid ethical issues that remain for embryonic stem cells, and has therefore been preferred source for cell transplantation and in liver assist devices (Hu and Li, 2015; Palakkan et al., 2013). *In vivo* injection of mesenchymal stem cells into the diseased liver differentiated to hepatocyte-like cells and unfavorable myofibroblasts at the site of injury. Commitment of mesenchymal stem cells from various sources to hepatocyte-like cells *in vitro* prior to *in vivo* administration overcomes the possibility of unfavorable myofibroblast generation (Palakkan et al., 2013). Recently, adipose tissue-derived stem cells encapsulated in alginate microspheres and transplanted to hepatectomized mouse had reportedly promoted hepatogenic differentiation by the microenvironment *in situ* (Chen et al., 2015). On the other hand, establishing protocols for obtaining clinically relevant number of fully differentiated adult hepatocytes remain challenging (Palakkan et al., 2013).

11.3.2 Preferred Cell Administration Sites

Like cell sources, route of administration plays a crucial role in hepatic repair and regeneration. The hepatic portal vein or artery has been conventional routes, comparatively less invasive than orthotopic cell transplantation for patients affected severely (Bhatia et al., 2014; Zhang et al., 2010). The vein carries blood from the gastrointestinal tract and spleen, accessing multiple vascular branches and hence is more preferred than hepatic artery. Such direct deliveries are highly efficient; on the other hand, risks include occlusion and fibrosis caused by portal hypertension and embolism of cells. In order to achieve delivery of effective cell number to the liver, other routes including spleen, kidney capsule, fat pad, and peritoneum have been investigated (Bhatia et al., 2014; Zhang et al., 2010).

11.3.2.1 Spleen

Spleen is the major alternate route, for the delivery of cells into the liver. Spleen has rich blood supply anatomically favorable as it has access to hepatic portal circulation and potentially accomplishes translocation of cells to hepatic sinusoids (Zhang et al., 2010). Intrahepatic transplantation of hepatocytes via spleen exhibited superior transgene expression compared to dorsal fat pad or peritoneal cavity administrations (Gupta et al., 1994).

11.3.2.2 Kidney Capsule

Hepatocytes transplanted through the vascular rich kidney capsule permitted insufficient number of cells with low survival rate due to its distance from the target site (Bhatia et al., 2014; Zhang et al., 2010). The survival was improved by transplanting under the bilateral kidney capsule spaces with matrigel (Ohashi et al., 2005). Matrigel comprises collagen IV, laminin, insulin-like growth factor 1, and epidermal growth factor that survives hepatocytes for 140 days forming small liver mass (Zhang et al., 2010).

11.3.2.3 Peritoneum

The easy anatomic accessibility, high vascularity, and provision for high cell number lodging are advantageous for cell and hepatic tissue construct transplantation via peritoneal cavity (Bhatia et al., 2014; Zhang et al., 2010, 2014). Various carriers encapsulated with cells have been reported to maintain survival and liver functions. The delivery of required cell numbers to the liver from the injection site remains a major concern (Zhang et al., 2010).

11.3.2.4 Fat Pad

Engraftment of cells for about 28 days was reported following delivery through both the dorsal and two anterior lateral fat pads. Though distanced from the target site and lack in complete functionality, some characteristic liver function such as glutamine synthetase production were exhibited by the hepatocytes in the dorsal fat pad microenvironment (Zhang et al., 2010).

The vicinal microenvironment largely affects the differentiation, proliferation, secretion, metabolism, and other functions of transplanted and endogenous cells. The diseased liver reduces the transplanted hepatocytes proliferative capability and regenerative potential of liver by adversely influencing the extracellular microenvironments (Zhang et al., 2010). As parenchymal architecture is lost in chronic liver failures, the unfavorable milieu does not support the engraftment of hepatocytes. Therefore, other possible routes of administration such as lymph node have been explored to generate ectopic liver mass that substitutes functioning (Komori et al., 2012). Hepatocytes transplanted under kidney capsule yielded engineered ectopic liver tissue with long-term functionality in mice (Ohashi et al., 2007).

11.4 Liver Support Devices

Liver support systems are primarily extracorporeal, employed to substitute the liver functions temporarily in patients with acute, acute-on-chronic, and end-stage chronic liver failure waiting for donor organ transplantation (Lee et al., 2015; Raschzok et al., 2015). The nonbiological liver support systems perform detoxification but lacks synthetic and metabolic functions. On the other hand, BALs potentially carry out all hepatic functions by using liver cells and bioreactors for simulation of liver functions extracorporeally (Lee et al., 2015; Raschzok et al., 2015; Sarika et al., 2015).

11.4.1 Nonbiological Liver Support Systems

The nonbiological support systems aim at purifying blood as temporarily bridging devices such as plasma separation adsorption and dialysis system (Prometheus), molecular adsorbent recirculating system (MARS), single-pass albumin dialysis, and selective plasma filtration therapy (Lee et al., 2015; Struecker et al., 2014). These systems carry out removal of water soluble, lipophilic, bilirubin, bile acids, medium chain fatty acids, aromatic amino acid metabolites by albumin dialysis, plasma filtration, and adsorption of accumulated toxins (Bhatia et al., 2014; Lee et al., 2015). The clearance of blood simultaneously protects brain, kidney, lung, and heart from damages caused by toxins. The most widely used system MARS consists of double circuit with one hemodiafilter and other with albumin to eliminate albumin-bound toxins. Similarly, Prometheus has double circuit for blood and plasma separated by albumin-permeable polysulfone membrane (Bhatia et al., 2014; Lee et al., 2015). Therefore, these nonbiological systems demonstrate detoxifying function but lack in synthetic and metabolic functions, giving rise to incorporation of biologically active cells and development of BALs that performs an array of functions (Bhatia et al., 2014).

11.4.2 Extracorporeal Bioartificial Liver Systems

The integration of viable hepatocytes with the 3D polymeric fibrous network that performs plasma perfusion and support cellular fate processes, has led to the development of ultimate liver support systems exhibiting multiple liver functions (Kulig and Vacanti, 2004). The BALs perform metabolic functions of liver such as ureagenesis, protein synthesis, gluconeogenesis, and enzymatic detoxification (Kulig and Vacanti, 2004; Raschzok et al., 2015). BALs that have been clinically evaluated include HepatAssist™ system, Extracorporeal Liver Assist Device (ELAD®), AMC-BAL (Academic Medical Center, Amsterdam, The Netherlands), and the MELS (Modular Extracorporeal Liver Support System, Charité, Berlin, Germany) (Raschzok et al., 2015; Struecker et al., 2014). The cell sources used in BALs include primary human hepatocytes, porcine hepatocyes, or hepatoma-derived cell lines (Raschzok et al., 2015). In HepatAssist, cryopreserved porcine hepatocytes are cultured across microporous membrane within modified dialysis cartridge to treat the plasma of patients (Struecker et al., 2014; Vacanti and Kulig, 2014). Subgroup of subfulminant and fulminant patients was survived by the BAL HepatAssist, proving the safety of this device. The ELAD system has been reported to improve bilirubin and ammonia levels and hepatic encephalopathy using C3A cell line for liver enzymatic activities (Lee et al., 2015; Vacanti and Kulig, 2014). However, the utilization of BALs clinically faces constraints due to lack of safe, reliable cell sources with profound proliferation, and multiple functions, thus paving the way for the exploration of bioengineering concepts to achieve better mass exchange (Lee et al., 2015).

11.5 Requirements-Driven Properties of Artificial Matrices for Liver Tissue Engineering

Engineering the liver tissue essentially involves the development of biocompatible, biodegradable 3D ECM analogous matrices to achieve cell adhesion, and cellular fate processes and functions (Vasanthan et al., 2012). Various scaffolds such as nanofibers, hydrogels, sponges, cryogels, and micro-carrier systems with different features have been investigated for the accommodation and delivery of viable liver cells (Davis and Vacanti, 1996; Jain et al., 2014). These scaffolds should ideally be fabricated to mimic the ECM and possess specific characteristics that meet out the challenging requirements for supporting hepatocyte viability, phenotype, and function retention (Davis and Vacanti, 1996).

The major challenge is to prevent the phenomenon of hepatocytes transdifferentiation to fibroblasts *in vitro*; such unfavorable differentiation leads to loss of functions (Bhandari et al., 2001; Jain et al., 2014). Hepatocytes are adhesion-dependent cells and require appropriate biological microenvironment to retain spheroidal morphology (Shang et al., 2014). The topography of 3D matrices, both morphology and dimension plays crucial role to establish the native tissue architecture, hepatocytes adhesion, migration, and proliferation (Figure 11.1) (Ananthanarayanan et al., 2011; Vasanthan et al., 2012). The nourishment of

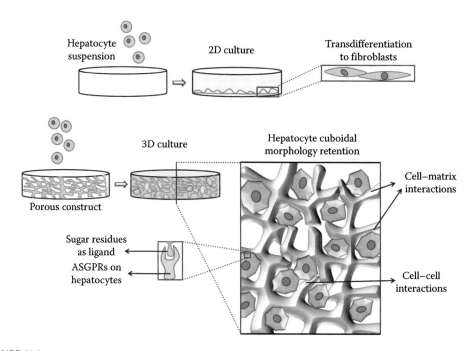

FIGURE 11.1
Hepatocytes cultured on two-dimensional substrates transdifferentiates to fibroblasts; 3D porous scaffolds with sugar residues promote cell–matrix and cell–cell interactions to maintain cuboidal morphology.

the lodged hepatocytes necessitates interconnected porous architecture with appropriate pore size that facilitates mass transport of nutrients and gases, metabolic exchange, diffusion of growth factor, and induces vascularization (Jain et al., 2014; Yang et al., 2001). In addition, the high surface-to-volume ratio provides high adhesion sites for hepatocytes and enhance engraftment of more cells seeded (Jain et al., 2014).

Another significant requirement is to accomplish hepatocyte–matrix interaction for the maintenance of differentiated state, proliferation, and functional activity of hepatocytes (Shang et al., 2014). The surface chemistry of adhesion ligands contributes to the binding of cells to the matrices. The incorporation of cell adhesive RGD motifs, sugar residues such as galactose, heparin, and glucose are some of the moieties used as ECM ligands on the surface of the scaffold for precisely directing the adhesion of hepatocyte (Jain et al., 2014). RGD motifs recognize the integrin receptors and galactose molecules exhibit high affinity toward asialoglycoprotein receptors presented by the hepatocytes, thereby mediates adhesion and functioning of hepatocytes (Figure 11.1) (Cho et al., 2006; Vasanthan et al., 2015). Galactose incorporation in both synthetic and natural polymers-based matrices influences the hepatocyte functions (Cho et al., 2006; Vasanthan et al., 2015).

The cellular behavior can also be controlled by the biomechanics of the matrices (Cassidy, 2014). Similar to the native liver tissue ECM, the mechanical stiffness gradients in the matrices mediates signal transduction via the cell adhesion ligands and cytoskeleton (Jain et al., 2014). The ECM surrounding the hepatocytes and endothelial cells are mechanically soft while being stiffer at the vicinity of cholangiocytes and stellate cells. Hepatic stem cells have been reported to differentiate into hepatocytes on soft surface and cholangiocytes on rigid surface, thus emphasizing the importance of matrix mechanical properties in regenerative strategies (Jain et al., 2014). Various scaffolds fabricated and investigated for their potential to support hepatocytes viability, proliferation, morphology, and functions have been summarized in Table 11.1.

11.5.1 Homotypic Hepatocyte Cultures

The last two decades have witnessed variety of modalities to address challenges that include engraftment of hepatocytes at the transplant site with viability, phenotype retention, and functional activity. The significance of high cell seeding density and 3D matrices on the hepatocellular functioning and morphology has been investigated by Dvir-Ginzberg et al. (2003). Vasanthan et al. (2015) have developed 3D porous poly(vinyl alcohol)/gelatin-blended hydrogel by freeze-thaw technique. The study demonstrated the synergistic effect of galactose and gelatin on the HepG2 proliferation, albumin secretion, and spheroidal morphology for 21 days. Thermosensitive, injectable, biodegradable poly(organophosphazene) hydrogel encapsulated rat hepatocytes spheroids exhibited higher viability, phenotype retention, synthesis of albumin and urea compared to single hepatocytes entrapment in 28-days culture (Park and Song, 2006).

Ohashi et al. (2007) utilized temperature responsive poly(N-isopropylacrylamide) substrates to yield uniformly continuous hepatic sheet of primary hepatocytes. The scaffold-free cellular sheet transplanted subcutaneously was engrafted and formed engineered hepatic tissues with liver-specific functions and stability for more than 200 days. Primary hepatocytes isolated from human α1-antitrypsin transgenic mice were transplanted into the urokinase-type plasminogen activator/severe combined immunodeficiency mice liver and actively repopulated the recipient liver in 2 months (Ohashi et al., 2012). The propagated hepatocytes were recovered to prepare hepatocyte sheets and transplanted subcutaneously into mice. The method exhibits clinical potential to obtain sufficient hepatocyte

TABLE 11.1

Various Biomaterial Designs and Homotypic/Heterotypic Cell Cultures Evaluated for Liver Tissue Engineering

Polymers	Substrate Design	Cells	Study Duration	Inference	References
Poly(styrene-*co*-maleic acid)/polystyrene	Galactose and RGD-modified fibrous scaffold	Hepatocytes	15 days	Spheroid formation and metabolic activity	Yan et al. (2015)
Gelatin, gum Arabic	Polysaccharide–protein packed bed matrix	Rat hepatocytes	7 days	Multicellular aggregation, structure, and functional gene expression	Sarika et al. (2015)
Thiolated heparin, diacrylated poly(ethylene glycol)	UV-induced gel layers	Rat hepatocytes	3 weeks	Retained growth factor, maintained differentiated, functional hepatocytes	Foster et al. (2015)
Silk sericin, alginate, chitosan	Microcapsules	HepG2 cells	7 days	Metabolically and functionally active	Nayak et al. (2014)
Alginate	3D porous bioscaffold	Human hepatocytes from metabolic–disordered children	14 days	Spheroid formation at 3 days and maximum metabolic activity at 7 days	Bierwolf et al. (2012)
Alginate/galactosylated chitosan	Porous sponge	Primary mouse hepatocytes	14 days	Improved spheroid formation and liver-specific function	Yang et al. (2001)
Galactosylated chitosan/HA	Hybrid sponge	Primary hepatocyte/endothelial cells	7 days	Hepatocyte-specific gene expression, urea production, and testosterone metabolism	Shang et al. (2014)
Alginate/galactosylated chitosan	Porous hydrogel	Hepatocytes/NIH3T3 fibroblasts	15 days	Enhanced liver-specific functions	Seo et al. (2006)
Galactosylated poly(vinylidene difluoride)	Membrane	Rat hepatocytes/NIH3T3 fibroblasts	15 days	Hepatocytes spheroids and functional maintenance	Lu et al. (2005)
Poly(DL-lactic acid) (PLA)	PLA-coated tissue culture dishes	Rat hepatocytes/hepatic stellate cells	2 months	Spheroids exhibited CYP-450 activity and albumin secretion	Riccalton-Banks et al. (2003)

number for potential value and also generate subcutaneously engineered liver tissues (Ohashi et al., 2012).

11.5.2 Co-Culturing of Heterotypic Cells

Hepatic tissue engineering strategies have developed various 3D scaffolds to provide appropriate substratum for the anchorage-dependent isolated hepatocytes, supplement with growth factors to enhance hepatocyte functioning and prevent dedifferentiation (Bhandari et al., 2001). An improvised approach provides a suitable environment by co-culturing parenchymal hepatocytes with other cells such as fibroblasts and stellate cells (Bhandari et al., 2001; Bhatia et al., 1999). Co-culture involves heterotypic cell–cell interactions mediated modulations for long-term phenotype retention and functioning of hepatocytes (Bhandari et al., 2001). Moreover, the paracine signaling interactions between the hepatocytes and nonparenchymal cells co-cultured with specific spatial pattern positively influences the hepatocytes function (Du et al., 2014).

Cellular multilayers with alternating cells and nano-scaled polyelectrolyte (PE) scaffolds resemble the complex liver sinusoidal structures *in vitro*. In addition, the multilayered cellular architecture improves the cell mass viability in liver assist systems. The layered architecture consisted of sequential deposition of oppositely charged ultrathin nanometer range PE layer and confluent cells monolayer. The chitosan cationic layer and DNA anionic layer interactions maintained hepatocytes morphology, cytoskeleton, and liver-specific functions. This nano-architecture scaffold supported the second layer of cells comprising hepatocyte–PE–hepatocyte layers, hepatocyte–PE–fibroblast cell layers, and hepatocyte–PE–endothelial cell layers in the constructs. This versatile construct has potential application in liver assist devices and cell-based therapies (Rajagopalan et al., 2006). Du et al. (2014) differentiated human iPSCs to hepatocytes and endothelial cells and encapsulated them in separate domains of multicomponent hydrogel fiber constructs. Endothelial cells in the construct enhanced the functions of hepatocytes *in vitro* and on implantation in mouse partial hepatectomy vascularization of the scaffold with host vasculature integration was demonstrated (Du et al., 2014). Vascularized cellular sheets were generated by co-culturing of human primary hepatocytes onto the fibroblast layer followed by subcutaneous implantation in mice. This engineered scaffold-free hepatocyte/fibroblast cell sheet exhibited enhanced vascularization, synthetic function, and glycogen storage compared to sheets with hepatocytes alone (Sakai et al., 2015).

11.5.3 Bioreactors

The conventional static cultures of hepatocytes restrict nourishment to the bulk of tissue-engineered constructs and lead to loss in metabolic functions (Zhang et al., 2014). The rapid decline of hepatocellular functions in monolayer static cultures has been prolonged by 3D aggregation or spheroids *in vitro* (Ananthanarayanan et al., 2011; Neiman et al., 2015). However, hepatocytes natively reside in close association with blood via vasculature controlling mass transfer of nutrients, substrates, and metabolites that poses challenge in static cultures (Neiman et al., 2015). Dynamic culture modalities that include perfusion cultures, spinner flasks, roller bottle cultures, and stirring bioreactors exhibit enhanced mass transfer of oxygen and nutrients thereby overcoming the demerits of static cultures (Neiman et al., 2015; Zhang et al., 2014). Physical shear stress exerted on the cultures by the dynamicity decreases the engraftment efficiency and hence is a concern while designing bioreactors (Zhang et al., 2014). Zhang et al. (2014) developed dynamic complex 3D system constituted by microgravity bioreactor, biodegradable poly-L-lactic–glycolic acid 50:50 (Synthecon) scaffold, and growth factor-reduced Matrigel for culturing neonatal mouse liver cells. Compared to the static culture, the dynamic hepatic tissue constructs maintained viability for 14 days *in vitro* and superior engraftment with function retention on transplantation *in vivo*.

11.6 Recellularization of Decellularized Matrices

Removal of cells from the tissue or organ by physical, chemical, or biological agents yields decellularized matrices with native 3D ultrastructure consisting of structural, functional proteins, and cell-specific secreted products (Crapo et al., 2011; Soto-Gutierrez et al., 2011; Zheng et al., 2015). These matrices are advantageous as scaffolds with inherent biological properties and mimetic microenvironment that promote cell–matrix interaction and retention of cell phenotype and function, thereby enabling tissue development (Soto-Gutierrez et al., 2011; Zheng et al., 2015). The perfusable vascular network in the scaffold assures nourishment for the tissue survival *in vivo* via blood supply. Various whole organ decellularization such as liver, lung, kidney, and heart have been performed from rodents, pigs, and goats. Soto-Gutierrez et al. adopted a less disruptive method to decellularize whole liver from Sprague–Dawley rats and different reseeding strategies with murine hepatocytes were investigated. The combination of enzymatic, detergent, and mechanical processes preserved the 3D ultrastructure, composition, and half of growth factor content, in addition to native microvascular network and biliary system. The recellularization attained better cell engraftment, liver-specific functions, which include synthesis of urea and albumin, cytochrome P450 induction (Soto-Gutierrez et al., 2011). Such whole organ approaches preserves the native vasculature that overcomes the major limitation of oxygen and nutrient transport in tissue-engineered constructs up to about 200 μm (Baptista et al., 2011; Shirakigawa et al., 2012; Uygun et al., 2010). Similarly, Uygen et al. demonstrated portal vein perfusion-mediated decellularization of ischemic rat livers and cultured 2 weeks *in vitro* following recellularization with rat hepatocytes. The recellularized rat liver was transplanted as auxiliary heterotropic graft with portal vein arterialization (Uygun et al., 2010). In a study by Mazza et al. (2015), the whole human liver and lobes were completely decellularized with preserved architecture and cubical scaffolds of dimension $5 \times 5 \times 5$ mm were repopulated using human cell lines, hepatic stellate cells (LX2), hepatocellular carcinoma (Sk-Hep-1), and hepatoblastoma (HepG2) for 21 days. The recellularized matrix showed cell viability, migration, proliferation, ECM modeling, and biocompatibility on xenotransplantation into immune competent mice, thereby promising bioartificial liver development (Mazza et al., 2015). Bruinsma et al. (2015) have attempted to improve hemocompatibility by reducing thrombogenicity of recellularized liver grafts. The construct was organized layer by layer self-assembly for effective immobilization of heparin in the graft without affecting recellularization and hepatocellular functions.

Other tissue sources apart from animal sources have been explored and necessitate thorough investigation of immune concerns to reach the clinics (Lin et al., 2004; Zheng et al., 2015). Decellularized porcine liver was recellularized with co-culture of Hfh and nonparenchymal human fetal stellate cells to engineer humanized liver organ. The matrix engrafted 40% of cells and exhibited active metabolism (Barakat et al., 2012). Zheng et al. (2015) have performed the preliminary trial of using splenic decellularized matrix for hepatocytes culturing. The study recorded the performance of recellularized splenic matrix compared to recellularized liver matrix using hepatocytes in dynamic culture for 6 days. Spleen has been known as ideal site for hepatocyte transplantation and extensively available clinically from patients with traumatic rupture, idiopathic thrombocytopenic purpura, and portal hypertension and donation after cardiac death. Hence, the functional assessment of decellularized matrices could emerge as indispensible source for scaffolding matrix in hepatic tissue regeneration (Zheng et al., 2015).

11.7 Bioprinting

The advent of bioprinting promises to overcome the difficulties in fabricating complex tissues, organoids, or the entire organs by precisely engineering the components including the intricately branched vasculature of tissues. 3D bioprinting techniques are computer-aided layer-by-layer additive fabrication of the tissue by respective cells and architecture similar to native (Struecker et al., 2014). Cell suspensions in biomaterials, mostly polymeric, have been used as bioink, which should ideally possess desired physical and biological properties such as rheology and cytocompatibility, respectively. This bottom-up approach permits the printing of cell spheroids, ECM components, and growth factors to exactly mimic the *in vivo* microenvironment that enhances cell–cell, cell–matrix interactions, and prevents dedifferentiation of hepatocytes (Derby, 2012). Skardal et al. (2015) have printed 3D construct using bioactive liver-specific hydrogel ink constituted by modular hyaluronic acid (HA), gelatin, and primary hepatocytes spheroids. The printable bioink and printed constructs were optimized and the final viable constructs demonstrated appreciable cell viability, and albumin and urea secretion for 14 days. Chang et al. (2010) have attempted the fabrication of microorgan within microfluidic platform by high throughput, precise patterning of layer-by-layer tissue constructs. The cell encapsulated alginate-based 3D printed constructs exhibited metabolic activity and can potentially be used as *in vitro* drug metabolism model.

11.8 Organogenesis in Organ Bud Transplant

Human iPSCs were cultured to liver buds (LBs) and further generated the vascularized functional human liver by Takebe et al. (2013). The iPSCs had first been differentiated to hepatic endodermal cells and subjected to recapitulation of early organogenesis by interacting with endothelial and mesenchymal cells, which yielded iPSC-induced LBs. The iPSC-LBs were further transplanted ectopically into immunodeficient mice, functional vasculature was stimulated and enhanced maturation into adult liver-like tissue has been reported. The same group has demonstrated the functional blood perfusion into the pre-formed vascular networks by live imaging and multiple hepatic functions of the generated liver tissue (Takebe et al., 2014). This entirely new regenerative approach would additionally facilitate developmental biology comprehension, disease modeling, and drug-screening platform (Takebe et al., 2014).

11.9 Concluding Remarks

The shortcomings existing in the current therapeutic scenario of liver diseases encourages exploration of tissue engineering approaches. The realization of tissue engineering potential warrants thorough investigation of various strategies in the preclinical and clinical trials. A wholesome approach that well addresses the multiple challenges of complex liver tissue such as hepatocytes phenotype, transdifferentiation to fibroblasts, synthetic and metabolic functions, and vasculature of clinically relevant liver graft size is yet to be achieved. However, the development in hepatic tissue engineering has evidenced improvization from nonbiological liver assist devices to bioartificial liver systems, from simple scaffolds to layer-by-layer intricate complex scaffolds, from homotypic to heterotypic cells culturing, static to dynamic cultures, recellularization of decellularized matrices, and the most promising rapid prototyping of biomaterials, cells, and growth factors with spatiotemporal positioning resembling the complex native tissue. Further, the generation of organoids and organogenesis from organ bud transplants are remarkable milestones in the progress of regenerative strategies toward the repair and restoration of functional hepatic diseases in clinics, which currently necessitates robust assessment *in vitro* and in preclinics.

References

Ananthanarayanan, A., Narmada, B.C., Mo, X., McMillian, M., Yu, H. 2011. Purpose-driven biomaterials research in liver tissue engineering. *Trends Biotechnol.* 29: 110–8.

Baptista, P.M., Siddiqui, M.M., Lozier, G., Rodriguez, S.R., Atala, A., Soker, S. 2011. The use of whole organ decellularization for the generation of a vascularized liver organoid. *Hepatology.* 53: 604–17.

Barakat, O., Abbasi, S., Rodriguez, G., Rios, J., Wood, R.P., Ozaki, C., Holley, L.S., Gauthier, P.K. 2012. Use of decellularized porcine liver for engineering humanized liver organ. *J Surg Res.* 173: e11–25.

Bhandari, R.N., Riccalton, L.A., Lewis, A.L., Fry, J.R., Hammond, A.H., Tendler, S.J., Shakesheff, K.M. 2001. Liver tissue engineering: A role for co-culture systems in modifying hepatocyte function and viability. *Tissue Eng.* 7: 345–57.

Bhatia, S.N., Balis, U.J., Yarmush, M.L., Toner, M. 1999. Effect of cell–cell interactions in preservation of cellular phenotype: Cocultivation of hepatocytes and nonparenchymal cells. *FASEB J.* 13: 1883–900.

Bhatia, S.N., Underhill, G.H., Zaret, K.S., Fox, I.J. 2014. Cell and tissue engineering for liver disease. *Sci Transl Med.* 6: 245sr2.

Bierwolf, J., Lutgehetmann, M., Deichmann, S., Erbes, J., Volz, T., Dandri, M., Cohen, S., Nashan, B., Pollok, J.M. 2012. Primary human hepatocytes from metabolic-disordered children recreate highly differentiated liver-tissue-like spheroids on alginate scaffolds. *Tissue Eng Part A.* 18: 1443–53.

Bruinsma, B.G., Kim, Y., Berendsen, T.A., Ozer, S., Yarmush, M.L., Uygun, B.E. 2015. Layer-by-layer heparinization of decellularized liver matrices to reduce thrombogenicity of tissue engineered grafts. *J Clin Transl Res.* 1: 48–56.

Cassidy, J.W. 2014. Nanotechnology in the regeneration of complex tissues. *Bone Tissue Regen Insights.* 5: 25–35.

Chang, R., Emami, K., Wu, H., Sun, W. 2010. Biofabrication of a three-dimensional liver microorgan as an *in vitro* drug metabolism model. *Biofabrication.* 2: 045004.

Chen, M.J., Lu, Y., Simpson, N.E., Beveridge, M.J., Elshikha, A.S., Akbar, M.A., Tsai, H.Y. et al. 2015. *In situ* transplantation of alginate bioencapsulated adipose tissues derived stem cells (ADSCs) via hepatic injection in a mouse model. *PLoS One.* 10: e0138184.

Chistiakov, D.A. 2012. Liver regenerative medicine: Advances and challenges. *Cells Tissues Organs.* 196: 291–312.

Cho, C.S., Seo, S.J., Park, I.K., Kim, S.H., Kim, T.H., Hoshiba, T., Harada, I., Akaike, T. 2006. Galactose-carrying polymers as extracellular matrices for liver tissue engineering. *Biomaterials.* 27: 576–85.

Crapo, P.M., Gilbert, T.W., Badylak, S.F. 2011. An overview of tissue and whole organ decellularization processes. *Biomaterials.* 32: 3233–43.

Davis, M.W., Vacanti, J.P. 1996. Toward development of an implantable tissue engineered liver. *Biomaterials.* 17: 365–72.

Derby, B. 2012. Printing and prototyping of tissues and scaffolds. *Science.* 338: 921–6.

Du, C., Narayanan, K., Leong, M.F., Wan, A.C.A. 2014. Induced pluripotent stem cell-derived hepatocytes and endothelial cells in multicomponent hydrogel fibers for liver tissue engineering. *Biomaterials.* 35: 6000–14.

Dvir-Ginzberg, M., Gamlieli-Bonshtein, I., Agbaria, R., Cohen, S. 2003. Liver tissue engineering within alginate scaffolds: Effects of cell-seeding density on hepatocyte viability, morphology, and function. *Tissue Eng.* 9: 757–66.

Foster, E., You, J., Siltanen, C., Patel, D., Haque, A., Anderson, L., Revzin, A. 2015. Heparin hydrogel sandwich cultures of primary hepatocytes. *Eur Polym J.* 72: 726–35.

Gupta, S., Vemuru, R.P., Lee, C., Yerneni, P.R., Aragona, E.A., Burk, R.D. 1994. Hepatocytes exhibit superior transgene expression after transplantation into liver and spleen compared with peritoneal cavity or dorsal fat pad: Implications for hepatic gene therapy. *Hum Gene Ther.* 5: 959–67.

Hu, C., Li, L. 2015. *In vitro* and *in vivo* hepatic differentiation of adult somatic stem cells and extraembryonic stem cells for treating end stage liver diseases. *Stem Cells Int.* 2015: 1–11.

Jain, E., Damania, A., Kumar, A. 2014. Biomaterials for liver tissue engineering. *Hepatol Int.* 8: 185–97.

Komori, J., Boone, L., DeWard, A., Hoppo, T., Lagasse, E. 2012. The mouse lymph node as an ectopic transplantation site for multiple tissues. *Nat Biotechnol.* 30: 976–83.

Kulig, K.M., Vacanti, J.P. 2004. Hepatic tissue engineering. *Transpl Immunol.* 12: 303–10.

Lee, S.Y., Kim, H.J., Choi, D. 2015. Cell sources, liver support systems and liver tissue engineering: Alternatives to liver transplantation. *Int J Stem Cells.* 8: 36–47.

Lin, P., Chan, W.C., Badylak, S.F., Bhatia, S.N. 2004. Assessing porcine liver-derived biomatrix for hepatic tissue engineering. *Tissue Eng.* 10: 1046–53.

Lu, H.F., Chua, K.N., Zhang, P.C., Lim, W.S., Ramakrishna, S., Leong, K.W., Mao, H.Q. 2005. Three-dimensional co-culture of rat hepatocyte spheroids and NIH/3T3 fibroblasts enhances hepatocyte functional maintenance. *Acta Biomater.* 1: 399–410.

Mazza, G.I., Rombouts, K., Rennie Hall, A., Urbani, L., Vinh Luong, T., Al-Akkad, W., Longato, L. et al. 2015. Decellularized human liver as a natural 3D-scaffold for liver bioengineering and transplantation. *Sci Rep.* 5: 13079.

Nayak, S., Dey, S., Kundu, S.C. 2014. Silk sericin–alginate–chitosan microcapsules: Hepatocytes encapsulation for enhanced cellular functions. *Int J Biol Macromol.* 65: 258–66.

Neiman, J.A., Raman, R., Chan, V., Rhoads, M.G., Raredon, M.S., Velazquez, J.J., Dyer, R.L., Bashir, R., Hammond, P.T., Griffith, L.G. 2015. Photopatterning of hydrogel scaffolds coupled to filter materials using stereolithography for perfused 3D culture of hepatocytes. *Biotechnol Bioeng.* 112: 777–87.

Ohashi, K., Kay, M.A., Yokoyama, T., Kuge, H., Kanehiro, H., Hisanaga, M., Ko, S., Nakajima, Y. 2005. Stability and repeat regeneration potential of the engineered liver tissues under the kidney capsule in mice. *Cell Transplant.* 14: 621–7.

Ohashi, K., Tatsumi, K., Tateno, C., Kataoka, M., Utoh, R., Yoshizato, K., Okano, T. 2012. Liver tissue engineering utilizing hepatocytes propagated in mouse livers *in vivo*. *Cell Transplant.* 21: 429–36.

Ohashi, K., Yokoyama, T., Yamato, M., Kuge, H., Kanehiro, H., Tsutsumi, M., Amanuma, T. et al. 2007. Engineering functional two- and three-dimensional liver systems *in vivo* using hepatic tissue sheets. *Nat Med.* 13: 880–5.

Palakkan, A.A., Hay, D.C., Anil Kumar, P.R., Kumary, T.V., Ross, J.A. 2013. Liver tissue engineering and cell sources: Issues and challenges. *Liver Int.* 33: 666–76.

Park, K.H., Song, S.C. 2006. Morphology of spheroidal hepatocytes within injectable, biodegradable, and thermosensitive poly(organophosphazene) hydrogel as cell delivery vehicle. *J Biosci Bioeng.* 101: 238–42.

Rajagopalan, P., Shen, C.J., Berthiaume, F., Tilles, A.W., Toner, M., Yarmush, M.L. 2006. Polyelectrolyte nano-scaffolds for the design of layered cellular architectures. *Tissue Eng.* 12: 1553–63.

Raschzok, N., Sallmon, H., Pratschke, J., Sauer, I.M. 2015. MicroRNAs in liver tissue engineering—New promises for failing organs. *Adv Drug Deliv Rev.* 88: 67–77.

Riccalton-Banks, L., Liew, C., Bhandari, R., Fry, J., Shakesheff, K. 2003. Long-term culture of functional liver tissue: Three-dimensional coculture of primary hepatocytes and stellate cells. *Tissue Eng.* 9: 401–10.

Sakai, Y., Yamanouchi, K., Ohashi, K., Koike, M., Utoh, R., Hasegawa, H., Muraoka, I. et al. 2015. Vascularized subcutaneous human liver tissue from engineered hepatocyte/fibroblast sheets in mice. *Biomaterials.* 65: 66–75.

Sarika, P.R., Sidhy Viha, C.V., Sajin Raj, R.G., Nirmala, R.J., Anil Kumar, P.R. 2015. A non-adhesive hybrid scaffold from gelatin and gum Arabic as packed bed matrix for hepatocyte perfusion culture. *Mater Sci Eng C Mater Biol Appl.* 46: 341–7.

Seo, S.J., Kim, I.Y., Choi, Y.J., Akaike, T., Cho, C.S. 2006. Enhanced liver functions of hepatocytes cocultured with NIH 3T3 in the alginate/galactosylated chitosan scaffold. *Biomaterials.* 27: 1487–95.

Shang, Y., Tamai, M., Ishii, R., Nagaoka, N., Yoshida, Y., Ogasawara, M., Yang, J., Tagawa, Y. 2014. Hybrid sponge comprised of galactosylated chitosan and hyaluronic acid mediates the coculture of hepatocytes and endothelial cells. *J Biosci Bioeng.* 117: 99–106.

Shirakigawa, N., Ijima, H., Takei, T. 2012. Decellularized liver as a practical scaffold with a vascular network template for liver tissue engineering. *J Biosci Bioeng.* 114: 546–51.

Skardal, A., Devarasetty, M., Kang, H.W., Mead, I., Bishop, C., Shupe, T., Lee, S.J. et al. 2015. A hydrogel bioink toolkit for mimicking native tissue biochemical and mechanical properties in bioprinted tissue constructs. *Acta Biomater.* 25: 24–34.

Soto-Gutierrez, A., Zhang, L., Medberry, C., Fukumitsu, K., Faulk, D., Jiang, H., Reing, J. et al. 2011. A whole-organ regenerative medicine approach for liver replacement. *Tissue Eng Part C Methods.* 17: 677–86.

Struecker, B., Raschzok, N., Sauer, I.M. 2014. Liver support strategies: Cutting-edge technologies. *Nat Rev Gastroenterol Hepatol.* 11: 166–76.

Takebe, T., Sekine, K., Enomura, M., Koike, H., Kimura, M., Ogaeri, T., Zhang, R.R. et al. 2013. Vascularized and functional human liver from an iPSC-derived organ bud transplant. *Nature.* 499: 481–4.

Takebe, T., Zhang, R.R., Koike, H., Kimura, M., Yoshizawa, E., Enomura, M., Koike, N., Sekine, K., Taniguchi, H. 2014. Generation of a vascularized and functional human liver from an iPSC-derived organ bud transplant. *Nat Protoc.* 9: 396–409.

Uygun, B.E., Soto-Gutierrez, A., Yagi, H., Izamis, M.L., Guzzardi, M.A., Shulman, C., Milwid, J. et al. 2010. Organ reengineering through development of a transplantable recellularized liver graft using decellularized liver matrix. *Nat Med.* 16: 814–20.

Vacanti, J.P., Kulig, K.M. 2014. Liver cell therapy and tissue engineering for transplantation. *Semin Pediatr Surg.* 23: 150–5.

Vasanthan, K.S., Subramanian, A., Krishnan, U.M., Sethuraman, S. 2012. Role of biomaterials, therapeutic molecules and cells for hepatic tissue engineering. *Biotechnol Adv.* 30: 742–52.

Vasanthan, K.S., Subramaniam, A., Krishnan, U.M., Sethuraman, S. 2015. Influence of 3D porous galactose containing PVA/gelatine hydrogel scaffolds on three-dimensional spheroidal morphology of hepatocytes. *J Mater Sci Mater Med.* 26: 5345.

Yan, S., Wei, J., Liu, Y., Zhang, H., Chen, J., Li, X. 2015. Hepatocyte spheroid culture on fibrous scaffolds with grafted functional ligands as an *in vitro* model for predicting drug metabolism and hepatotoxicity. *Acta Biomater.* 28: 138–48.

Yang, J., Chung, T.W., Nagaoka, M., Goto, M., Cho, C., Akaike, T. 2001. Hepatocyte-specific porous polymer-scaffolds of alginate/galactosylated chitosan sponge for liver-tissue engineering. *Biotechnol Lett.* 23: 1385–9.

Zhang, S., Zhang, B., Chen, X., Chen, L., Wang, Z., Wang, Y. 2014. Three-dimensional culture in a microgravity bioreactor improves the engraftment efficiency of hepatic tissue constructs in mice. *J Mater Sci Mater Med.* 25: 2699–709.

Zhang, W., Tucker-Kellogg, L., Narmada, B.C., Venkatraman, L., Chang, S., Lu, Y., Tan, N. et al. 2010. *Adv Drug Deliv Rev.* 62: 814–26.

Zheng, X.L., Xiang, J.X., Wu, W.Q., Wang, B., Liu, W.Y., Gao, R., Dong, D.H., Lv, Y. 2015. Using a decellularized splenic matrix as a 3D scaffold for hepatocyte cultivation *in vitro*: A preliminary trial. *Biomed Mater.* 10: 045023.

Section V

Additive Manufacturing-Based Tissue Engineering

12

Laser-Assisted Bioprinting for Tissue Engineering

Olivia Kérourédan, Hélène Desrus, Murielle Rémy,
Jérôme Kalisky, Jean-Michel Bourget, Joëlle Amédée-Vilamitjana,
Jean-Christophe Fricain, Sylvain Catros, and Raphaël Devillard

CONTENTS

12.1 Laser-Induced Forward Transfer for Laser-Assisted Bioprinting

12.1.1 The History of Laser-Induced Forward Transfer

The first experiments using a laser-induced forward transfer (LIFT) procedure were done by Bohandy et al., in the 1980s (Bohandy et al., 1986, 1988) to deposit Cu and Ag over silicon and fused silica using excimer or Nd:YAG lasers. The laser pulse was focalized onto a donor substrate coated with the metal of interest and induced a vaporization of the coating. Then, the material was recondensed on a receiving substrate. LIFT was first used to transfer metals (Bohandy et al., 1986), subsequently it was extended to oxides deposits (Fogarassy et al., 1989). In the 2000s, LIFT was adapted to print biomecules (Fernández-Pradas et al., 2004), proteins (Barron et al., 2004a), deoxyribonucleic acid (DNA) (Colina et al., 2005), hydrogels (Unger et al., 2011), and cells (Auger et al., 1998; Barron et al., 2004a,b; Ringeisen et al., 2004; Doraiswamy et al., 2006; Lin et al., 2010; Hopp, 2012; Guillotin et al., 2010; Catros et al., 2011a).

Following the pioneering experiments using LIFT, several methods have emerged, among which matrix-assisted pulsed-laser evaporation direct-writing (MAPLE-DW) and absorbing film-assisted LIFT (AFA-LIFT) are the most popular.

MAPLE-DW was developed from LIFT and MAPLE in 1999 by Piqué et al. (1999a). MAPLE is a process inspired by the pulsed-laser deposition (PLD) method (Eason, 2006) and permits to deposit thin films of molecules (notably organic/polymer materials) that cannot be processed by PLD. MAPLE involves the deposition of a material that had been mixed or dissolved in particulate form into a solvent matrix material. The solution is coated onto a substrate or frozen (to counteract the volatility of the solvent) to form a target. Then the matrix is evaporated by several laser pulses and releases the printing solution. The energy relieved by the evaporation of the matrix propels the material toward a receiver substrate. Finally, the donor material is printed as a thin layer on the receiver substrate.

MAPLE-DW is a variant of MAPLE with the direct-write capabilities of LIFT. This technique is based on the use of a matrix in the donor substrate that promotes laser energy absorption and transfer (Chrisey et al., 2003; Ringeisen et al., 2004; Young et al., 2004). The matrix is homogeneously mixed to the donor material, forming a solution. This solution is coated as a thin layer on a donor slide. Then, a pulsed laser is focused through this substrate to evaporate the matrix and transfers the donor material on a receiver substrate, facing the donor substrate. MAPLE-DW allowed the printing of metals (Modi et al., 2001), organic materials (Piqué et al., 1999b), and biomaterials (Ringeisen et al., 2002a), among which are enzymes, proteins, cells, and tissues (Wu et al., 2003). For cell bioprinting, the matrix can be a culture medium or an adhering surface such as a hydrogel or extracellular matrix (Ringeisen et al., 2004; Hopp, 2012).

AFA-LIFT acronym was given by Hopp et al., in 2005 (Hopp et al., 2005) and it designated the same technique as biological laser printing (BioLP) (Barron et al., 2004c) or dynamic release layer LIFT (DRL-LIFT) (Tolbert et al., 1993). The purpose of this technique was to avoid direct laser exposure of the donor material, thanks to an absorbing layer and to make energy conversion more efficient by limiting pulse-to-pulse variations. In the AFA-LIFT procedure, the absorbing layer is usually a thin metallic layer (50–100 nm) deposited on the donor substrate by vacuum evaporation. Metals, ceramics, polymers, and liquids can be transferred without damage with AFA-LIFT. However, residual absorbing layer contamination of the deposited material can be observed if the absorbing layer is not completely evaporated by the process (Smausz et al., 2006). Using an absorbing layer with ultraviolet (UV) radiation had been experimented.

To reduce this contamination issue, a triazene polymer layer was used as an absorbing layer of UV laser in an AFA-LIFT setup (Fardel et al., 2007; Banks et al., 2008). It was shown that this polymer-absorbing layer limited particle contamination on the receiving substrate. However, due to the low temperature of decomposition of the triazene polymer, there are a limited number of donor materials that can be used with this absorbing layer (Nagel et al., 2007). For biomaterials printing, a metallic absorbing layer has been widely used (Fernández-Pradas et al., 2004; Hopp et al., 2005; Catros et al., 2011b) and Doraiswamy et al. (2006) have demonstrated the deposition of biomaterials with a triazene layer.

12.1.2 General and Physical Principles Involved in LIFT Technologies

LIFT is a technique initially used for microelectronic applications (Chakraborty et al., 2007; Thomas et al., 2007; Baum et al., 2013). It consists in transferring an element of matter from a substrate toward another substrate, thanks to a laser pulse. Using a laser-assisted bioprinting (LAB) setup, the element of matter is under the liquid form and is called "bioink."

The temporal evolution of the LIFT-printing process can be observed using time-resolved imaging (TRI) (Figure 12.1). Various steps can be identified. At the beginning of the process, the liquid surface is deformed by a bump, which grows gradually with time. Then,

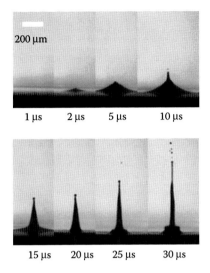

FIGURE 12.1
Experimental images of LIFT temporal evolution (t = 0 corresponds to the laser pulse). At 0.4 μs there is a bubble formation, then until 1.2 μs the bubble is growing. The bubble collapses and jet formation occurs from 1.5 to 4 μs. From 4 to 95 μs the jet grows until it breaks off into droplets at 105 μs. At 1000 μs only a bump of the liquid surface persists. (Images are extracted from Duocastella, M. et al. 2008. *Appl Phys A.* 93(2): 453–56.)

the deformation collapses progressively and a jet of liquid is formed. Later, the jet gets longer and becomes narrower until it breaks off into multiple droplets.

The physical principle consists in the following processes described elsewhere (Young et al., 2002; Duocastella et al., 2009; Guillemot et al., 2010b; Petit, 2011; Ali et al., 2014). Briefly, the laser pulse is absorbed by the absorbing material at the donor interface, leading to the formation of a gas bubble. The bubble diameter oscillates and grows until it reaches a maximum diameter and progressively deforms the liquid interface. This bubble dynamic is described by the Rayleigh–Plesset equation in a finite liquid volume (Thoroddsen et al., 2009).

The internal pressure forces gradually diminishes with the bubble expansion. With this expansion, there is no more equilibrium between internal and external forces and this leads to the bubble collapsing and jet formation. The jet becomes higher and thinner and breaks off into droplets; this disruption is caused by the Rayleigh–Plateau instability.

Three different jetting regimes can be identified, depending on the laser energy and the bioink viscosity (Souquet, 2011; Ali et al., 2014) (Figure 12.2). In the subthreshold regime, there is only a surface deformation and no jet is formed. This regime is encountered for low energy, high viscosity, and high-bioink thickness. In the jetting regime, the jet is well defined until it breaks off into droplets. This regime can be observed for intermediate values of energy, viscosity, and bioink thickness. In the plume regime, a panache of liquid explodes. This regime can be observed when high-pulse energy, low-bioink viscosity, and low-bioink thickness are used.

12.1.3 Material and Methods for LAB

A LAB setup is based on a laser beam focalized on a ribbon (donor substrate) and a receiving substrate. A typical setup is represented in Figure 12.3.

Different laser pulses could be used, depending on the type of process. An absorbing layer must be used on the donor substrate when a nanosecond laser is employed in

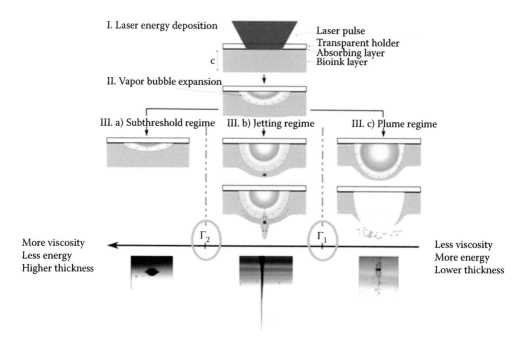

FIGURE 12.2
Scheme of the different LAB regimes. (Reproduced with permission from Nanomedicine as agreed by Future Medicine Ltd. This figure is extracted from Guillemot, F. et al. 2010b. *Nanomedicine*, 5(3): 507–15.)

the setup. Indeed, the formation of a cavitation bubble is needed to initiate the deposition process (Duchemin et al., 2002) and the laser intensity is not sufficient with a nanosecond pulse to create the bubble without an absorbing layer (Noack and Vogel, 1999). A laser with a femtosecond pulse duration can be either used with or without the absorbing layer (Dinca et al., 2008). Moreover, the nature of the absorbing layer can lead the laser

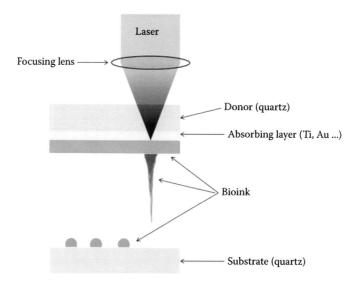

FIGURE 12.3
Laser-assisted bioprinting (LAB) setup.

wavelength choice, if the material is more absorbent for a particulate wavelength (Souquet, 2011). Furthermore, wavelengths in the near infrared are often preferred over UV to avoid alteration of the donor material in biological properties, that is, potential distortion of DNA under UV action (Catros et al., 2009). Various types of lasers had been used for bioprinting: KrF excimer laser for proteins deposition (248 nm, 15 ns) (Dinca et al., 2008); excimer lasers for mammalian cells deposition (193 nm, 30 ns) (Doraiswamy et al., 2006); dye laser-based femtosecond excimer laser for proteins deposition (500 fs, 248 nm) (Dinca et al., 2008); Nd:YAG laser for endothelial cells (ECs) deposition (1064 nm, 30 ns) (Catros et al., 2011b); and quadrupled Nd:YAG laser for protein and cell deposition (266 nm, 5 ns) (Barron et al., 2004c).

The donor substrate is usually made of quartz, as it must be transparent to the laser wavelength in order to enable the light to get through the ribbon. The donor substrate comprises a laser-absorbing layer, which is vaporized by the laser pulse, resulting in a jet of liquid bioink that is transferred on the receiving substrate. This thin absorbing layer of several dozen nanometers can be made of gold (Schultze and Wagner, 1991), titanium (Guillotin et al., 2010), silver (Smausz et al., 2006), or triazene polymer (Fardel et al., 2007; Dinca et al., 2012). The metallic absorbing layer is deposited on the ribbon by a sputter coater (Hopp, 2012).

The receiver substrate is usually made of quartz and it can be covered by a thin collagen layer (Chrisey et al., 2003) for cell-printing experiments. This collagen layer softens the cell landing during printing and constitutes a support for cell development after printing. The laser displacement on the ribbon is controlled by galvanometric mirrors (sometimes named scanner) or stage displacement of the ribbon. The receiver substrate can also be a living tissue such as an open wound (Keriquel et al., 2010).

The bioink can be made of cells suspended into a culture medium (Lin et al., 2010), DNA (Zergioti et al., 2005a), proteins (Piqué et al., 2002), or a biomaterial (Zergioti et al., 2005a). Different procedures have been described to deposit the bioink onto the ribbon. A micrometric pipette can be used (Catros et al., 2011b), as well as a micrometric blade coater (Ali et al., 2014) in order to spread a thin layer of several tenths of microns. Also, a tank of several hundreds of microns in depth can be used as a ribbon in case of LAB without absorbing layer. The laser bioink is prepared with usual chemistry tools such as milligram weighing scale, milliliter pipettes, and magnetic stirrer. Cell bioink is prepared under sterile conditions.

An example of laser bioprinter is the LAB workstation of BioTis research group (U1026, Inserm, Bordeaux, France). It consists of a laser driven with galvanometric mirrors, a positioning system to move the donor substrate, a dedicated software to print desired complex patterns and to control laser printing parameters (Catros et al., 2011b). The Nd:YAG laser (Navigator I, Newport Spectra Physics) has a pulse duration of 30 ns at 1064 nm for a repetition rate ranged from 1 to 100 kHz. The five-axe motorized stages system (NovaLase, SA, Canéjan, France) is composed of three axes dedicated to the donor substrate displacement with a resolution up to 1 μm for x, y axis and up to 5 μm for z axis (axis in the laser propagation direction). The two other axis are driven by a donor carousel with an angular resolution of 1°. This carousel, allowing the use of five different donors, permits to achieve multicolor printing.

It is essential for bioprinting to control a large set of parameters, among which are the laser pulse energy, the distance between donor and receiver, the bioink viscosity, and the position of the focused laser beam relatively to the air/bioink interface or the bioink thickness. Indeed, the printed diameter, linked with the maximum high reached by the printing jet, can vary if these parameters are modified (Dinca et al., 2008). Also, the viability of the printed cells is altered depending on the pulse energy (Catros et al., 2011b).

12.2 Applications of LAB for Tissue Engineering

12.2.1 Contribution of LAB in Biofabrication and Tissue Engineering

The definition of bioprinting technology has been formulated as "the use of computer-aided transfer processes for patterning and assembling living and non-living materials with a prescribed 2D or 3D organization in order to produce bioengineered structures serving in regenerative medicine, pharmacology and basic cell biology studies" (Guillemot et al., 2010a). Bioprinting is certainly a shift in paradigm as compared to other available approaches of tissue engineering. Its principle is to organize the individual elements of the tissue during its fabrication through the layer-by-layer deposition of cells and bio-materials. It allows to reproduce the environment and creates a structure of precise and reproducible shape. This bottom-up approach is compatible with an automation of the procedure for tissue production and can work in a 100% sterile environment. Moreover, as tissue engineering is an expensive technology, automation will allow reduction of costs and better quality and reproducibility of the products. Rapid prototyping can also offer solutions for quick testing of new shape or biomaterial.

LAB is based on LIFT technology. As discussed in Section 12.1, the original application for LIFT was metal transfers. It was modified for its considerable potential for biological applications. It can print a large class of biological materials including peptides, DNA, bio-materials, and cells, with a cell-level resolution. As opposed to ink-jet and extrusion-based printers, this technique is free of orifice, allowing for printing at high-cell density without risk of clogging. The control over cell density and three-dimensional (3D) organization of the tissue will eventually contribute toward engineering of more complex organ in a physiological architecture.

From a macro and micro point of view, organ architecture is defined by the layout of cells with different functions in their individually designed extracellular matrix (ECM). They are in close interactions with each other and precisely organized in three dimensions.

Engineering of biological tissues *in vitro* requires the use of appropriate combination of cells and biomaterials in order to mimic both cell microenvironment and tissues microar-chitecture in the body. Miniaturization of tissue-engineered structures will allow for the fabrication of organotypic structures with a physiologically relevant size and a potential functionality.

During tissue development and remodeling, the local microenvironment of cells defines their behavior and phenotype. This environment includes gradients of soluble and insolu-ble factors as well as physical forces. Dynamic reciprocity created between form and func-tion is relevant to the justification of engineering a multicellular architecture reproducing a physiological histoarchitecture of human organs.

Bioprinting aims at creating 3D biological structures, layer by layer, from the bottom. The reproduction of the microarchitecture of living tissue, first at a cell level, remains a challenge. LAB allows precise printing of different types of cells, using high-cell density and at the same time high-spatial organization. The high resolution achievable by LAB allows to respect this spatial organization and study cell–cell and cell–material interac-tions. Moreover, LAB offers possibilities to create gradients of printed materials to manip-ulate the microenvironment.

Even if reproducing the local cell microenvironment is considered as the ultimate target to obtain artificial organs and tissues, cell patterning is also very important for *in vitro* experiments. For example, Schiele et al., demonstrated the potential of LAB for applications in tissue engineering, studies of tumorigenesis, cancer drug screening, studies of cell differentiation, analysis of interactions between cell–cell, cell–drug, and cell–biomaterial, for instance, (Schiele et al., 2010; 2011).

12.2.2 Bioprinting of Biomaterials and Cells

In tissue engineering, laser printing technologies have been used to print viable cells with a cell-level resolution and a desired 3D architecture with the aim of mimicking the histological organization of organs.

Odde et al., have first reported a technique, using a near-infrared diode laser, to print embryonic chick spinal cord cells and deposit them onto a glass slide to form small patterns of cells. This deposition process was called "laser-guided direct-writing" (Odde and Renn, 1999). After this first application, Wu et al., have developed two systems: MAPLE and MAPLE direct-write (MDW), to print thin layers of biomaterials (Wu et al., 2001).

MDW was first performed to produce patterns of proteins and *Escherichia coli*, with a micrometric resolution (Ringeisen et al., 2002a). These prokaryotes were the first cells to be printed with success by LIFT. They preserved their viability and functionality after printing but reproducibility and resolution were limited.

Ringeisen et al., demonstrated accurate dispensing of active proteins at the picoliter scale using this laser transfer technique. Their results indicated that the active site of proteins was not damaged by the laser process and that this system can be employed successfully to elaborate a powerful protein microarray (Ringeisen et al., 2002b). The same research group showed that the mammalian cells can be transferred onto hydrogel substrate by the same technique and a matrix material to absorb the laser pulse and initiate printing (Ringeisen et al., 2004). Embryonal carcinoma cell line has been printed with viability proportional to the thickness of the hydrogel on the collector slide. Modified-LIFT experiments have demonstrated high preservation of cell viability after printing. The next challenge was the creation of 3D cell constructs using this printing technology (Stratakis et al., 2009).

Barron et al., have modified MAPLE-DW to precisely and quickly deposit mammalian cells and this novel laser-based printing technique was named "biological laser printing" (BioLP). BioLP was used to form patterns of human osteosarcoma and rat cardiac cells, near single-cell resolution, with near 100% viability. BioLP was presented as a technology allowing printing of multiple cell types, large-scale cell arrays, preliminary experiments on creating multilayer cell constructs and finally, transfer of genetically modified bacteria for biosensor applications. BioLP enabled smaller drop sizes, higher resolution, and increased reproducibility compared to other laser technologies (Barron et al., 2004c).

Several other groups showed near-100% post-printing cell viability for different types of absorbing layers and cells (Hopp et al., 2005; Othon et al., 2008; Koch et al., 2009). Many cell types and biomaterials have been successfully printed using LAB. Chen et al., utilized BioLP to pattern bovine aortic endothelial cells (BAECs) onto a cell-adherent hydrogel substrate, with near-100% viability post-printing (Chen et al., 2006). Doraiswamy et al., have demonstrated deposition of hydroxyapatite, MG63 osteoblast-like cells, and ECM using MAPLE-DW. Cell viability and capacity for proliferation were preserved when MG63 were co-deposited with bioceramic scaffold materials (Doraiswamy et al., 2007). Lin et al., have studied how laser fluence impacts cell viability after printing and cell-recovery ability in MAPLE-DW using *Saccharomyces cerevisiae* cells. Viability of yeast cells was decreasing while increasing laser fluence and some of the MAPLE-DW process-induced cell damage was reversible (Lin et al., 2009). With regard to human primary cells, several applications and consistent types of cells have been addressed: Human umbilical vein endothelial cells (HUVECs), human umbilical vein smooth muscle cells (HUVSMCs) (Wu and Ringeisen, 2010; Gaebel et al., 2011), Human mesenchymal stem cells (hMSCs) (Koch et al., 2009; Martin Gruene et al., 2010; Gaebel et al., 2011), adipose-tissue-derived stem cells (ADSCs) endothelial colony-forming cells (ECFCs) (Gruene et al., 2011), as well as bone-marrow-derived human osteoprogenitors (HOPs) (Catros et al., 2011a). This list proves the versatility of the process and the possibility to combine several types of cells to investigate cell-to-cell cooperation *in vitro*.

It is noteworthy that these cells have been systematically embedded in specific bioinks such as culture medium alone, in combination with sodium alginate, thrombin, combination of hyaluronic acid and fibrinogen, or a combination of blood plasma and sodium alginate (Gruene et al., 2011). Culture medium supplemented with sodium alginate, or hydrogels such as collagen type I and Matrigel have been used as well.

Therefore, LAB gives the possibility to print patterns of biomaterials before printing cells onto the patterned biomaterial for the creation of stem cell niches. The aim of future studies may be to organize several components such as cells, ECM-like materials, and growth factors at different scale of histology to analyze the behavior of several combinations (Piqué et al., 1999c; Ringeisen et al., 2002b; Chrisey et al., 2003). This patterning of biomaterials by LAB can be used for the fabrication of 3D structures and therefore can lead to applications in regenerative medicine.

Another approach could be to combine different rapid prototyping technologies for scaffold fabrication prior to cell seeding by LAB (Pirlo et al., 2006). Combination of multiple approaches will allow a better control over tissue architecture than what can be achieved in scaffold-based constructs (Schiele et al., 2009). Precise cell deposition technologies permit to control cell fate and behavior and to guide cells at the desired site of the structure by directly inserting chemical or biological factors onto substrate. This process can also permit to organize and use traction forces from cells to induce a 3D conformation of the constructs (Kuribayashi-Shigetomi et al., 2012).

12.2.3 Bioprinting of Other Biological Elements, DNA, and Peptides

Transmembrane proteins are major cellular components of cellular microenvironment, playing fundamental roles in the control of functions of cell adhesion and migration. Enzymes, antibodies, and membrane receptors can be printed by LIFT as spots of protein arrays. A pulsed-laser beam has been used by Serra et al., to print droplets of the *Treponema pallidum* protein antigen on a glass slide. This single-protein microarray was produced through LIFT to assess the effect of the deposition technique on protein integrity and reactivity (Serra et al., 2004).

DNA and protein microarrays are powerful tool in biology in areas such as genomics and proteomics. They can be used to detect variations in protein sequence and allow diagnosis, evaluation, and drug development (Stratakis et al., 2009). Heterogeneous microbead patterns have been fabricated on a bead-by-bead basis to support new opportunities for development of medical sensors and actuators, biosensors, lab-on-a-chip platforms, as well as cell-culture systems. Indeed, LIFT is a powerful technology capable of patterning micrometer-diameter beads into predefined patterns. High-precision placement of physiologically relevant microbead subunits into patterns has demonstrated broad implication for biomedical applications (Phamduy et al., 2012). Karaiskou et al., have fabricated lambda-phage DNA microarray, on glass substrates by LIFT. Zergioti et al., have developed the microprinting of DNA and protein patterns, using ultrafast UV LIFT (Zergioti et al., 2005b). They demonstrated the maintenance of their properties and biological functions and showed that they can actually be used as biosensors (Stratakis et al., 2009). LIFT has also been used for the transfer of salmon DNA-containing droplets. This double-stranded DNA was transferred from a liquid film onto poly-L-lysine slides by means of a pulsed Nd:YAG laser (Fernández-Pradas et al., 2004). The adherence of DNA onto the substrates was demonstrated by fluorescence analyses and proved that the titanium thin film can be used as the absorbing layer. Colina et al., showed that LIFT printing did not significantly damage the transferred DNA (Colina et al., 2005). They showed that microarrays produced through LIFT are comparable to other approaches such as pin microspotting regarding intensity and stability of the signal as well as gene discrimination. Dinca et al., used nanosecond LIFT to generate high-density peptide arrays on modified glass surfaces (Dinca et al., 2008). Taken together, these studies established the usefulness of LIFT techniques for microarray fabrication using DNA.

12.2.4 Intake of LAB in 3D Printing Strategies

3D printing of tissue constructs *in vitro* remains a challenge. Tissue engineering for tissue repair requires the management of vascularization and histological complexity. LAB does not seem to be appropriated for building large-volume constructs, since the usual volume of a droplet is around 1 pL (Guillemot et al., 2010c). Nevertheless, some materials such as hydrogels and biopapers can provide volume in this layer-by-layer approach and generates larger constructs.

Nahmias et al., showed that HUVEC can be patterned in 2D and 3D with a micrometer precision using laser-guided direct writing (LGDW) (Nahmias et al., 2005). Patterning of HUVEC on matrigel results in self-assembly of ECs into vascular structures along the desired pattern. Patz et al., demonstrated that B35 neuronal cells can be transferred onto a polymerized matrigel substrate using MDW (Patz et al., 2006). Othon et al., printed olfactory ensheathing cells in 3D lines providing a favorable environment for neurite outgrowth in this original spinal cord injury models (Othon et al., 2008).

Some authors suggested to support the layer-by-layer assembly of biological components such as cells and ECM with biopapers, which provide a mechanical support and offer to the cells a specific microenvironment. Biopapers consist of thin films (few hundred microns) of solid biomaterials inserted between successive layers of bioprinted cells. Cells are patterned within the material with respect to the diffusion limit of oxygen (200 μm in living tissues), in order to prevent hypoxia. Another advantage of this method is that biopapers can limit the migration of patterns after printing.

Catros et al., have demonstrated that the position of the cells in a 3D construct, using a sandwich combining polycaprolacton (PCL) biopapers and osteosarcoma cell line MG63 printed onto them by LAB, had a significant effect on cell proliferation *in vitro* and *in vivo* (Catros et al., 2012). Also, Wu et al., used poly-lactide-*co*-glycolide (PLGA)/hydrogel (type I collagen or matrigel) biopapers to print HUVEC (Pirlo et al., 2012). This material was stackable and might be useful for 3D printing.

Different materials can be used in combination with LAB for the generation of 3D structures, which have potential applications in biological and/or medical fields. LAB could be associated with various other tissue engineering methods.

12.2.5 *In Vivo* Bioprinting

LAB could lead to different applications in medical fields and to innovative therapeutic solutions as *in vivo* bioprinting.

Koch et al., printed skin cell (fibroblasts/keratinocytes) and hMSC using LAB because those cell types have shown a high potential in human skin regeneration (Koch et al., 2009). Collagen-embedded fibroblasts and keratinocytes were 3D printed as a simple model of skin tissue. They suggested that these tissue-engineered constructs could be used for *in vivo* testing after implantation on model animal (Koch et al., 2012). To do so, Michael et al., have created a skin substitute by LAB. They organized fibroblasts and keratinocytes on a stabilizing matrix (Matriderm®) and implanted these skin constructs *in vivo*, in mice. They demonstrated that this LAB-produced cell construct can be remodeled *in vivo* (Michael et al., 2013). Gaebel et al., prepared a cardiac patch seeded with HUVEC and hMSC in a defined pattern, using LIFT cell printing technique, for cardiac regeneration. They demonstrated feasibility of transplantation of a LAB tissue-engineered constructs *in vivo*, on the myocardial infarcted heart of a rat model (Gaebel et al., 2011). Therefore, LAB technology allows tissue regeneration, patterning of cells, and promotion of vasculogenesis. It has been proposed that layer-by-layer bioprinting increases seeding efficiency in porous materials (Catros et al., 2011a). The results showed that LAB permits to print and organize nHA and HOPs in 2D and 3D. They demonstrated that the layer-by-layer approach was relevant to encapsulate cells between PCL biopapers. Moreover, this method allows preservation of cell viability as well as capacity to proliferate.

LAB was used to create *in vitro* 3D constructs, suggesting a second step of *in vivo* implantation. Nevertheless, another approach consists in direct *in situ* bioprinting: In the early 1980s, the development of computer-assisted medical interventions (CAMIs) arises from converging evolutions of a variety of domains including physics, medicine, materials, electronics, informatics, and robotics. CAMIs provide a tool that allows the clinician to use multimodality data in a rational and quantitative way in order to plan, simulate, and execute minimally invasive medical interventions more accurately and safely (Nof, 2009). Rapid prototyping in regenerative medicine allow tissue engineers to precisely control scaffold structure and guide cells in the formation of a functional tissue. Bioprinting technologies have been applied to CAMIs for *in vivo* printing (Keriquel et al., 2010). This study aimed at filling a critical size calvarial bone defect in mouse by printing nanohydroxyapatite directly into the skull. A workstation was therefore adapted and dedicated to *in vivo* bioprinting experiments. Their results demonstrated that *in vivo* printing is possible and represents a significant advancement in CAMIs. This is a novel approach of bioprinting consisting in the layer-by-layer deposition of a biomaterial *in vivo* and *in situ*. There are currently several clinical applications for the regeneration of superficial organs, but future developments of the printing setups and methods are needed for the *in vivo* and *in situ* regeneration of internal organs.

Increasing the resolution, for example, by studying patterning at a cell-level resolution, may promote faster tissue organization such as improved vasculogenesis, which in turn supports quicker tissue formation and regeneration.

These cells can be printed onto a large variety of biomaterials; alone or combined. The association of biomaterials and prevascularization by LAB could allow the fabrication of functional transplants for tissue regeneration. This technology could permit to bypass the *in vitro* construction process by printing directly on the patient to diminish contamination risks or implantation delay.

12.2.6 Example of Lab Application for Bone Tissue Engineering

12.2.6.1 Vascularization in Bone Tissue-Engineered Constructs

Development of microvasculature and microcirculation is critical for bone tissue engineering (Novosel et al., 2011). To resolve the issue of a reduced vascular component, the reproduction of local microenvironment and the organization of cells are regarded as ultimate goals.

Due to the growing demand for vascularized constructs, a large number of research has been done to develop functional vascularized bone tissue *in vitro* (Grellier et al., 2009a). Bone formation requires an active process of angiogenesis, which involves communication between ECs and osteoblastic progenitors. *In vitro* studies showed that ECs in coculture with osteoblasts are able to organize in capillary-like structures that can remain stable in culture (Grellier et al., 2009). In addition, the complexity of these structures is often confirmed by the presence of a vascular lumen and by collagen type I expression in perivascular region, a major component of ECM (Hofmann et al., 2008).

Within the body, most cells are found no more than 100–200 µm from a capillary, which provides diffusion of oxygen and nutrients, and waste products elimination, to support and maintain viable tissue (Folkman and Hochberg, 1973). Promoting vascularization of engineered tissues is critical for supporting cell organization and maintaining tissue function.

To this aim, building 3D biological structures using bioprinting have been suggested.

Using bottom-up approach, functional microscale tissue building blocks can be assembled into 3D microscale tissue constructs. The design of microscale components combined with the capability to link them together to generate larger structures represents a promising way to build vascularized 3D constructs.

12.2.6.2 Generation of Coculture Models by LAB for Bone Regeneration

LAB is able to print all cell types and is a useful tool to create coculture models. For example, some authors developed cocultures by LAB in order to promote vascularization. Wu et al., fabricated branch/stem structures of HUVECs and HUVSMCs, using BioLP (Wu and Ringeisen, 2010). When HUVSMCs and HUVECs are printed in close contact with each other, they develop cell–cell junctions around lumen-like structures.

The approach developed in our group, which more specifically focused on bone regeneration, combines the use of osteoblastic and endothelial precursors both obtained from stem cells of the apical papilla (SCAPs) and organized in a specific pattern, to promote synergy in cell differentiation and reorganization. We also associated multiple mesenchymal stem cells in coculture to analyze the spontaneous cells organization (Figure 12.4).

Bone healing is a complex process precisely driven by local mechanical and chemical factors. Cytokines produced by the osteoblasts guide the recruitment of niche stem cells to promote healing. With the help of LAB, we investigated the behavior of controlled bioprinted patterns of mesenchymal stem cells at different stages of osteoblastic differentiation to evaluate the optimal patterns for bone regeneration and the effect of cell-to-cell interactions before the construction of layer-by-layer 3D construct. For this purpose, we printed specific patterns of mesenchymal cells (D1-Td Tomato) onto a monolayer of dental stem cells, the SCAPs on collagen, according to a pattern of 250×1000 (250 µm between spots, 1000 µm between segments). D1-Td are multipotent mouse bone-marrow stromal precursors, which can be considered as more mature than the SCAPs. Pattern evolution

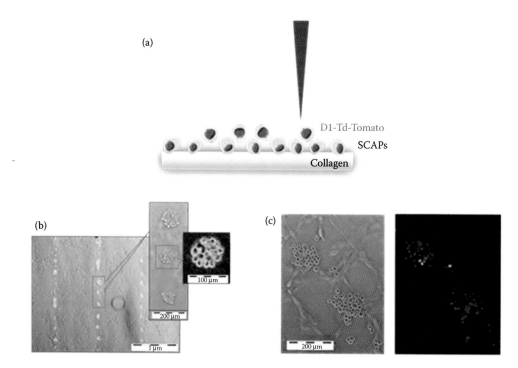

FIGURE 12.4
Generation of coculture model by LAB (a) Schematic representation of the experimentation; (b) Laser printing of D1-Td-Tomato mesenchymal cells (bioink concentration = 100 millions/mL), with a laser energy of 29 μJ and a pattern 250 × 1000 μm (250 μm between each spot, 1000 μm between each segment), featuring a concentration of 20–30 cells per droplet. Phase-contrast microscope images of cells printed onto a monolayer of SCAPs and collagen; (c) Phase-contrast and fluorescence microscope images of two printed spots.

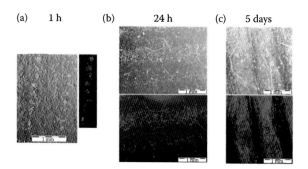

FIGURE 12.5
Phase-contrast and fluorescence microscope images of D1-Td-Tomato mesenchymal cells after being transferred by LAB, in coculture with SCAPs. Preservation of printed patterns as a function of time post-printing (a) 1 h, (b) 24 h, and (c) 5 days.

was followed by time-lapse imaging in order to evaluate the conservation of the pattern through time (Figure 12.5) and if the presence of a monolayer of SCAPs could promote or inhibit the alignment of D1-Td.

The results indicate that it could be possible to guide the formation and growth of cellular constructs with predictable patterns without interaction of the underlying cells.

The final goal will be to reproduce alveolar bone structure to improve the vascularization of graft after transplantation, and then promote bone regeneration. Indeed, the superposition of layers with such cellular architecture with different angle could lead to a better mechanical resistance and allow angiogenesis through the mimicking alveolar bone structure. For this purpose, strategies have to be developed in order to assemble several layers and elaborate tailor-made 3D constructs. This could lead to the development of innovative therapeutic solutions.

12.3 Clinical Implications and Conclusions

Two major challenges in tissue engineering are mimicking final cell organization of tissues to regenerate a functional tissue and preserving viability of 3D constructs thicker than 300 μm before implantation through the process of maturation. Accurate cell bioprinting and prevascularization of engineered tissues are promising approaches that can be both allowed by LAB. Moreover, LAB could lead to many different applications such as clinical use in implants, *in vitro* models, in pharmacokinetic studies, as model systems for bone-related diseases. Laser-based bioprinting techniques have been used for analyzing cellular interactions, cancer studies, tissue formation and regeneration, cell differentiation, biomaterial studies, and drug screening and toxicity testing. These technologies have singular advantages for the development of *in vitro* tools but also for clinical applications. Generation of cardiac patches by LIFT for the treatment of myocardial infarction could improve wound healing and functional preservation (Gaebel et al., 2011). Additionally, this technology has been utilized for complex tissues such as bioprinting skin with its various ECM and cellular components (Koch et al., 2012). LAB, an emerging technology in tissue engineering, allows to reproduce *in vitro* cell microenvironment by controlling shape and density of cell patterns and gradients. Combined with other tissue engineering methods, LAB technology is an innovative tool for fundamental research, tissue engineering, and repair. Finally, while great progress have been made in the development of cell chips and microarrays produced by LAB, original applications will certainly arise in the following years such as automated robotics process, allowing for transition of LAB workstations from the bench to bedside.

References

Ali, M., Pages, E., Ducom, A., Fontaine, A., Guillemot, F. 2014. Controlling laser-induced jet formation for bioprinting mesenchymal stem cells with high viability and high resolution. *Biofabrication.* 6:045001.

Auger, F. A., Rouabhia, M., Goulet, F., Berthod, F., Moulin, V., Germain, L. 1998. Tissue-engineered human skin substitutes developed from collagen-populated hydrated gels: Clinical and fundamental applications. *Med Biol Eng Comput.* 36: 801–12.

Banks, D. P., Grivas, C., Zergioti, I., Eason, R. W. 2008. Ballistic laser-assisted solid transfer (BLAST) from a thin film precursor. *Opt Express.* 16: 3249–54.

Barron, J. A., Ringeisen, B. R., Kim, H., Spargo, B. J., Chrisey, D. B. 2004a. Application of laser printing to mammalian cells. *Thin Solid Films.* 453–454: 383–7.

Barron, J. A., Spargo, B. J., Ringeisen, B. R. 2004b. Biological laser printing of three dimensional cellular structures. *Appl. Phys. A* 79: 4–6.

Barron, J. A., Wu, P., Ladouceur, H. D., Ringeisen, B. R. 2004c. Biological laser printing: A novel technique for creating heterogeneous 3-dimensional cell patterns. *Biomed Microdevices.* 6: 139–47.

Baum, M., Kim, H., Alexeev, I., Piqué, A., Schmidt, M. 2013. Generation of transparent conductive electrodes by laser consolidation of LIFT printed ITO nanoparticle layers. *Appl Phys A.* 111: 799–805.

Bohandy, J., Kim, B. F., Adrian, F. J. 1986. Metal deposition from a supported metal film using an excimer laser. *J Appl Phys.* 60: 1538–9.

Bohandy, J., Kim, B. F., Adrian, F. J., Jette, A. N. 1988. Metal deposition at 532 Nm using a laser transfer technique. *J Appl Phys.* 63: 1158.

Catros, S., Fricain, J. C., Guillotin, B., Pippenger, B., Bareille, R., Amédée, J., Guillemot, F. 2009. *High-Throughput Biological Laser Printing For Bone Tissue Engineering.* Presented at the 2nd World Termis Congress, Seoul, South Korea.

Catros, S., Fricain, J. C., Guillotin, B., Pippenger, B., Bareille, R., Remy, M., Lebraud, E., Desbat, B., Amédée, J., Guillemot F. 2011a. Laser-assisted bioprinting for creating on-demand patterns of human osteoprogenitor cells and nano-hydroxyapatite. *Biofabrication.* 3: 025001.

Catros, S., Guillemot, F., Nandakumar, A., Ziane, S., Moroni, L., Habibovic, P., van Blitterswijk C. et al. 2012. Layer-by-layer tissue microfabrication supports cell proliferation *in vitro* and *in vivo*. *Tissue Eng Part C Methods.* 18: 62–70.

Catros, S., Guillotin, B., Bacáková, M., Fricain, J. C., Guillemot, F. 2011b. Effect of laser energy, substrate film thickness and bioink viscosity on viability of endothelial cells printed by laser-assisted bioprinting. *Appl Surf Sci.* 257: 5142–7.

Chakraborty, S., Sakata, H., Yokoyama, E., Wakaki, M., Chakravorty, D. 2007. Laser-induced forward transfer technique for maskless patterning of amorphous V2O5 thin film. *Appl Surf Sci.* 254: 638–43.

Chen, C. Y., Barron, J. A., Ringeisen, B. R. 2006. Cell patterning without chemical surface modification: Cell–cell interactions between printed bovine aortic endothelial cells (BAEC) on a homogeneous cell-adherent hydrogel. *Appl Surf Sci.* 252: 8641–5.

Chrisey, D. B., Piqué, A., McGill, R. A., Horwitz, J. S., Ringeisen, B. R., Bubb, D. M., Wu, P. K. 2003. Laser deposition of polymer and biomaterial films. *Chem Rev.* 103: 553–76.

Colina, M., Serra, P., Fernández-Pradas, J. M., Sevilla, L., Morenza, J. L. 2005. DNA deposition through laser induced forward transfer. *Biosens Bioelectron.* 20: 1638–42.

Dinca, V., Farsari, M., Kafetzopoulos, D., Popescu, A., Dinescu, M., Fotakis, C. 2008. Patterning parameters for biomolecules microarrays constructed with nanosecond and femtosecond UV lasers. *Thin Solid Films.* 4,516: 6504–11.

Dinca, V., Patrascioiu, A., Fernández-Pradas, J. M., Morenza, J. L., Serra, P. 2012. Influence of solution properties in the laser forward transfer of liquids. *Appl Surf Sci.* 258: 9379–84.

Doraiswamy, A., Narayan, R. J., Harris, M. L., Qadri, S. B., Modi, R., Chrisey, D. B. 2007. Laser microfabrication of hydroxyapatite-osteoblast-like cell composites. *J Biomed Mater Res A.* 80A: 635–43.

Doraiswamy, A., Narayan, R. J., Lippert, T., Urech, L., Wokaun, A., Nagel, M., Hopp, B. et al. 2006. Excimer laser forward transfer of mammalian cells using a novel triazene absorbing layer. *Appl Surf Sci.* 252: 4743–7.

Duchemin, L., Popinet, S., Josserand, C., Zaleski, S. 2002. Jet formation in bubbles bursting at a free surface. *Phys Fluids* 14: 3000.

Duocastella, M., Fernández-Pradas, J. M., Serra, P., Morenza, J.L. 2008. Jet formation in the laser forward transfer of liquids. *Appl Phys A.* 93(2): 453–56.

Duocastella, M., Fernández-Pradas, J. M., Morenza, J. L., Serra, P. 2009. Time-resolved imaging of the laser forward transfer of liquids. *J Appl Phys.* 106: 084907.

Eason, R. 2006. *Pulsed Laser Deposition of Thin Films: Applications-Led Growth of Functional Materials.* Hoboken, NJ, USA: John Wiley & Sons, Inc.

Fardel, R., Nagel, M., Nüesch, F., Lippert, T., Wokaun, A. 2007. Fabrication of organic light-emitting diode pixels by laser-assisted forward transfer. *Appl Phys Lett.* 91: 061103.

Fernández-Pradas, J. M., Colina, M., Serra, P., Domínguez, J., Morenza, J. L. 2004. Laser-induced forward transfer of biomolecules. *Thin Solid Films*. 453–454: 27–30.

Fogarassy, E., Fuchs, C., Kerherve, F., Hauchecorne, G., Perriere, J. 1989. Laser-induced forward transfer of high-Tc YBaCuO and BiSrCaCuO superconducting thin films. *J Appl Phys*. 66: 457–9.

Folkman, J., Hochberg, M. 1973. Self-regulation of growth in three dimensions. *J Exp Med*. 138: 745–53.

Gaebel, R., Ma, N., Liu, J., Guan, J., Koch, L., Klopsch, C., Gruene, M. et al. 2011. Patterning human stem cells and endothelial cells with laser printing for cardiac regeneration. *Biomaterials*. 32: 9218–30.

Grellier, M., Bordenave, L., Amédée, J. 2009a. Cell-to-cell communication between osteogenic and endothelial lineages: Implications for tissue engineering. *Trends Biotech*. 27: 562–71.

Grellier, M., Granja, P. L., Fricain, J. C., Bidarra, S. J., Renard, M., Bareille, R., Bourget, C., Amédée, J., Barbosa, M. A. 2009b. The effect of the co-immobilization of human osteoprogenitors and endothelial cells within alginate microspheres on mineralization in a bone defect. *Biomaterials*. 30: 3271–8.

Gruene, M., Deiwick, A., Koch, L., Schlie, S., Unger, C., Hofmann, N., Bernemann, I., Glasmacher, B., Chichkov, B. 2010. Laser printing of stem cells for biofabrication of scaffold-free autologous grafts. *Tissue Eng Part C: Meth*. 17: 79–87.

Gruene, M., Pflaum, M., Deiwick, A., Koch, L., Schlie, S., Unger, C., Wilhelmi, M., Haverich, A., Chichkov, B. N. 2011a. Adipogenic differentiation of laser-printed 3D tissue grafts consisting of human adipose-derived stem cells. *Biofabrication*. 3: 015005.

Gruene, M., Unger, C., Koch, L., Deiwick, A., Chichkov, B. 2011b. Dispensing pico to nanolitre of a natural hydrogel by laser-assisted bioprinting. *Biomed Eng Online*. 10: 19.

Guillemot, F., Mironov, V., Nakamura, M. 2010a. *Bioprinting Is Coming of Age*. Report from the International Conference on Bioprinting and Biofabrication in Bordeaux (3B'09). *Biofabrication*. 2: 010201.

Guillemot, F., Souquet, A., Catros, S., Guillotin, B. 2010b. Laser-assisted cell printing: Principle, physical parameters versus cell fate and perspectives in tissue engineering. *Nanomedicine*. 5(3): 507–15.

Guillemot, F., Souquet, A., Catros, S., Guillotin, B., Lopez, J., Faucon, M., Pippenger, B. et al. 2010c. High-throughput laser printing of cells and biomaterials for tissue engineering. *Acta Biomater*. 6: 2494–500.

Guillotin, B., Souquet, A., Catros, S., Duocastella, M., Pippenger, B., Bellance, S., Bareille, R. et al. 2010. Laser assisted bioprinting of engineered tissue with high cell density and microscale organization. *Biomaterials*. 31: 7250–6.

Hofmann, A., Ritz, U., Verrier, S., Eglin, D., Alini, M., Fuchs, S., Kirkpatrick, C. J., Rommens, P. M. 2008. The effect of human osteoblasts on proliferation and Neo-vessel formation of human umbilical vein endothelial cells in a long-term 3D co-culture on polyurethane scaffolds. *Biomaterials*. 29: 4217–26.

Hopp, B. 2012. Femtosecond laser printing of living cells using absorbing film-assisted laser-induced forward transfer. *Opt Eng*. 51: 014302.

Hopp, B., Smausz, T., Kresz, N., Barna, N., Bor, Z., Kolozsvári, L., Chrisey, D. B., Szabó, A., Nógrádi, A. 2005. Survival and proliferative ability of various living cell types after laser-induced forward transfer. *Tissue Eng*. 11: 1817–23. doi: 32.

Keriquel, V., Guillemot, F., Arnault, I., Guillotin, B., Miraux, S., Amédée, J., Fricain, J. C., Catros S. 2010. *In vivo* bioprinting for computer- and robotic-assisted medical intervention: Preliminary study in mice. *Biofabrication*. 2: 014101.

Koch, L., Deiwick, A., Schlie, S., Michael, S., Gruene, M., Coger, V., Zychlinski, D. et al. 2012. Skin tissue generation by laser cell printing. *Biotechnol Bioeng*. 109: 1855–63.

Koch, L., Kuhn, S., Sorg, H., Gruene, M., Schlie, S., Gaebel, R., Polchow, B. et al. 2009. Laser printing of skin cells and human stem cells. *Tissue Eng Part C Meth*. 16: 847–54.

Kuribayashi-Shigetomi, K., Onoe, H., Takeuchi, S. 2012. Cell origami: Self-folding of three-dimensional cell-laden microstructures driven by cell traction force. *PloS One*. 7: e51085.

Lin, Y., Huang, G., Huang, Y., Tzeng, T. R., Chrisey, D. B. 2010. Effect of laser fluence in laser assisted direct writing of human colon cancer cell. *Tissue Eng Part C Meth.* 16: 202–8.

Lin, Y., Huang, Y., Wang, G., Tzeng, T. R. J., Chrisey, D. B. 2009. Effect of laser fluence on yeast cell viability in laser-assisted cell transfer. *J. Appl Phy.* 106: 043106.

Michael, S., Sorg, H., Peck, C. T., Koch, L., Deiwick, A., Chichkov, B., Vogt, P. M., Reimers, K. 2013. Tissue engineered skin substitutes created by laser-assisted bioprinting form skin-like structures in the dorsal skin fold chamber in mice. *PLoS ONE.* 8: e57741.

Modi, R., Wu, H. D., Auyeung, R. C. Y., Gilmore, C. M., Chrisey, D. B. 2001. Direct writing of polymer thick film resistors using a novel laser transfer technique. *J Mater Res.* 16: 3214–22.

Nagel, M., Hany, R., Lippert, T., Molberg, M., Nüesch, F. A., Rentsch, D. 2007. Aryltriazene photopolymers for UV-laser applications: Improved synthesis and photodecomposition study. *Macromol Chem Phys.* 208: 277–86.

Nahmias, Y., Schwartz, R. E., Verfaillie, C. M., Odde, D. J. 2005. Laser-guided direct writing for three-dimensional tissue engineering. *Biotechnol Bioeng.* 92: 129–36.

Noack, J., Vogel, A. 1999. Laser-induced plasma formation in water at nanosecond to femtosecond time scales: Calculation of thresholds, absorption coefficients, and energy density. *IEEE J Quantum Electron.* 35: 1156–67.

Nof, S. Y., 2009. *Springer Handbook of Automation.* Berlin, Heidelberg: Springer Science & Business Media.

Novosel, E. C., Kleinhans, C., Kluger, P. J. 2011. Vascularization is the key challenge in tissue engineering. *Adv Drug Deliv Rev.* 63: 300–11.

Odde, D. J., Renn, M. J. 1999. Laser-guided direct writing for applications in biotechnology. *Trends Biotechnol.* 17: 385–9.

Othon, C. M., Wu, X., Anders, J. J., Ringeisen, B. R. 2008. Single-cell printing to form three-dimensional lines of olfactory ensheathing cells. *Biomed Mater.* 3: 034101.

Patz, T. M., Doraiswamy, A., Narayan, R. J., He, W., Zhong, Y., Bellamkonda, R., Modi, R., Chrisey, D. B. 2006. Three-dimensional direct writing of B35 neuronal cells. *J Biomed Mater Res B Appl Biomater.* 78: 124–30.

Petit, J. 2011. Déformations et Instabilités D'interfaces Liquides Pilotées Par La Diffusion D'une Onde Laser En Milieux Turbides (Deformations and instabilities of liquid interfaces driven by the diffusion of a laser wave in turbid media). PhD diss., Université Sciences et Technologies–Bordeaux I.

Phamduy, T. B., Raof, N. A., Schiele, N. R., Yan, Z., Corr, D. T., Huang, Y., Xie, Y., Chrisey, D. B. 2012. Laser direct-write of single microbeads into spatially-ordered patterns. *Biofabrication.* 4: 025006.

Piqué, A., Chrisey, D. B., Auyeung, R. C. Y., Fitz-Gerald, J., Wu, H. D., McGill, R. A., Lakeou, S., Nguyen, V., Duignan, M. 1999a. A novel laser transfer process for direct writing of electronic and sensor materials. *Appl Phys A.* 69: S279–84.

Piqué, A., Chrisey, D. B., Auyeung, R. C. Y., Lakeou, S., Chung, R., McGill, R. A., Wu, P. K., Duignan, M. T., Fitz-Gerald, J. M., Wu, H. D. 1999b. Laser direct writing of circuit elements and sensors. *SPIE LASE.* 3618: 330–9.

Piqué, A., McGill, R. A., Chrisey, D. B., Leonhardt, D., Mslna, T. E., Spargo, B. J., Callahan, J. H., Vachet, R. W., Chung, R., Bucaro, M. A. 1999c. Growth of organic thin films by the matrix assisted pulsed laser evaporation (MAPLE) technique. *Thin Solid Films.* 355–356: 536–41.

Piqué, A., Weir, D. W., Wu, P. K., Pratap, B., Arnold, C. B., Ringeisen, B. R., McGill, R. A., Auyeung, R. C. Y., Kant, R. A., Chrisey, D. B. 2002. Direct-write of sensor devices by a laser forward transfer technique. *SPIE LASE.* 361–8.

Pirlo, R. K., Dean, D. M. D., Knapp, D. R., Gao, B. Z. 2006. Cell deposition system based on laser guidance. *Biotechnol J.* 1: 1007–13.

Pirlo, R. K., Wu, P., Liu, J., Ringeisen, B. 2012. PLGA/hydrogel biopapers as a stackable substrate for printing HUVEC networks via BioLP. *Biotechnol Bioeng.* 109:262–7.

Ringeisen, B. R., Chrisey, D. B., Piqué, A., Young, H. D., Jones-Meehan, J., Modi, R., Bucaro, M., Spargo, B. J. 2002a. Generation of mesoscopic patterns of viable *Escherichia coli* by ambient laser transfer. *Biomaterials.* 23: 161–6.

Ringeisen, B. R., Kim, H., Barron, J. A., Krizman, D. B., Chrisey, D. B., Jackman, S., Auyeung, R. Y. C., Spargo, B. J. 2004. Laser printing of pluripotent embryonal carcinoma Cells. *Tissue Eng.* 10: 483–91.

Ringeisen, B. R., Wu, P. K., Kim, H., Piqué, A., Auyeung, R. Y. C., Young, H. D., Chrisey, D. B., Krizman, D. B. 2002b. Picoliter-scale protein microarrays by laser direct write. *Biotechnol Prog.* 18: 1126–9.

Schiele, N. R., Chrisey, D. B., Corr, D. T. 2011. Gelatin-based laser direct-write technique for the precise spatial patterning of cells. *Tissue Eng C: Meth.* 17: 289–98.

Schiele, N. R., Corr, D. T., Huang, Y., Raof, N. A., Xie, Y., Chrisey, D. B. 2010. Laser-based direct-write techniques for cell printing. *Biofabrication.* 2: 032001.

Schiele, N. R., Koppes, R. A., Corr, D. T., Ellison, K. S., Thompson, D. M., Ligon, L. A., Lippert, T. K. M., Chrisey, D. B. 2009. Laser direct writing of combinatorial libraries of idealized cellular constructs: Biomedical applications. *Appl Surf Sci.* 255: 5444–7.

Schultze, V., Wagner, M. 1991. Laser-induced forward transfer of aluminium. *Appl Surf Sci.* 52(4): 303–9.

Serra, P., Fernandez-Pradas, J. M., Berthet, F. X., Colina, M., Elvira, J., Morenza, J. L. 2004. Laser direct writing of biomolecule microarrays. *Appl Phys A.* 79(4–6): 949–952.

Smausz, T., Hopp, B., Kecskeméti, G., Bor, Z. 2006. Study on metal microparticle content of the material transferred with absorbing film assisted laser induced forward transfer when using silver absorbing layer. *Appl Surf Sci.* 252: 4738–42.

Souquet, A. 2011. Etude Des Processus Physiques Mis En Jeu Lors de La Microimpression D'éléments Biologiques Assistée Par Laser (Study of the physical processes involved in laser-assisted microprinting of biological elements). PhD diss., L'universite Bordeaux 1. http://www.theses. fr/2011BOR14232. Accessed August 2, 2016.

Stratakis, E., Ranella, A., Farsari, M., Fotakis, C. 2009. Laser-based micro/nanoengineering for biological applications. *Prog Quantum Electron.* 33(5): 127–63.

Thomas, B., Alloncle, A. P., Delaporte, P., Sentis, M., Sanaur, S., Barret, M., Collot, P. 2007. Experimental investigations of laser-induced forward transfer process of organic thin films. *Appl Surf Sci.* 254: 1206–10.

Thoroddsen, S. T., Takehara, K., Etoh, T. G., Ohl, C. D. 2009. Spray and microjets produced by focusing a laser pulse into a hemispherical drop. *Phys Fluids.* 21: 112101.

Tolbert, W. A., Lee, I. Y. S., Doxtader, M. M., Ellis, E. W., Dlott, D. D. 1993. High-speed color imaging by laser ablation transfer with a dynamic release layer: Fundamental mechanisms. *J Imag Sci.* 37: 411–21.

Unger, C., Gruene, M., Koch, L., Koch, J., Chichkov, B. N. 2011. Time-resolved imaging of hydrogel printing via laser-induced forward transfer. *Appl Phys A.* 103: 271–7.

Wu, P. K., Ringeisen, B. R. 2010. Development of human umbilical vein endothelial cell (HUVEC) and human umbilical vein smooth muscle cell (HUVSMC) branch/stem structures on hydrogel layers via biological laser printing (BioLP). *Biofabrication.* 2: 014111.

Wu, P. K., Ringeisen, B. R., Callahan, J., Brooks, M., Bubb, D. M., Wu, H. D., Piqué, A., Spargo, B., McGill, R. A., Chrisey, D. B. 2001. The deposition, structure, pattern deposition, and activity of biomaterial thin-films by matrix-assisted pulsed-laser evaporation (MAPLE) and MAPLE direct write. *Thin Solid Films.* 398–399: 607–14.

Wu, P. K., Ringeisen, B. R., Krizman, D. B., Frondoza, C. G., Brooks, M., Bubb, D. M., Auyeung, R. C. Y. et al. 2003. Laser transfer of biomaterials: Matrix-assisted pulsed laser evaporation (MAPLE) and MAPLE direct write. *Rev Sci Instrum.* 74: 2546.

Young, D., Auyeung, R. C. Y., Piqué, A., Chrisey, D. B., Dlott, D. D. 2002. Plume and jetting regimes in a laser based forward transfer process as observed by time-resolved optical microscopy. *Appl Surf Sci.* 197–198: 181–7.

Young, H. D., Auyeung, R. C. Y., Chrisley, D. B., Dlott, D. D. 2004. Jetting behavior in the laser forward transfer of rheological systems. Patent US6815015 B2.

Zergioti, I., Karaiskou, A., Papazoglou, D. G., Fotakis, C., Kapsetaki, M., Kafetzopoulos, D. 2005a. Time resolved Schlieren study of sub-pecosecond and nanosecond laser transfer of biomaterials. *Appl Surf Sci.* 247: 584–9.

Zergioti, I., Karaiskou, A., Papazoglou, D. G., Fotakis, C., Kapsetaki, M., Kafetzopoulos, D. 2005b. Femtosecond laser microprinting of biomaterials. *Appl Phys Lett.* 86(16): 163902.

Section VI

Translational Aspects of Tissue Engineering

13

Tissue-Engineered Medical Products

Ohan S. Manoukian, Jonathan Nip, Olajide Abiola, Aadarsh Gopalakrishna, and Sangamesh G. Kumbar

CONTENTS

13.1 Introduction

The human body is an amazingly complex organism, consisting of several individual organ systems working together in a dynamic fashion. Underneath it all lies the cell, the basic functional unit of structure, physiology, and organization in all living things; the foundation of tissue engineering (TE). For decades, scientists have researched vigorously to unlock the regenerative potential harnessed within undifferentiated cells. As the population continues to age, acute and chronic injuries/pathologies are in need of safe and effective therapeutic alternatives.

Currently, the "gold standard" of most orthopedic treatments is considered to be the autograft (e.g., bone or tissue taken from one part of a patient's body and transplanted into another) or allograft (e.g., bone or tissue taken from another individual and transplanted into the patient). Worldwide, autografts or allografts are used in approximately 2.2 million orthopedic procedures annually, with approximately 1.5 million musculoskeletal grafting procedures in the United States alone (Giannoudis et al., 2005), generating more than $2.5 billion a year (Desai, 2007). Despite their popularity, autograft usage is limited by donor site morbidity and supply, while allograft usage is limited by host immunogenic response and potential for disease transmission (De Long et al., 2007; Desai, 2007; Toolan, 2006). Because of these shortcomings, the need for potential alternative or complementary solutions has become of particular academic and commercial research interest. The development of technologies, products, and treatments utilizing TE strategies hold promise for and are emerging as significant, viable alternatives.

More than two decades ago, the rapidly growing field of TE was considered as an interdisciplinary field that applies the principles of engineering and the life sciences toward the development of biological substitutes that restore, maintain, or improve tissue function (Heineken and Skalak, 1991). Even prior to defining the field, early research was focused heavily on artificial skin, in an effort to treat severe burn victims. As early as 1981, a bilayer artificial skin consisting of silicone and porous collagen cross-linked chondroitin was successfully used in the treatment of extensive burn injury (Burke et al., 1981). As the field of TE expanded, research interest and investment grew exponentially, garnering interest from academia and commercial partners alike. As a result of rapidly expanding research and significant developments, tissue-engineered medical products (TEMPs) began making their way into commercial markets. One of the earliest TEMPs to reach the commercial market was Interpore's Pro-Osteon calcium phosphate bone graft substitute in 1993 (Persidis, 1999). Since then, several products have made their way into commercial markets with many more in various stages of development.

Much of the current TEMP are based upon bioengineered scaffold materials, used to facilitate cell growth, alone or in combination with various TE strategies. Researchers and engineers manufacture acellular tissue matrices via mimicking natural extracellular matrix (ECM) framework using artificial products, or by removing cellular components from tissues to produce a collagen matrix. Synthetic biomaterials used for TE must be biodegradable (degradation products can be safely removed via metabolic pathways), biocompatible (the scaffold supports cell adhesion, proliferation, migration, and differentiation), and limit inflammation (prevents rejection and necrosis). These characteristics are induced by examining specific parameters such as scaffold material, dimensions, pore size, and porosity. If engineered ideally, over time these matrices degrade and are replaced by native ECM and tissue. Commercially, synthetic scaffolds are usually polyesters of naturally occurring alpha-hydroxy acids such as poly(lactic-co-glycolic acid) (PLGA), mineral components of a natural organs such as hydroxyapatite, or a composite of organic collagenous proteins in conjunction with inorganic components. Tissue scaffolds retaining native ECM framework and vasculature are derived from bovine or human donors and processed via sterilization and decellularization to yield a biologically compatible material. Autologous cells, however, are often derived from the recipients' own tissue, where a biopsy of the tissue cells are either dissociated and expanded in culture or modified with growth factors and reimplanted into the host with an appropriate scaffold.

Currently, TE is revolutionizing the surgical industry as a plethora of different organ repairs are utilizing TE concepts; this chapter will touch upon TE applications specifically in bone, cartilage, tendon, tissue interface, skin, and nerves. Each class of tissue types has developments of new medical products that uniquely incorporate TE concepts to augment the body's natural-healing abilities. These include bone morphogenetic proteins (BMPs), porous nano-hydroxyapatite/polyamide (PA) 66 ceramic composites, bovine type I collagen matrix scaffolds, agarose–alginate hydrogels, polycaprolactone (PCL), poly-L-lactic acid (PLLA), and many more. These materials have applications in repairing many of the different tissue types that will be addressed in this chapter. The concepts of TE unique to each tissue type will be discussed throughout this chapter. A brief description of components of each tissue, according to its unique structure, function, and composition will be provided. Common injuries, complication of current gold standards to treat these injuries, TEMP that address these problems, and clinical studies evaluating their efficacy and efficiency in repairing the damaged tissues will also be dealt with. We will also evaluate the efficacy and safety of a few TEMPs in the market.

13.2 Bone

Bones are the dynamic framework upon which the human body is built; they serve a series of mechanical and homeostatic functions such as supporting movement, storing inorganic minerals, and synthesizing blood cells. There are a total of 213 bones in our body, of which 80% is cortical bone (a sense and solid material surrounding the marrow space) and 20% is trabecular bone (a honeycomb-like network interspersed in the marrow space). These structures are formed by a combination of endochondral and/or membranous composite deposition of 50%–70% inorganic minerals and 20%–40% extracellular organic matrix. The mineral component is derived of a crystal lattice called hydroxyapatite [$Ca_{10}(PO_4)_6(OH)_2$] with small amounts of carbonate, magnesium, and acid phosphate; while the organic content is composed of 85%–90% collagenous proteins, mostly type I collagen, with several noncollagenous proteins including osteocalcin, osteopontin, and osteonectin (Boskey and Coleman, 2010). The composites are deposed as cylindrical rays called concentric lamellae that collectively form Haversian systems. During childhood and adolescence, our bones exhibit longitudinal growth along the epiphyseal and metaphyseal plates and radial growth around the marrow channel (Clarke, 2008).

Throughout life, our bones are constantly adapting its architecture in response to stress and strain by replacing old bone with newly synthesized bone matrix. An adventitious feature, this process occurs in four steps: activation, resorption, reversal, and formation. During activation, multinucleated preosteoclasts (derived from bone marrow monocyte–macrophages) are recruited to the site where they interact with the bone matrix via its rat genome database (RGD) (arginine, glycine, and asparagine) integrin receptor to create a suction seal. Quickly following attachment, the activated osteoblasts secrete hydrogen ions via a H^+ ATPase proton pump/chloride channel and cathepsin K enzyme to dissolve the bone mineral and digest the protein matrix, respectively; creating the Howship's lacunae and contributing to its characteristic ruffled border. Growth factors are released through the resorption process that results in the subsequent activation of osteoclast and osteoblast by receptor activator of nuclear factor kappa-B (RANK)-RANK ligand—osteoprotegrin system interaction further depicted in Figure 13.1 (Vukicevic et al., 2014). Finally, the osteoblast release vesicles that concentrate calcium and phosphate matrix of which they are ultimately buried within to become osteocytes. This phenomenon prevents the buildup of microdamage that would otherwise greatly decrease the integrity of our bone tissues. In times of trauma and/or load failure, the integrity of these heterogeneous constructs can become disrupted and result in fractures or chronic bone loss. If left untreated, significant bone dysfunction can prove to be detrimental to our wellbeing. Bone repair encapsulates a cascade of events involving the regulation of various growth factors, cytokines, hormones, and mesenchymal stem cells (MSCs). Through a process known as endochondral ossification, these MSCs are differentiated to osteoblast and function as ECM depository units.

According to the Bone and Joint Initiative of the United States, the numbers of spinal fusion procedures have since double from 204,000 in 1998 to 457,000 in 2011. The US National Center for Health Statistics reported annual incidence of 492,000 fractures of tibia, fibula, and ankle (Antonova et al., 2013). Tibia and fibula fractures annually result in 77,000 hospitalizations accounting for 569,000 hospital days and 825,000 physician office visits (Miller and Askew, 2007). In the event that bone repair is unsuccessful, a nonunion can occur that leads to significant morbidity and functional deficit, which constitutes 2%–10% of all tibial fractures. Treatment consists of removal of ineffective or infected hardware and bone stabilization, and biological stimulation. In the Unites States, approximately

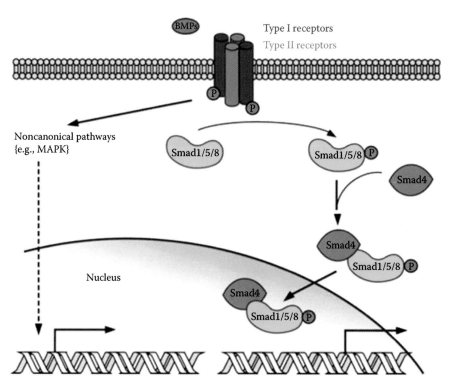

FIGURE 13.1
BMPs signal via the Smad-dependent pathway (canonical) or various non-Smad-dependent pathways. In the canonical BMPs bind type I or II receptors, forming a heterotetrameric complex. Receptor activation allows the phosphorylation of R-Smads (Smad1/5/8). Phosphorylated R-Smads associate with co-Smad (Smad 4). The complex translocates to the nucleus to regulate gene expression. Various noncanonical pathways, including MAP kinase, can also lead to the regulation of gene expression. (Reprinted from *J Orthop Transl.*, 4, Cecchi, S., Bennet, S. and Arora, M., Bone morphogenetic protein-7: Review of signaling and efficacy in fracture healing, Copyright 2015, with permission from Elsevier.)

2.2 million long bone nonunions and spinal fusions are fixated with plates, screws, and autologous bone tissue. The concocted bone matrix serves as a natural reservoir for collagen type I, insulin-like growth factor (IGF)-1, transforming growth factor (TGF)-β, acidic fibroblast growth factor, vascular endothelial growth factor, and platelet-derived growth factor. However, this gold standard repair is often associated with limited donor availability, increased postoperative pain, increased intraoperative blood loss, and extended operative time (Bishop and Einhorn, 2007). Ultimately, these complications can lead to ineffective treatment resulting in delayed or incomplete bone unions. A rapidly growing alternative treatment is bone grafting using allografts. They serve as adequate substitutes of autografts but carry the risk of disease transmission. To overcome these disadvantages, researchers have looked at tissue-engineered synthetic bone grafts, ceramic composites, and BMPs as an alternate solution for tibial nonunions and spinal fusions. Clinicians utilize engineered bone grafts and BMPs as means of augmenting bone's regenerative potential through natural repair processes such as endochondral ossification. These engineered constructs enhance the proliferation and induction of undifferentiated mesenchymal cells into matrix depositing osteoblast. BMPs specifically facilitate the translation of necessary growth factors involved in the induction of osteoblast, while bone graft's unique microstructure facilitates osteoconductive mechanisms, or the influx of various physiological

TABLE 13.1

Definition of Terms and Common Examples

Term	Definition	Example
Osteoconduction	The process by which an implanted scaffold passively allows ingrowth of host vasculature, cells, and tissue	Resorption of calcium sulfate or phosphate cements
Osteoinduction	The process by which exogenous growth factors promotes differentiation of host MSCs to form chondroblasts and osteoblasts that form new bone	BMPs
Osteogenesis	The synthesis of new bone by donor cells derived from either the host or graft donor	Various autografts, stem cell transplants
Fracture nonunion	A bone fracture that is at least 9 months old in which there have been no signs of healing for 3 months (US FDA definition)	
Growth factor	A naturally occurring protein or hormone that stimulates cellular differentiation, proliferation, and/or growth	TGF beta, IGF
Mitogen	A growth factor that specifically induces cellular mitosis	BMPs, vascular endothelial growth factors, fibroblast growth factors
Ceramic	An inorganic compound formed at high temperatures that contains metallic and nonmetallic elements with a crystalline structure	Alumina, zirconium, hydroxyapatite, calcium phosphates

Source: Reprinted from Roberts, T.T. and Rosenbaum, A.J. 2012. *Organogenesis*, 8(4): 114–124. With permission from Taylor & Francis Group.

elements needed for bone repair as defined in Table 13.1 (Bishop and Einhorn, 2007). This section will focus on two options in particular: porous nano-hydroxyapatite/PA 66 ceramics (n-HA.PA66) and BMP-7 or osteogenic protein-1 (OP-1) (Xiong et al., 2014).

BMPs are potent osteoblast-differentiation factors that coordinate bone growth during development, they are a subfamily of the TGF-β superfamily. BMPs were discovered to harbor bone induction properties through molecular biology techniques and sequencing of bovine molecular clones, which led to the discovery of each BMP coding sequence in human homologues. By inserting a vector encoding human BMP into mammalian cell host, the BMP molecule was able to be amplified and experimented (Cecchi et al., 2016). Studies utilizing this technique discovered that recombinant human BMP (rhBMP) were produced by osteoprogenitor cells, osteoblast, chondrocytes, and platelets. They function to impair bone defects via induction of pluripotent cells into osteoblast, chondrocytes, blood vessels, thereby facilitating the synthesis of ECM; as shown when implanted with a collagen scaffold and bone fragments composite (Sampath et al., 1992). The mechanism by which BMP's work involves binding to type I and type II serine/threonine kinase receptors, thus creating dimers and influencing the transcription of vital proteins as depicted in Figure 13.1 (Lissenberg-Thunnissen).

There are a total of 15 BMPs whose characteristics are listed in Table 13.2, two of which, BMP2 and BMP7, have shown through laboratory, animal, and human clinical trials, to

TABLE 13.2

BMPs with Musculoskeletal Function

Identification	Description
BMP-2	Bone and cartilage morphogenesis, osteoinduction, osteoblast differentiation, apoptosis
BMP-3	Negative regulator of bone morphogenesis
BMP-3b	Negative regulator of bone morphogenesis
BMP-4	Cartilage, teeth, and bone morphogenesis
BMP-5	Limb development, cartilage, and bone morphogenesis
BMP-6	Osteoblast differentiation, chondrogenesis
BMP-7	Cartilage and bone morphogenesis
BMP-8	Bone and cartilage morphogenesis
BMP-9	Bone morphogenesis
BMP-11	Axial-skeleton patterning
BMP-12	Ligament and tendon development
BMP-13	Cartilage development
BMP-14	Chondrogenesis, angiogenesis

Source: Reprinted from *J Orthop Translat.*, 4, Cecchi, S., Bennet, S. and Arora, M., Bone morphogenetic protein-7: Review of signaling and efficacy in fracture healing, 28–34, Copyright 2015, with permission from Elsevier.

utilize its osteoinductive qualities in accelerating bone regeneration and fracture healing (Bishop and Einhorn, 2007; Burkus et al., 2002; Friedlaender et al., 2001).

This section will focus on rhBMP-7/OP-1 in particular, which was created by Stryker and credited by the Food and Drug Administration (FDA) on October 17, 2001. Commercially, OP-1 is combined with a purified bovine type I collagen scaffold to provide the implant with osteoconductive properties. It is now available for use in recalcitrant long-bone non-unions, where autograft is unfeasible and alternative treatments have failed. The nature of OP-1 resides in its osteoinductive ability to facilitate bone growth and formation. It actively recruits stem cells from the surrounding tissue and initiates the bone formation cascade by providing the primordial signals necessary for the differentiation of MSCs into osteochondrogenic lineage cells and osteoblast precursor cells (Termaat et al., 2005). This process involves binding of the BMP-7 growth factor to a type II serine/threonine kinase receptor (BMPR-II) followed by recruitment and phosphorylation of the type I serine/threonine kinase receptor (BMPR-I). The activated BMPR-I subsequently proceeds to phosphorylate and activate intracellular effector proteins Smad1, Smad5, and Smad8. The activated receptor-regulated Smad1/5/8 protein unit forms a complex with Smad4 and translocates into the nucleus where it functions as a transcription factor. Other osteoinductive signaling pathways that BMP-7 utilizes include interaction with p38 mitogen-activated protein (MAP) kinase pathway and phosphatidylinositol 3-kinase (PI3K) and Protein Kinase B (AKT) pathway (Termaat et al., 2005). The pathways discussed above converge to facilitate differentiation of MSCs to osteoblast by regulating the runt-related transcription factor 2 (Runx2) and Osterix genes. The Runx2 is the earliest differentiation maker of the osteoblastic lineage and is required for the formation of chondrocytes, which is noted within 5–7 days post-BMP-7 implantation. After 9–12 days, capillaries invade the area and the chondrocytes become calcified, hypertrophied, and subsequently replaced by osteoid or mineralized bone deposition from surrounding osteoblast. By day 14–21, the mineralized bone is remodeled and filled with bone marrow (Termaat et al., 2005). This reconstruction process facilitated by BMP-7 is very similar to the physiological endochondral bone formation that occurs naturally, and confirms its regulatory role in bone healing.

OP-1 was certified through Friedlaender et al.'s prospective randomized clinical trial in which 122 patients, from February 1992 to August 1996, at one of 17 medical centers in the United States were treated for tibial nonunion. Based on the 1988 FDA guidance document, the use of OP-1 was approved for 9 month duration of a nonunited tibial fracture with no evidence of progressive healing over the previous 3 months (Friedlaender et al., 2001). Each of the 122 patients that met the assessment criteria, underwent intramedullary (IM) rod fixation with OP-1 augmentation in a bovine type I collagen carrier, while the rest were IM rod fixated with bone autograft. Results were assessed clinically, immunologically, and radiologically. Clinical assessment involved the presence of pain at fracture site and ability to bear weight. Immunological assessment utilized an enzyme-linked immunosorbent assay (ELISA) to screen for antibodies against OP-1 and type 1 collagen after 9 and 24 months following surgery. The results of the study showed that OP-1 is a clinically safe osteogenic implant whose rate of success are comparable to autograft by the assessment standards mentioned above (Bishop and Einhorn, 2007; Friedlaender et al., 2001). Since Friedlaender et al.'s prospective randomized clinical trial, a large number of clinical trials investigating applications of BMPs at various anatomical sites have provided evidence supporting the use BMPs for treating many bone defects. These are listed in Table 13.3 (Termaat et al., 2005). These defects include open tibial fractures and posterolateral lumbar fusions. According to a nationwide population-based database to assess the utilization of BMP in spinal fusion surgery, the adjusted annual number of procedures with BMP has increased from 1116 in 2002 to 79,294 in 2011, representing 26.9 of all spinal fusions (Singh et al., 2014).

When choosing a bone graft substitute, one must ensure its materials exhibit strong osteogenesis, biocompatibility, and bioactivity. Furthermore, the structure must maintain its integrity, integrate with host tissue, and provide enough mechanical strength to meet the fundamental support requirements necessary thoroughout the healing period. Based on these ideals, Sichuan University found hydroxyapatite (HA) to possess the osteoconductivity of native bone and PA to provide excellent mechanical properties as well as biocompatibility of type I collagen; and therefore combined the two materials. The composite was prepared by thermal-press molding that yielded high compressive strength and an excellent porous structure as depicted in Figure 13.2 (Xu et al., 2014).

PA is a synthetic polymer of a type made by linkage of an amino group of one molecule with a carboxylic acid group of another. The n-HA crystals mimic bone composition by being encased in PA, which is similar in structure to endogenous collagen through its network of carboxyl and amide groups. When combined together, the composite exhibits strong molecular interactions of hydrogen bonds and electrostatic forces between the ionic groups of the composite created the macrostructure illustrated in Figure 13.3 (Xiong et al., 2014).

This contributes to its excellent compressive strength, and strong mechanical properties; all characteristics of natural bone (Zhang et al., 2014).

Characterization of the 6:4 ratio porous n-HA/PA66 demonstrated a bending, tensile, and compression strength of 95, 79, and 117 MPa, respectively, which is comparable to natural bone (80–100, 60–120, and 50–140 MPa separately). The elastic modulus of the n-HA/PA66 composite was measured to be 5.6 GPa (natural bone 3–25 GPa) (Xu et al., 2010). When optimized to a specific porosity of 75%–80% and average pore diameter of 500 μm, the synthetic graft has shown to successfully repair bone defects (Wang et al., 2007; Xiong et al., 2014). Wang et al. conducted studies that have shown the compound to be biocompatible, osteoconductive with host bone, and osteoinductive of human mesenchymal stem cells (hMSCs)

TABLE 13.3

Clinical Studies on the Application of BMPs at Various Anatomical Sites with an Indication of Nonunion

Authors	Type of Study	Level of Evidence	No. of Cases of BMPs	Indication (Anatomical Site of Nonunion)	Union Rates (%)	Reoperation (%)
Friedlaender et al. (2001)	Prospective randomized controlled (BMP-7 vs. ABG)	II	63	Tibial	75–81	5
Dimitriou et al. (2005)	Prospective observational (BMP-7)	IV	25	Tibial–femoral–humeral–forearm	92.3	12
Kanakaris et al. (2009)	Prospective observational (BMP-7)	IV	30	Femoral	86.7	13
Giannoudis and Tzioupis (2005)	Retrospective cohort study (BMP-7)	IV	395	Femoral–tibial–clavicle–ankle–radius–scaphoid–ankle–humerus–olecranon	82	n/a
Desmyter et al. (2008)	Retrospective cohort study	IV	62	Tibial	84.9	14
Calori et al. (2008)	Prospective randomized controlled (BMP-7 vs. PRP)	III	5	Femoral	100	6.2

Source: Reprinted from *J Orthop Translat.*, 4, Cecchi, S., Bennet, S. and Arora, M., Bone morphogenetic protein-7: Review of signaling and efficacy in fracture healing, 28–34, Copyright 2015, with permission from Elsevier.

Note: ABG—autogenous bone grafting; BMP—bone morphogenetic protein.

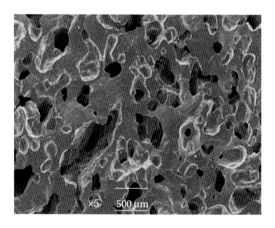

FIGURE 13.2
Scanning electron microscopy micrographs of porous n-HA.PA66. (Reprinted from Hui Xu et al. 2014. *Int J Polymer Sci.* With permission from Hindawi.)

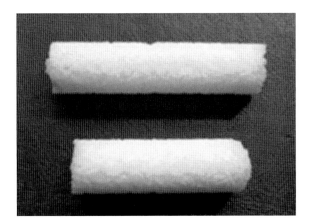

FIGURE 13.3
Columnar n-HA/PA66. (Reprinted from Hui Xu et al. 2014. *Int J Polymer Sci*. With permission from Hindawi.)

into osteogenic cells. The cross-linked composite exhibits good biocompatibility and bio-activity, primarily due to its unique nanoparticle size and shape, as well as high porosity, which promotes cell adhesion, proliferation, and differentiation (Xiong et al., 2014). These characteristics give porous n-HA/PA66 composite the ability to integrate itself within host bone tissue, which has to be shown through rabbit tibial implantation using the composite. Biological efficacy of the composite evaluated via laboratory and animal studies showed that the composite had no cytotoxicity, no sensitization effect, and no pyrogenic reactions. In clinical practice, the exposed bone tissue is filled with the porous n-HA/PA66 composite and stabilized with an internal fixation. Radiological assessment revealed that 25% of grafting zones were replaced by new bone within 2–3 months, after 6–9 months new bone formation rose to 50%. Within 1.5 years, the defects were completely filled with new bone (Xiong et al., 2014). None of the patients experienced major side effects such as graft rejection, aseptic inflammation, or infections. Therefore, clinical studies have shown that the n-HA/PA66 composite to be cost effective, safe, and efficient.

The process of fixing fractures can be complex and result in associated risk factors such as excessive bone loss, instability, and secondary tissue injury. Many biological and synthetic materials have been explored for their therapeutic potential. Ceramics, synthetic, and biological ingredients have proved to provide efficacious solutions for the treatment of bond defects. However, the literature shows both bone grafts and BMPs have their shortcomings. BMPs are great for long-bone fractures and spinal fusion, proving to be as efficient as autologous bone grafts; but they have short biological half-lives and are 6.7% more expensive than the alternate option. Also, patients who undergo BMP therapy are at a greater risk of developing an immunogenic response and ectopic bone formation in response to the supra-physiological dose of BMP often used by clinicians (Dahabreh et al., 2009). Despite these drawbacks, clinical use of BMP-7 is still recommended as it efficaciously accelerates bone repair resulting in shorter surgery time and faster discharge of the patient (Garrison et al., 2007; Lissenberg-Thunnissen et al., 2011). Bone autografts can repair a wide variety of defects, but are limited to the amount of bone tissue available in donor site and may provoke host immune reaction, respectively (Dahabreh et al., 2009). The n-HA/P66 composite solves the issue of donor tissue availability that is necessary for autograft implantation. Several medical device companies have taken advantage of

HA and HA hybrids in the design of various bone substitutes for regenerative applications. Stryker created the OP-1/BMP-7 line of products consisting of OP-1 Putty for spinal fusion and OP-1 Implant for fracture repair, which stimulate the recruitment of natural bone-healing processes. In an effort to create a long-lasting, nonbiologic substitute for bone, Zimmer commercialized an HA-based synthetic product known as IngeniOs HA®. Similarly, Geistlich Biomaterials developed Bio-Oss® specifically directed for bone substitute for regenerative dentistry applications. Based upon their optimal biocompatibility, osteoinduction, and integration, these biological and synthetic materials are an efficacious and cost-effective alternative to treating bone defects. Many bone grafts that contain the characteristic osteoconductive, osteoinductive, and osteogenic properties necessary to foster bone healing are listed in Tables 13.4 and 13.5 (Roberts and Rosenbaum, 2012).

13.3 Cartilage

Cartilage tissue, particularly articular cartilage (AC), is immensely important for joint mobility and providing a lubricative surface that allows repetitive load transfer over a length of time. Consisting primarily of hyaline cartilage, it has the ability to distribute loads that no other tissue or current device can fully replicate (Temenoff and Mikos, 2000). It is a very thin tissue that makes it vulnerable to degeneration from multiple factors including trauma, disease, and weight overloading (Adam et al., 1998). Injuries are classified into three categories: superficial matrix disruption, partial thickness defects, and full thickness defects. In superficial matrix disruption defects, blunt trauma shallowly damages the ECM. Partial thickness defects occur when damage breaks the cartilage tissue but does not harm subchondral bone. Full thickness defects occur when damage disrupts both the cartilage tissue and the underlying subchondral bone. In these cases, bone marrow cells are naturally recruited to regenerate cartilage tissue, but this will be of the much weaker fibrocartilage rather than the stronger native hyaline cartilage (Matsiko et al., 2013). Human chondrocytes are capable of naturally repairing injured cartilage if the injury is a superficial matrix disruption but cannot correctly repair the damage if the injury is a partial thickness defect or a full thickness defect (Zhu et al., 2015). As a result, external intervention is required to repair these defects.

Cartilage is a vital tissue in the human body that functions in various capacities, which are needed for the body to operate, including supporting the mechanical aspects of the body such as joint functionality as well as being a vital component in bone development. Other functions include force transmission, shock absorption, joint stability, lubrication, and proprioception (Schwartz et al., 2014). Problems with repairing cartilage include its avascular nature that gives it a very limited natural regenerative capability (Ravindran et al., 2015). Cartilage is composed of mainly proteoglycans and collagen with very little blood perfusion. This lack of blood perfusion means that it is very difficult for nutrients and cells to reach those areas to heal. Currently, there are methods being investigated that are shown to provide the same structural and functional properties of healthy cartilage to aid patients with damaged tissue, such as patients with osteoarthritis (OA), inflammation, and even cancer. Methods of this sort include microfracture, mosaicplasty, and autologous chondrocyte implantation but they all have poor outcomes (Jiang et al., 2011). Microfracture is a repair method in which holes are created in the subchondral plate to stimulate the formation of new AC. However, this method creates tough fibrocartilage

TABLE 13.4

Bone Substitutes: Properties and Commercial Product Examples

Graft	Forms	Resorption Rate	Compressive Strength	Common Products	Notes
Calcium sulfate	Pellets, powders, mixable injectable forms	Fast (4–12 weeks)	≈ [a]cancellous bone	Osteoset, BonePlast, OsteoMax, Stimulan[b]	Resorbs faster than bone; may be associated with high rates of serous wound drainage [102]
Calcium phosphate	Injectable pastes, moldable semisolid cement	Slow (6 months to 10 years)	4–10 × > cancellous bone	Norian SRS, α-BSM, BoneSource, Mimix CopiOs[c]	Available in standard and fast-setting forms
Tricalcium phosphate	Granules, various implantable solid shapes: blocks, cubes, wedges, cylinders	Slow (6–18 months)	≈ cancellous bone	Allogram-R, Cellplex, Cerasorb M, Chron OS, Conduit, TheiLok, Vitoss[d]	Notably brittle
Coralline hydroxyapatite	Porous or solid blocks or granules; ceramic and non-ceramic forms	Slow, often incomplete (6 months [non-ceramic form] to 10+ years [ceramic form])	≈ cancellous bone	Pro Osteon[e]	Notably brittle. Non-ceramic hydroxyapatite is readily absorbed; in ceramic form, residual material present for years

Source: Reprinted from Roberts, T.T. and Rosenbaum, A.J. 2012. *Organogenesis*, 8(4): 114–124. With permission from Taylor & Francis Group.

[a] ≈ Approximately equal.

[b] Osteoset (Wright Medical Technology), Bone Plast (Biomet), 2012. OsteoMax (Orthofix), Stimulan (Biocomposites).

[c] Norian SRS (Synthes, Paoli, Pennsylvania), α-BSM (DePuy, Warsaw, Indiana), BoneSource (Stryker), Mimix (Biomet), CopiOs (Zimmer Spine).

[d] Allogram-R (Biocomposites, Cellplex (Wright Medical Technology, Arlington, Tennessee), Cerasorb M (Ascension Orthopaedics), Chron OS (Synthes), Conduit (DePuy), TheiLok (Therics), Vitoss (Orthovita).

[e] Pro Osteon (Biomet).

TABLE 13.5

Properties, Functions, and Cost of Various Forms of Bone Grafts and Substitutes

Graft	Osteoconductive	Osteoinductive	Osteogenic	Structural	Disadvantages
Autograft					
Cancellous	+++	+++	+++	+	Donor site morbidity, increased OR time, increased blood loss
Allograft					
Cancellous	+	+/−[b]	−	+	Potential infection transmission, no osteogenic potential, potential host rejection
Demineralized bone matrix	+	++	−	−	No structural properties, potential host rejection
Synthetic Ceramics					
Calcium sulfate	+	−	−	++	Rapid resorption (faster than bone growth), osteoconductive properties only
Calcium phosphate	+	−	−	+++	Osteoconductive properties only
Tricalcium phosphate	+	−	−	++	Osteoconductive properties only
Other					
rhBMPs	+/−[a]	+	+	−	Expensive, limited FDA approval, limited indications, increasing evidence of neurovascular complications when used in the spine

Source: Reprinted from Roberts, T.T. and Rosenbaum, A.J. 2012. *Organogenesis*, 8(4), 114–124. With permission from Taylor & Francis Group.

[a] Excludes preparation costs.

[b] +, typically with fresh allografts; −, typically with frozen-preserved allografts.

instead of the native hyaline cartilage needed to maintain joint fluidity (Berta et al., 2015). In addition, deterioration of the repair site is expected after 2–5 years and is not a favorable long-term solution (Gobbi et al., 2014). Mosaicplasty is a method that uses multiple autologous osteochondral cylinders that are implanted to repair osteochondral defects. This method is limited in its use from a lack of available resources to produce them and its inability to repair large-sized defects (Ma et al., 2015). Another method includes autologous chondrocyte transplantation, which involves the injection of *in vitro* expanded chondrocyte cell suspension within the lesion site, thus providing the cells necessary for cartilage regeneration. Problems that microfracture and autologous chondrocyte transplantation have include mechanically inferior repair tissue, uneven distribution of autologous cells, and small inclusion criterion of patients.

To combat these issues, two products have been engineered and tested for the safety and efficacy as a novel method to chondral defect repairs. Histogenics in Waltham, Mass created NeoCart®, an autologous cartilage tissue implant consisting of bovine type I collagen matix scaffold with autogenous chondrocytes. The implant is unique in that it is fabricated from the patient's own cells. A minimally invasive arthroscopy retrieves a small cartilage sample from the patient, which is then cultured and allowed to proliferate. Thus, the patient's own cartilage cells form a hyaline-like cartilage tissue, which is then seeded on a collagen scaffold. In a randomized clinical trial, 30 diagnostically eligible patients underwent either NeoCart implantation or microfracture repair. Preliminary findings suggested that the NeoCart implant significantly decreased knee pain and improved function much better than microfracture repair (Crawford et al., 2012). The Tissue Bank of France, in Lyon, France, developed a novel agarose–alginate hydrogel scaffold named *CARTIPATCH*. An autologous chondrocyte cell solution is suspended in the Cartipatch scaffold. The cell implanted hydrogel is squeezed through pre-drilled holes until it completely layers the defect. Clinically, 17 patients underwent the procedure and their outcomes were evaluated via a series of subjective and objective assessment methods including magnetic resonance imaging (MRI), histology, and arthroscopy. Upon a 2-year follow up post-implantation, MRI analysis of 11 patients showed perfect tissue integration, and arthroscopy analysis revealed repaired tissue to be leveled with normal adjacent cartilage in 10 patients. Moreover, histological analysis of eight biopsied tissues consisted of predominantly hyaline-like cartilage. Therefore, cell-Cartipatch composite is a safe and efficacious method of treating chondral and osteochondral defects by augmenting the current autologous chondrocyte implant method (Selmi et al., 2008).

OA is a degenerative joint disease, which currently affects approximately 27 million Americans (Ouzzine et al., 2012). In OA, the cartilage that provides a smooth, gliding surface for joint motion breaks down causing immense pain, swelling, and joint immobility. This breakdown is often a result of poor vascularization and matrix mineralization, and can be caused by a combination of genetic traits, weight, and repetitive injury or over use. As OA worsens over time, bones may break down and the body's inflammatory response begins to further damage the cartilage. Due to the avascular and aneural nature of cartilage tissue, normal mechanisms of tissue repair through recruitment of cells and nutrients to the site of tissue destruction are not feasible (Ouzzine et al., 2012). Current treatments for OA include medications like acetaminophen or NSAIDs, physical therapy, or surgical procedures like cortisone injections, bone realignments, and joint replacement surgery. Acetaminophen and NSAIDs are only used for symptomatic treatment of the disease, reducing inflammation and swelling, but can neither reverse the disease process nor heal the damage (Flood, 2010). Chondrogenic ECM scaffolds have been made using collagen and chitosan matrices seeded with human MSCs. The scaffolds can also be used in combination with various substances through exposure in the supporting medium solution to help the seeded cells develop. These can include growth factors including TGF β1, TGF β3, IGF, and bone morphogenic protein (BMP). Combinations may also be used and it has been noted that a mix of TGF β3 and BMP2 is much more successful at promoting chondrogenesis than using singular factors (Nirmal and Nair, 2013). Another important feature is the absence of vascularization in the resulting tissue during the formation process. Thus, this concept can be applied to potential devices in the future to allow easier regeneration of damaged cartilage tissue (Ravindran et al., 2015).

Three-dimensional (3D) scaffolds of various compositions are currently being investigated due to their beneficial biocompatibility, biomimetic, and bioactive properties. PCL is one of the most widely accepted polymers for use in making 3D scaffolds due to its high biocompatibility, biodegradability, and mechanical properties (Pham et al., 2006). However, PCL is limited in its application because of an absence of surface cell-recognition sites that are caused by its hydrophobic nature (Ciardelli et al., 2005). Thus, a study conducted at George Washington University investigated the use of cold atmospheric plasma (CAP) to give the scaffold a more bioactive and cell-favorable surface (Zhu et al., 2015). CAP is an ionized gas kept at room temperature composed of reactive oxygen and nitrogen species, and photons as well as electrostatic and electromagnetic fields. Plasma-assisted surface modifications can be used for numerous applications such as cleaning, etching, sterilization, activation, or coating. In plasma-assisted activation, a surface can be modified to be made more bioactive by deposition of various functional group coatings. An O_2 plasma can deposit hydroxyl, carboxyl, and ketone groups, while an N_2 plasma can deposit amine, amide, and nitro groups. Exposure of a scaffold to this gas modifies the scaffold surface to display a more biomimetic and bioactive surface than before. This particular study focused on the use of an electrospun PCL scaffold embedded with PLGA microspheres to promote the growth and development of human MSCs. PCL and PLGA have already been shown in the literature to be biocompatible and biomimetic and so is able to provide a solid foundation on which to create a novel scaffold suitable for use in tissue regenerative engineering (Yang et al., 2015). The materials are able to mimic the same biochemical processes that are naturally occurring in the human body and thus elicit similar cellular responses by native tissue to the materials used in the implant. The study showed an increase in MSC proliferation and chondrogenic differentiation of those MSCs on the scaffolds treated with CAP (Zhu et al., 2015). This was done through analyzing the amount of glycosaminoglycans, a vital component in cartilage ECM, and collagen that were secreted by the implanted cells. Plasma modification has a great potential for enhancing the viability of existing devices that already are able to foster successful regeneration of cartilage tissue. This can be applied to any cartilage tissue construct and can be shaped in such a way to maximize performance.

Tissue-engineered devices can be designed to accurately mimic entire structures in the human body. As an example, the trachea is one of the many areas of the body where healthy cartilage is vital to its performance and can be modified using a tissue-engineered device. The structure and mechanical properties of the cartilage are vital for maintaining the airways. In this organ, hyaline cartilage provides mechanical strength to the tube and prevents its collapse during respiration. It also helps to maintain the structure of the trachea as it rotates, flexes, and extends in everyday movements. The tracheal tube can collapse due to varying causes, the most common of which include endotracheal intubation and tracheostomy, and is most concerning in premature infants and young children who need intubation (Park et al., 2015). The trachea can also be damaged from trauma, infections, congenital defects, or cancers. Surgical resection of affected segments and anastomosis of the remaining ends is currently the medical standard today, but this can only be performed if the airway does not exceed half of the total length in adults and a third of the total length in children (Jungebluth et al., 2012). Transplantation of an allograft requires lifelong immunosuppression and usually results in necrosis leading to infection and subsequent death. Scaffold implants have great potential in correcting tracheal defects while avoiding many of the complications affecting current treatment methods today.

Scaffolds made from biocompatible and bioactive materials are suitable for repairing damaged tracheal cartilage tissue. Scaffolds have been made using poly(L-lactide-*co*-caprolactone) (PLCL) and gelatin made from porcine skin and combined with gelatin sponges infused with TGF-β1 to provide sustained release of the growth factor. The scaffolds were created using indirect 3D-printing method to give them adequate mechanical properties comparable to native tracheal tissue. Sustained release of the growth factor TGF-β1 promoted proliferation of the chondrocytes and production of the necessary ECM to support the cells. This combination successfully enhanced cartilage regeneration as well as sustained degradation of the gelatin sponge to provide structural support during the development phase of the cartilage tissue (Park et al., 2015). This system may be used in the future as an alternative to the methods currently used today.

13.4 Tendon

Tendon rotator cuff repairs are a rapidly developing procedure in the United States, performed 250,000 times every year. They account for nearly 32 million orthopedic musculoskeletal injuries annually (Colvin et al., 2012). With it grows the necessity for innovative solutions as 20%–90% of surgical cases exhibit re-tearing of the tendon depending on patient age, tear size, muscle atrophy and degeneration, tendon quality, repair technique, and postoperative rehabilitation protocol (Derwin et al., 2009). Scientists are motivated by the great success found in scaffold fabrication for augmenting tissue regeneration (Lambers Heerspink et al., 2015). Currently, the gold standard patella tendon autograft is limited by several factors including duration of symptoms, shoulder dominance, the type of tear (partial vs. full thickness), and patient factors such as age, comorbidities, and activity level. To date, treatment options are categorized into surgical repair and nonoperative management. Surgical repair indications are usually acute, full thickness traumatic tears of a once healthy rotator cuff to prevent muscular atrophy with tendon degeneration and retraction. They are preformed arthroscopically or open (standard or "mini open"). Conservative management employs subacromial steroid infiltration, physiotherapy, and analgesic medication. Chronic, symptomatic rotator cuff tears are usually managed with conservative management for up to 6–12 weeks; however, they often fail to restore functional capability and structural integrity to that of native tissue. This causes abnormal healing and leaves the injury site ridden with scar tissue and subpar tendon-to-bone integration; therefore, increasing the risk of re-tearing the structure (Zhang et al., 2012). Problems as such can be attributed to the complex anatomy of joints and the hypovascular nature of tendons that restricts mineral influx to the injury site thereby limiting overall healing potential. As a solution, scientists have turned to alternative options through TE to combat the debilitating effect of rotator cuff tears coupled with the high incidence of failure associated with existing graft choices (Zhang et al., 2012). The ideal scaffold must match the mechanical properties and highly organized nanoscale structure of native tendon, degrade at an optimal rate to allow for gradual replacement of host tissue, and integrate with both the tendon and surrounding tissues for full physiological function (Zhang et al., 2012).

Two materials in particular, GraftJacket® a decellularized dermal allograft matrix derived from human skin, and X-repair a slowly degrading and biocompatible synthetic polymer named PLLA, have shown to provide mechanical strength and biocompatibility necessary for rapid healing. GraftJacket uses skin transplants and processes them to produce a sheet containing collagen, fibronectin, proteoglycans, hyaluronan, and elastin, all essential components of skin tissue. These engineered biological and synthetic polymer-based grafts recapitulate the nanostructure of native tendon ECM; by exhibiting tightly packed parallel collagen fiber bundles of various diameter, high aspect ratio (ratio of length to width) to ensure uniform distribution of stress, high surface area to volume ratio, low density, and high permeability and porosity (Zhang et al., 2012). The aforementioned characteristics directly contribute to the human tendon's physiological function of stabilizing and guiding joint motion, transmitting physiological loads, and maintaining anatomical alignment of the skeleton (Jung et al., 2009).

The GraftJacket is a cellular human dermal matrix fabricated by Wright Medical Technology, in Arlington, Tennessee. It is processed by a patented technique that removes epidermal and dermal cells from the donated skin, the acellular graft is then freeze dried to prevent formation of ice crystals and to retain the native extracellular architecture and vascularization (Longo et al., 2010). The resulting graft is composed of closely packed parallel fiber bundles of collagen types I, III, IV, VII, elastin, chondroitin sulfate, proteoglycans, and fibroblast growth factor. Specialized to treat tendon repairs and ligament augmentation, this biomaterial naturally induces the repopulation and revascularization of the soft tissue (Derwin et al., 2006). An *in vitro* study comparing the growth and proliferation of tenocytes on ECM-derived biological scaffolds (GraftJacket, Restore, CuffPatch, TissueMend, Permacol) showed that Graftjacket and Restore induced cell growth and proliferation, promoted vascularization, and decreased inflammation better than their slowly degrading competitor grafts CuffPatch, TissueMend, and Permacol (Longo et al., 2010). Furthermore, biomechanical assessment of the GraftJacket was tested via cycle loading and stress to failure of cadaveric supraspinatus tendon. Results showed that load-to-failure strength of the control was 273 ± 116 N, the median failure strength test was 254 N, with a range of 145–518 N. The load-to-failure strength of the supraspinatus with GraftJacket augmentation was 325 ± 74 N, with a median value of 309 N and a range of 257–479 N. The maximum load was statistically significantly greater in the graft group than control, and stress to failure testing confirmed the strength and stability of GraftJacket (Omae et al., 2012).

A randomized clinical study involving 45 patients assessed the safety and efficacy of GraftJacket in treating massive rotator cuff tears via minimally invasive approach. When employing the suggested Maxforce Extreme bridging technique, the augmented treatments using the GraftJacket exhibited a statistically significant mean modified UCLA score increase from 18.4 preoperatively to 27.5 postoperatively with no adverse events at 2 years follow-up (Wong et al., 2010). In second study by Bond *et al.*, 16 patients were treated for a massive rotator cuff tears with arthroscopic implantation of a GraftJacket allograft. At a mean follow-up of 26.7 months, 15 of 16 patients were satisfied with the procedure. Statistically significant improvements were noted in pain, forward flexion, and external rotation strength. MRI scans showed full incorporation of the graft into the native tissue in 13 patients (Longo et al., 2010). A chronic Achilles tendon rupture repair study was also conducted using a GraftJacket scaffold, the results showed early return to normal activities within approximately 15 weeks. They consist of satisfactory plantaflextion, with no re-ruptures or recurrent pain after 20 months postoperative (Longo et al., 2010).

The synthetic graft X-repair is an ultrathin patch developed by Synthasome Inc. in of San Diego and Soft Tissue Regeneration Inc., New Haven, Connecticut. The product received its US FDA 501(k) clearance in 2009 for the surgical repair of massive tendon, ligament, and other soft tissue repairs. The scaffold design is a mesh complex fabricated of PLLA to accentuate the tensile strength, stiffness, and cellular facilitation of the human tendon. Surgeons drape the X-repair patch over the lesion site and anchor it with sutures to allow the tendon, bones, and nearby tissues time to heal. Preclinical studies on canines and cadaveric shoulder models showed that X-repair effectively augments surgically repaired rotator cuff injuries by enhancing its ability to sustain heavier loads with minimal displacement, as shown in Figure 13.4 and Table 13.6 (Derwin et al., 2006; McCarron et al., 2012).

A clinical study determining the functional and structural outcomes for arthroscopic repair of large to massive (two to three tendon) rotator cuff tears with X-repair was conducted and analyzed by radiography and clinical assessments. The study inducted

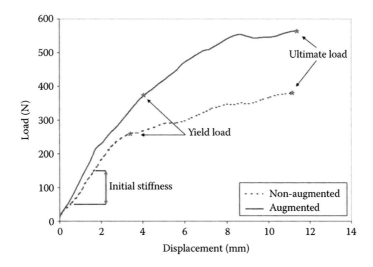

FIGURE 13.4
Pair of representative load-displacement curves for non-augmented and augmented constructs in anterior supraspinatus region of rotator cuff during load-to-failure test. Initial stiffness was defined as the slope of the load-displacement curve between 50 and 150 N. Yield load was defined as the load at which the stiffness of the construct dropped to 50% of the initial stiffness or less. Ultimate load was defined as the maximum load achieved during testing. (Reprinted from *J Shoulder Elbow Surg.*, 21(12), McCarron, J.A. et al., Reinforced fascia patch limits cyclic gapping of rotator cuff repairs in a human cadaveric model, 1680–1686, Copyright 2011, with permission from Elsevier.)

18 patients (average age, 66 years; range 52–89 years) who were clinically diagnosed with large rotator cuff tears. The synthetic patch was secured with sutures along the musculotendinous junction and medial tuberosity of the humorous as illustrated in Figure 13.5.

Postoperatively, ultrasound confirmed that the intervention exhibited a 78% success rate with two repairs failing at 2 months, one failing at 6 months, and another failing at 42 months. Each patient also regained the ability to mobilize the joint based upon the American Shoulder and Elbow Surgery assessment scale, the average score increased from 44 to 73 during the 42-month span. Although a small and rather complex cohort of patients, the study successfully showed clinical and structural improvement of large to massive rotator cuff tear and re-tear repairs with the X-repair scaffold (Proctor, 2014). In recent years, efficient cost-effective solutions for the management of irreparable rotator cuff injuries have been under rapid investigation. This is primarily to meet the inevitable increase in rate of rotator cuff injuries accompanying the aging population, which Figure 13.6 depicts illustrating results of an investigation in Japan discovering that the percentage of rotator cuff tears per generation increased with age (Yamamoto et al., 2010).

Currently, there are many commercial graft materials in the market as depicted in Table 13.7, of which both GraftJacket and X-repair show great promise in healing rotator cuff injuries. Their strong mechanical properties in conjunction with nanostructured design underscore their ability to restore tendon physiological function. Although the studies investigating X-repair yielded encouraging results, there are concerns regarding X-repair's PLLA degradation products as high levels of lactic acid may impair cellular function and tissue integration (Thangarajah et al., 2015). Meyer et al. revealed the effect of high concentrations of up to 50 mM of lactic acid and glycolic acid ceasing osteoblastic, tenocytes, and myofibroblast proliferation, which are vital processes for tendon repair (Meyer et al., 2012). Therefore it is imperative that long durations of functional studies

TABLE 13.6

Biomechanical Differences between X-Repair-Augmented and Non-Augmented Rotator Cuff Repairs

	Sample Size	Non-augmented (mean ± SD)	Augmented (mean ± SD)	Mean Difference (±SD) (Augmented–Non-augmented)	Mean % Increase (Augmented–Non-augmented)	P Value	Power
Initial Stiffness (Slope of Load-Displacement Curve between 50–150 N)							
Anterior supraspinatus	7	100 ± 14 N/mm	115 ± 17 N/mm	15 ± 16 N/mm	16%	0.059	0.419
Posterior supraspinatus	6	81 ± 13 N/mm	96 ± 26 N/mm	18 ± 30 N/mm	24%	0.21	0.131
Superior infraspinatus	7	130 ± 31 N/mm	113 ± 14 N/mm	–17 ± 30 N/mm	–10%	0.187	0.149
Yield Load (Load at which Stiffness of Specimen Dropped to ≤50% of Initial Stiffness)							
Anterior supraspinatus	7	280 ± 54 N	441 ± 136 N	150 ± 161 N	59%	0.048	0.473
Posterior supraspinatus	6	220 ± 18 N	342 ± 68 N	121 ± 66 N	56%	0.007	0.937
Superior infraspinatus	7	260 ± 107 N	482 ± 163 N	222 ± 94 N	92%	<0.001	0.999
Ultimate Load (Maximum Load Achieved during Testing)							
Anterior supraspinatus	7	358 ± 68 N	673 ± 209 N	295 ± 177 N	76%	0.005	0.951
Posterior supraspinatus	6	279 ± 32 N	437 ± 78 N	156 ± 56 N	56%	0.001	1
Superior infraspinatus	7	406 ± 100 N	694 ± 191 N	288 ± 120 N	72%	<0.001	1

Source: Reprinted from *J Shoulder Elbow Surg.*, 21(12), McCarron, J.A. et al., Reinforced fascia patch limits cyclic gapping of rotator cuff repairs in a human cadaveric model, 1680–1686, Copyright 2011, with permission from Elsevier.

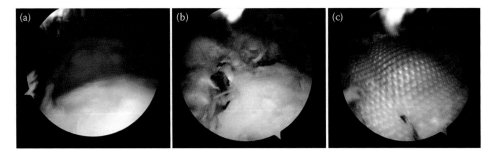

FIGURE 13.5
Right shoulder viewed from lateral portal. (a) Massive tear with retraction to level of glenoid. (b) Rotator cuff repaired to greater tuberosity at articular margin viewed before insertion of synthetic patch. (c) Synthetic patch secured with two medial sutures placed near the musculotendinous junction and two laterally secured with two separate knotless anchors more lateral on the tuberosity such that there was medial to lateral tension, ensuring that load was imposed on the device and load sharing with the tendon occurred. (Reprinted from *J Shoulder Elbow Surg.*, 23(10), Proctor, C.S., Long-term successful arthroscopic repair of large and massive rotator cuff tears with a functional and degradable reinforcement device, 1508–1513, Copyright 2014, with permission from Elsevier.)

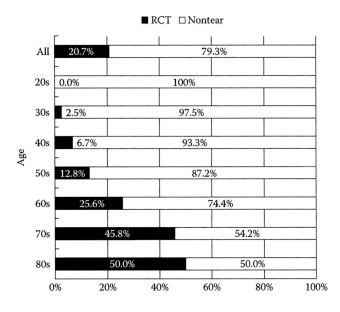

FIGURE 13.6
Percentage of the "RCT group" and "Nontear group" in each generation, the RCT group included of 20.7% of all subjects and the prevalence increased with age. (Reprinted from *J Shoulder Elbow Surg.*, 18(1), Yamamoto, A. et al. Prevalence and risk factors of a rotator cuff tear in the general population, 116–120, Copyright 2009, with permission from Elsevier.)

be performed to assess the degradation influences of these synthetic products on tissue regeneration and tendon-to-bone integration. All considered, graft implantation has shown to be an effective and safe option in enhancing the functional capacity of the regenerated tendon; both X-repair and GraftJacket have great potential for treating massive and irreparable rotator cuff tears.

TABLE 13.7
Clinical Studies Investigating Scaffolds Used for Augmentation of Rotator Cuff Repairs

Type of Scaffold	Study	Level of Evidence	Tear Size	Sample Size	Follow-up Period (Range)	Failure Rate on USS/MRI	Functional Outcome	Adverse Events
Porcine small intestinal mucosa	Iannotti et al. (2006)	2 (prospective RCT)	Large and massive (≥ 4 cm)	CG: 15, AG:15	14 months (12–26.5 months)	CG: 6/15 AG: 11/15	No difference between groups using PENN	AG: 3/15 postoperative inflammatory reaction
	Phipatanakul and Petersen (2009)	4 (case series)	Massive tears (≥ 5 cm)	11	26 months (14–38 months)	5//9	Significant improvement in UCLA and ASES scores	3/11 postoperative inflammatory reaction
	Walton et al. (2007)	3 (case control)	–	CG: 16, AG: 15	24 months	CG: 7/12 AG: 6/10	AG had significantly less lift-off strength, and significantly less strength in internal rotation and adduction than the CG	AG: 4/10 postoperative inflammatory reaction
Porcine dermal collagen patch	Badhe et al. (2008)	4 (case series)	Tears ≥ 5 cm	10	4.5 y (3–5 years)	2//10	Significant improvement in constant score	None
Porcine dermal extracellular tissue matrix	Gupta et al. (2013)	4 (case series)	Full thickness supraspinatus tear with ≥ 5 cm retraction/full thickness 2 tendon tear	26	32 months (24–40 months)	1//26	Significant improvement in ASES and SF-12 scores	None
Acellular dermal matrix	Bond et al. (2008)	4 (case series)	Tears that were ≥ 5 cm or involved 2 tendons, or both	16	26.7 months (12–38 months)	3//16	Significant improvement in UCLA and constant scores	None

(Continued)

TABLE 13.7 (*Continued*)

Clinical Studies Investigating Scaffolds Used for Augmentation of Rotator Cuff Repairs

Type of Scaffold	Study	Level of Evidence	Tear Size	Sample Size	Follow-up Period (Range)	Failure Rate on USS/MRI	Functional Outcome	Adverse Events
	Barber et al. (2012)	2 (prospective RCT)	Large (≥3 cm) 2-tendon tears	CG: 20, AG: 22	24 months (12–38 months)	CG: 9/15 AG: 3/20	AG exhibited significantly better ASES and constant scores	None
	Gupta et al. (2012)	4 (case series)	Full thickness rotator cuff tear with > 5 cm retraction	24	36 months (29–42 months)	1/24	Significant improvement in ASES and SF-12 scores	None
Absorbable collagen and nonabsorbable polyproplene patch	Ciampi et al. (2014)	3 (cohort study)	Full thickness, 2-tendon tear with < 2 cm postoperative residual retraction	Collagen: 49, polypropylene: 52, CG: 51	36 months	Collagen: 24/49 polypropylene: 9/52 CG: 21/51	Pathological histocompatibility scores at 36 months were significantly higher for the polypropylene group. Elevation and strength of the polypropylene group were significantly higher than those of the other groups	None
Absorbable PLLA	Proctor (2014)	4 (case series)	Large to massive (2 or 3 tendons) tears with ≥ 3 cm retraction	18	42 months (35–47 months)	3/18	Significant improvement in ASES score	None
	Lenart et al. (2015)	4 (case series)	Massive tear (complete detachment of at least 2 tendons)	16	1.5 years (1.2–1.7 years)	8/13	Significant improvement in ASES and PENN scores	None

Source: Reprinted from Thangarajah, T. et al. 2015. *Orthop J Sports Med*, 3(6). With permissions from Sage Journals.

Note: AG, augmentation group; ASES, American Shoulder and Elbow Surgeons; CG, control group; MRI, magnetic resonance imaging; PENN, PENN shoulder score; RCT, randomized controlled trial; USS, ultrasound scan; SF-12, Short Form-12; UCLA, University of California, Los Angeles.

13.5 Tissue Interface

The human body is an entire system of different tissues and substances that are enmeshed together to make the body function. It is impossible for a single tissue to viably sustain the mechanisms of the body independently. Thus, when working with tissue regenerative engineering, it is vital that the relationships between each type of tissue are maintained. For example, skeletal muscle must attach to a tendon while the tendon attaches to the bone. Skeletal muscle cannot provide mobility unless it is properly attached to the bone structure. Cartilage is vital for joint health and mobility and is always found at the ends of articulating joints. It is important that engineered AC tissue have a proper interface with the articulating bone to maintain its protective properties. With these examples in mind, it is crucial to always consider how an engineered device will interact with adjacent tissues, and ensure that the interface between different tissues is comparable to native tissues. Relationships between common tissue interfaces that are being investigated in current research can be seen in Figure 13.7. Learning how to create a synchronous unit of different types of tissues is the next phase in the field of TE (Spalazzi et al., 2008).

A very common defect that occurs in the human body is osteochondral defect, which damages both cartilage and subchondral bone (Gadjanski and Vunjak-Novakovic, 2015). Osteochondral defects have limited natural healing ability due to the lack of communication between cartilage and bone as well as the avascular nature of the cartilage tissue. If not treated, the wound may cause significant mobility impairment and decrease in the patient's overall quality of life. In cases where an implant or a tissue-engineered device is needed to repair bone, it is essential that an integrated system between cartilage and bone is created in order to repair the damaged area to the fullest extent. Advances in TE methods open up new options for treating osteochondral and other defects. The various components of the system include cells, the supporting scaffold, and the bioreactor itself to support and maintain proper cellular differentiation and proliferation. Regardless of the technique, the main methodology of developing a functioning cartilage to bone interface is to be able to recreate key aspects of the *in vivo* development through *in vitro* techniques using an approach called biomimetic TE (Gadjanski and Vunjak-Novakovic, 2015). The environment is controlled to cue cells to develop as desired while creating stratification of tissue types through a gradient of applied growth factors and the surrounding scaffold or environment. The scaffold material would degrade over time and foster tissue development in its place (Dua et al., 2014).

In one particular study, hydroxyapatite nanoparticles were used to promote tissue development at a bone–cartilage interface that was seeded using bone marrow stem cells. The nanoparticles were used to enhance tissue attachment of cartilage tissue developed using a hydrogel to bone tissue developed using an agar scaffold (Dua et al., 2014). After the constructs were developed, it was found that the hydroxyapatite-containing constructs exhibited a greater amount of calcium phosphate, an important indicator of bone growth, than constructs without hydroxyapatite. The use of hydroxyapatite also increased the interfacial shear stress by about 62% between the two tissues (Dua et al., 2014). This happened as early as 7 days after the start of culture and was observed throughout the entire 28 days of the experiment. Thus, the incorporation of hydroxyapatite helps to maintain the interface between developing cartilage and bone tissue during the early stages of maturation when it is most needed. Tissue development occurs naturally after that point with increased shear strength as a result. The use of hydroxyapatite also correlated with an increased amount of alkaline phosphatase activity in the transition zone, an important

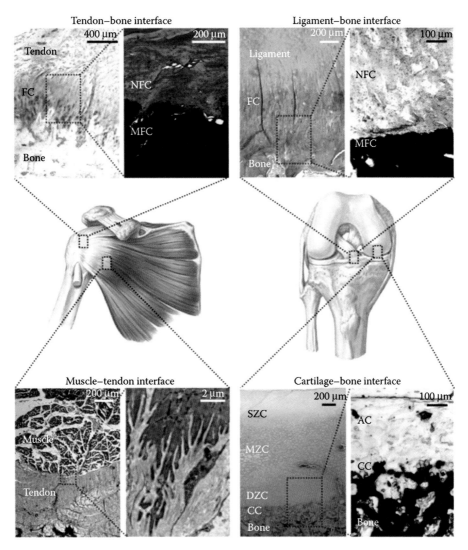

FIGURE 13.7
Common orthopedic tissue–tissue interfaces. Ligaments, such as the ACL in the knee and tendons, such as the supraspinatus tendon in the shoulder connect to bone via an FC transition, which can be further subdivided into non-mineralized (NFC) and mineralized (MFC) regions. The muscle–tendon junction (Modified Goldner's Masson Trichrome) consists of an interdigitating band of connective tissue. AC, which can be subdivided into surface (SZC), middle (MZC), and deep (DZC) zones, connects to subchondral bone via a transitional calcified cartilage region.

indicator of functioning osteoblasts migrating into the zone. Increased calcium phosphate ECM deposits from functioning osteoblasts in the transition zone were observed when hydroxyapatite nanoparticles were used. The interface strength between bone and cartilage was thus increased and able to handle a greater shear stress load than without.

To help address the issue of developing tissues next to each other, multiphasic scaffolds are being developed. It is very difficult to accurately recreate a heterogeneous network of tissues while using a homogenous scaffold because each type of tissue requires a specific set of conditions to optimally grow (Han et al., 2010). By using multiphasic scaffolds, it is

possible to provide the optimal environments to different tissues and create a heterogeneous transition that allows different native tissues to attach to each other. Bone tissue can
be grown attached to cartilage tissue, or ligament tissue can be grown attached to bone tissue. Devices based on this theory recognize the need to integrate varying tissues together
as they are in the human body and allow for more complex interfaces between tissues than
homogenous devices can achieve (Kon et al., 2010).

One study that was done demonstrated that multiphasic cartilage to bone scaffold units
can be made using differing ratios of type 1 collagen and magnesium–hydroxyapatite. The
scaffold is designed as a porous 3D trilayer composite with different phases to accommodate a transition of different tissue types. Each section was separately synthesized using
collagen taken from an atelocollagen solution for the mineralized end and a type 1 collagen solution for the non-mineralized end. The collagen fibers were further treated with
H_3PO_4. The mineralized gradient was created by increasing concentrations of $Ca(OH)_2$
and $MgCl_2$ to nucleate hydroxyapatite nanoparticles into the collagen fibers. The ratios are
altered along the length of the scaffold depending on the desired tissue type, where one
end was composed of pure type 1 collagen while the other end was composed of 70% magnesium–hydroxyapatite (Kon et al., 2010). What resulted was a solid integration between
cartilage and bone that included hyaline-like cartilage and structured bone tissue located
next to the native bone and cartilage tissues. The grafts showed complete resorption of the
implanted materials and no inflammatory reactions were observed in the experimental
sites. Histological comparisons to untreated control sites all showed a marked increase of
reconstructed tissue that anchored well to the adjacent tissue while keeping bone tissue
growth out of the upper cartilaginous layer, as desired.

Multiphasic scaffolds are also used in the repair of ligament tissue. Ligaments are an
important component to the musculoskeletal system that is often injured, the anterior cruciate ligament (ACL) being a well-known example of this. Homogenous grafts have been
usually used to replace damaged ligaments but they do not address how to repair the
functional soft-hard tissue unit of the ligament (Qu et al., 2015). The functional unit of a
ligament is a multi-tissue group that consists of interface areas between the ligament and
the bone tissue. However, what does form when a graft is used is a disorganized mass of
fibrovascular tissue that provides a weak attachment to the bone and lowers the expected
patient outcomes and mobility (Qu et al., 2015). Mechanically and biologically competent
scaffolds can be used in place of a ligament to heal an injury. Multiphasic scaffolds made
using integrated tissue types have been made using materials including polylactide fibers
in polymethyl methacrylate plugs and braided polylactide-co-glycolide microfibers posi-
tioned at the ends of the graft to encourage bone development there (Cooper et al., 2005).

It is possible to release growth factors like basic fibroblast growth factor (bFGF) by introducing them through a multiphase construct made from a polylactide acid and collagen
scaffold with gelatin hydrogels on the periphery that released fibroblast growth factors
over time (Kimura et al., 2008). bFGF is a common growth factor used to promote the
regeneration of a wide variety of tissues including ligaments, bone, and skin. The hydrogels were formed using mixes of glutaraldehyde and gelatin left to crosslink, after which
the resulting sheet was treated with glycine aqueous solution preventing any further
reactions. The bFGF was incorporated into the hydrogel through immersion in solution.
Polylactide acid scaffolds were created by weaving strands together to form plain braids,
around which was wrapped a collagen membrane reinforced with polylactide acid microspheres for mechanical strength. These structures were then combined with the gelatin
hydrogel and then implanted as a ligament transplant. Compared to control samples,
bFGF release systems demonstrated significant increases of over 15–20 N in failure load

and 5–10 N/mm in stiffness compared to the control groups (Thangarajah et al., 2015). The amount of collagen produced in the ligament scaffold site was also increased compared to the control groups.

The fibrocartilaginous (FC) interface between ligament and bone presents a challenge because, although it is optimized to handle the tensile and compressive loading stresses and is critical for this function, it is not consistently uniform throughout the entire interface (Qu et al., 2015). The elastic modulus of bone is greater than that of a ligament, so the transition of mechanical properties inducted through the fibrocartilage regions of the ligament is crucial for shielding the soft tissues from damage at high stresses and strains and is another reason why interface design is crucial to any successful tissue-engineered device. Multiphasic designs were created using polylactide-glycolic acid (Spalazzi et al., 2008) or poly-e-caprolactone (Qu et al., 2015) that fostered the formation of stratified tissue types, which exhibited graded mechanical properties along its entire length. The designs include distinct yet continuous segments that are optimized for tissue and cell types specific to each region of the interface tissue. For the interface between ligament and bone, the segment furthest away from the point of attachment to bone consists of fibroblasts used for soft tissue formation to adhere to muscle tissue. The next closest segment is designed for fibrochondrocytes and fibrocartilage formation, while the segment attaching the tissue unit to the host bone is optimized for osteoblast and bone tissue formation (Jung et al., 2009). The resulting stratified tissue scaffold demonstrated superior mechanical properties over single phasic designs and allow for free spatial control over the cellular construct and promote regeneration of a fully functional tissue transition. The design successfully imitates an actual ligament–bone interface unit with the scaffold tissue nearest the bone displaying the highest elastic modulus and yield strength (Qu et al., 2015).

One such scaffold for ligament repair is the L-C Ligament Created by Soft Tissue Regeneration Inc. This scaffold is made of PLLA and functions to regenerate and repair torn ligament tissue, primarily the ACL. The ACL is fibrous rope stabilizing the posterior end of the femur base to the anterior portion of the tibial head. This vital structure keeps the tibia from pushing forward during retraction of the knee. In times of intense physical activity, abrupt movements can damage this structure causing extreme pain, loss of knee stabilization, and limited range of motion. Injuries as such are categorized by degree of ligament tear notated as grade 1, 2, or 3 sprains; in which a grade 1 strain is mildly damaged ligament and a grade 3 strain being a completely torn ligament. Common treatment options include ACL reconstruction with an autograft; controversy surrounds the use of allografts for ACL repair due to the high risk of disease transmission and graft rejection. Therefore, synthetic grafts such as the L-C ligament hopes to confront these problems while reducing operating time and eliminating donor site morbidity (Freeman et al., 2007). The L-C ligament uses a braided rope structure that mimics the biomechanical behaviors as native ACL tissue. The twisting of the scaffold strands affords it a greater strength and abrasion resistance than less intertwined structures (Freeman et al., 2007). Clinical trials are currently being conducted in Europe, and due to success in small studies, a new 60 patient randomized trial has already begun.

13.6 Skin

Skin is the body's largest organ, covering every external facet of the human body and has many functions, both protective and cosmetic. It is vital as the first line of defense against antigens, toxins, and other factors that could harm the tissues beneath. Wounds to the skin can be categorized into different groups based on depth including epidermal, partial thickness, deep partial thickness, and full thickness. The severity of the wounds also strongly impacts the amount of scar tissue that is created during the healing process. Thus, there are various methods that have been or are being developed that repair and functionalize skin after damage has been caused. These methods include different compounds and materials to encourage and facilitate skin regeneration, including collagen, human amniotic membrane, and skin grafts, among others. When skin damage is extensive, as happens during second and third degree burns, skin substitute devices may be used. Burns of these calibers damage the dermal and hypodermal layers of the skin, respectively. The injuries can cause loss of fluids, loss of temperature control, pain, immunodepression, bacterial infection, and even permanent disability (Varkey et al., 2015). Skin substitutes provide the same protective benefits as typical skin including barrier function, hydration, and minimal inflammatory response, and toxicity (Arasteh et al., 2015). In addition, an ideal skin substitute should provide adequate mechanical compatibility and degradability to avoid disrupting the surrounding wound as well as being able to mimic the ECM, which is vital for cell migration, proliferation, differentiation, and signaling (Arasteh et al., 2015). The mechanical properties of a skin repair device are important because mechanical stresses are a major signaling factor for cell differentiation while the stiffness of a device determines how well it is able to withstand stresses while the new tissue is developing (Arasteh et al., 2015).

The current gold standard for major skin repair is to use skin grafts. The effectiveness of this is due to the presence of vital cells, ECM, and regenerative and healing factors they naturally provide (Arasteh et al., 2015). However, this method is limited in its use by limited donor sites, donor site scarring, risk of infection, and potential pain (Chandika et al., 2015). As a result, research is constantly being done to discover new ways for skin to be remade in an effort to circumvent the limitations encountered by skin grafting.

One particular method for tissue-engineered skin is effective as a single stage treatment for defects like burns and ulcers. This method uses a modification of porous scaffolds created using collagen and glycosaminoglycans, which are used to make human skin equivalents (HSEs) that included epidermal cells to mimic native skin. A benefit to this method is that the scaffolds used in the making of the HSEs are made under quality standards that allow for reliable replication and integration into the wound area (Paul et al., 2015). The scaffolds allow for host cell infiltration and vascularization and are also resistant to degradation by wound collagenases. However, using collagen scaffolds by themselves are not enough due to their failure to provide an effective surface for anchoring keratinocytes for skin epidermization as well as their often excessive porosity. These problems have been circumvented using clotted human plasma to fill in excessive porosities while pre-seeded fibroblasts. Human plasma is a substance rich in cytokines and growth factors that also functions as a carrier for keratinocytes. Flooding a skin scaffold with human plasma indicated reduced pore sizes and created a smooth surface conductive toward keratinocyte infiltration and adhesion (Paul et al., 2015). This engineered epidermis is then able to mesh well and interface with the surrounding native epidermis. Using scaffolds of this nature reduces the need for donor skin grafts while also ensuring that the engineered epidermis interfaces well with native epidermis, all of which promotes a shorter recovery time for the patient.

Collagen is a major component of skin ECM, so finding methods for utilizing its properties in skin regeneration has been a target of many researchers in developing new TE applications for skin. Fish collagen has been used as an excellent alternative to bovine and porcine collagen due to its more similar characteristics to human collagen as well as having no risk of disease transmission compared to other sources of collagen (Chandika et al., 2015). It has to be modified by cross-linking and combining it with various polymers to prevent the collagen from degrading too quickly. An example of this includes a cross-linking of collagen with sodium alginate and chitooligosaccharides. Alginate occurs naturally in seaweed and provides a scaffold with increased toughness and stiffness. It also has the benefit of stimulating macrophages, resulting in an increase in the level of inflammatory cytokines including tumor necrosis factor and α-interleukin-6, both of which are beneficial for the healing process. The porous scaffold structure that was created using these materials was shown to be an effective means of mimicking the required physical, mechanical, and biological properties of native skin tissue (Chandika et al., 2015). Cell adhesion was improved with the addition of the chitooligosaccharides and tissue development was successfully fostered by the combined effects of these materials used in the scaffold.

The use of bilayer scaffolds in skin regeneration has been shown to be similar to native skin with both dermal and epidermal components in their structure (Varkey et al., 2015). This type of scaffold was further modified using human amniotic membrane, which has been beneficial for healing large ulcers and combined with fibroin to create a bilayer scaffold that proved to enhance the viability of the cells implanted into them. Amniotic membrane is composed of a monolayer of epithelial cells projected from a basement membrane full of collagen, fibronectin, and laminin (Arasteh et al., 2015). The basement membrane acts as a mechanical support that promotes epithelium cell proliferation and maturation as well as inhibiting cell apoptosis. In addition to being readily available, the properties of amniotic membrane make it a unique material for use in skin-regeneration applications. Using these properties, the bilayer scaffold was successful in improving the integration of cultured cells with the scaffold matrix and the surrounding tissue and has great promise in future applications.

Skin grafts are currently used in the clinical setting to treat disorders associated with many diseases. One such disorder is diabetes-related foot ulcers; it is a growing problem in the United States affecting more than 5 million Americans. Diabetic foot ulcers are the leading cause of hospitalization among individuals suffering with diabetes and accounts for 85% of lower extremity amputations. This is due to the slow healing rate and failure of current treatment methods. Currently, treatment methods involve application of moist dressings and infection control; these methods require many months of treatment. In an effort to streamline the healing process, researchers have investigated different attributes of native skin to create a skin graft that augments the healing process. Circulating the market are two FDA-approved bioengineered skin substitutes named Apligraf and Dermagraft. Both consist of human fibroblast-derived cells cultivated onto a scaffold. Apligraf uses a bovine type I collagen matrix as a base, which Dermagraft uses as a bioresorbable polyglactin mesh. They specifically treat chronic diabetic foot ulcers by producing cytokines and growth factors necessary for assisting the patient's own epithelial cells in regenerating the lesion area faster and with less scar tissue. Evaluations of both scaffolds were conducted via randomized clinical studies, which tested each dermal implantation against the current gold standard procedures. Results showed that the implants significantly healed more foot ulcers than the gold standard. No adverse effects were noted when using the implants, and both have proven to be a safe and effective solution to chronic diabetic foot ulcers (Marston et al., 2003; Zelen et al., 2014). A formal comparison of Apligraf versus Dermagraft in treating diabetic foot ulcers (DFUs) has not been conducted but may benefit physicians deciding which treatment to use. Other devices currently in the market can be seen in Table 13.8.

TABLE 13.8

List of Commercially Available Skin Substitutes on the Market

Skin Substitute	Composition	Comments
Biobrane™	Outer epidermal analog—ultrathin silicone film; inner dermal analog—3D nylon filament with type I collagen peptides	Temporary wound dressing that is removed when wound is healed or when autograft skin is available
TransCyte™	Nylon mesh seeded with neonatal human foreskin fibroblasts that are destroyed before grafting	Temporary wound dressing upon which autografts are placed
Integra™	Dermal analog—bovine collagen and chondroitin-6-sulfate glycosaminoglycan; epidermal analog—silicone polymer	Silicone layer is removed upon vascularization of dermis, and replaced by a thin layer of autograft
Alloderm™	Human allograft skin that has been screened for transmissible pathogens, with all epidermal components and dermal cells removed	Grafted like dermal autograft and covered with a thin autograft
Dermagraft™	Bioabsorbable polygalactin mesh matrix seeded with human neonatal fibroblasts and cryopreserved	Matrix facilitates reepithelialization by the patient's own keratinocytes
Apligraf™	Bovine collagen gel seeded with neonatal foreskin fibroblasts and keratinocytes	Wound dressing with two different cell types
OrCel™	Type I collagen matrix seeded with neonatal foreskin fibroblasts and keratinocytes	
Epicel™	Sheets of autologous keratinocytes attached to petrolatum gauze support	Wound dressing with autologous cells
StrataGraft™	Full thickness skin substitute with dermal and fully differentiated epidermal layers	Made with naturally immortalized NIKS® keratinocyte cell line; contains two different cell types
Tiscover™ (A-Skin)	Autologous full thickness cultured skin for healing of chronic, therapy resistant wounds	Contains two different cell types
Permaderm™	Autologous tissue-engineered skin consisting of epidermal and dermal cells	Contains two different cell types
denovoDerm™	Autologous dermal substitute	To be used in combination with split-thickness skin grafts
denovoSkin™	Autologous full thickness substitute consisting of dermal and epidermal layers	Contains two different cell types

13.7 Nerve

The peripheral nervous system (PNS) is a network of collagenous bundles outside the central nervous system (CNS), comprising the brain and spinal cord, which conduct sensory and motor communication to and from the CNS. Neurons are the functional unit of the vast network; they consist of dendrites that carry electrical impulses to the cell body, and a long axon that transfers the impulse toward the synaptic cleft, via action potentials. The microanatomy of nerves is a complex hierarchy of structures in which individual myelinated and unmyelinated axons or nerve fibers covered in an endoneurial sheath containing capillaries and collagen fibers assume a bundled arrangement of fascicles encased by a perineurial sheath. Individual nerve fascicles are grouped together and collectively encased by another connective tissue layer called the epineurium that includes types I and III collagen fibrils and elastic fibers (Topp and Boyd, 2006). The PNS

TABLE 13.9

Nerve Injury Classification in Increasing Severity

Grade	Name	Features
Type 1	Neuropraxia	Damage to local myelin only
Type 2	Axonotmesis	Division of intraneural axons only
Type 3	Axonotmesis	Division of axons and endoneurium
Type 4	Axonotmesis	Division of axons, endo-, and perineurium
Type 5	Neurotmesis	Complete division of all elements including epineurium
Type 6	Mixed	Combination of types 2–4

Source: Reprinted from Grinsell, D. and Keating, C.P. 2014. *BioMed Res Int.*, vol. 2014. With permissions from Hindawi.

is subdivided into sensory, motor, and mixed functions that allow for complex movements and sensory behaviors.

Twenty million Americans suffer from peripheral nerve injury (PNI) caused by trauma and medical disorders (Lundborg, 2003). Nerve injuries result in approximately $150 billion spent in annual healthcare dollars in the United States (Taylor et al., 2008). These injuries are classified in Table 13.9 and can lead to sensory and motor functional defects, which can result in paralysis of the affected limb or neuropathic pain. Therefore, the goal of nerve repair is to reinnervate the target organs with minimal loss of sensory and motor fibers, while minimizing time of rejuvenation. Upon PNI, axons degenerate proximally as well as distally. Distal to the injury zone, Wallerian degeneration is initiated as a measure to alleviate abnormal axon regeneration, starting with axonal breakdown. Macrophages are recruited to the area and axonal and myelin debris are phagocytosed, leading to myelin tube collapse. Regeneration at the proximal stump begins within 24–48 h, as a growth cone protrudes from the axonal stump and grows in a direct path to the target organ (Griffin et al., 2013). However, axonal regeneration is an extremely slow process that occurs at a rate of approximately 1 mm/day, requiring at least 12–18 months for muscle reinnervation and initial functional recovery (Pfister et al., 2011). In the case of a critical-sized nerve defect, where the lesion extends too far away from the proximal end of the intact axon, regeneration to the distal stump is vitally slow and there is a great risk of traumatic neuroma formation, which not only renders the neuron ineffective, but is often very painful (Grinsell and Keating, 2014).

Surgical intervention of nerve defects currently utilizes autograft/allograft nerve graft transplantation therapy as the gold standard technique for a nerve gap greater than 3 cm, as end-to-end suture cannot adequately repair the injury with minimal tension (Scherman et al., 2004). Nerve grafts are characterized as single, cable, trunk, interfascicular, or vascularized. Single graft conjoins nerve gaps with a segment of a donor nerve with similar diameter while cable grafts are used to span between large diameter nerves. Trunk grafts use a donor segment from a sensory nerve to repair gaps in a proximal nerve, which differs from the interfascicular nerve graft that interposes groups of fascicles between the damaged nerve and the graft itself. Vascularized nerve grafts consist of both the donor nerve with its accompanying vasculature to avoid the initial period of ischemia postsurgical repair (Grinsell and Keating, 2014). The autograph technique utilizes a patient's superficial nerve such as the sural or superficial radial nerve and repurposes them as a graft to connect the severed ends (Lundborg, 2003). For more extensive injuries, allograft techniques offer a greater amount of nerve tissue; utilizing immunosuppressed cadaveric and animal nerve graphs to restore nerve function (Ghasemi-Mobarakeh et al., 2011; Siemionow and Sonmez, 2007).

Clinically, these autografts have several disadvantages, including multiple surgical steps, sensory loss at the donor site, and toxicity of immunosuppression. For allografts, host acceptance and possibility of disease transmission are limiting factors (Siemionow and Sonmez, 2007). Therefore, it would be extremely beneficial to create a bioengineered solution that matches or surpasses the performance of autograft/allograft (Pfister et al., 2011; Siemionow and Sonmez, 2007). Several synthetic and biologically derived porous structures have been used successfully as nerve growth conduits (NGCs) (Jiang et al., 2010; Johnson and Soucacos, 2008; Kim et al., 1998). However, the rate of successful nerve regeneration has been far lower than the "gold standard" autografts (Grinsell and Keating, 2014). Briefly, we will focus on the use of tissue-engineered products Neurolac® and *Avance*® nerve graft as alternative approaches to promote nerve regeneration. To adequately assess the effectiveness of a NGC, it is important to observe its electrical conductivity, biodegradability, biocompatibility, and functionality (Balint et al., 2014).

Neurolac, a nerve guide scaffold created by Polyganics B.V. (Groningen, The Netherlands) is composed of poly(dl-lactide-ε-caprolactone), a copolymer of lactic acid and caprolactone monomers. The polymer was prepared by ring-opening polymerization of lactide with ε-caprolactone using stannous octoate (Sn(Oct)2) as a catalyst. The nerve guides were manufactured by dipcoating from a chloroform solution (Meek and Den Dunnen, 2009). They have customized dimensions for pore size, length, internal diameter, and wall thickness. A randomized, multicenter clinical investigation found that the PCL component yields many adventitious properties compared to competing scaffolds including a decrease in toxic acidic degradation products and a transparent conduit for ease of surgical placement. The scaffold also degrades within 1 year, allowing adequate time for nerve tissue regeneration (Bertleff et al., 2005). An alternate study conducted between 2007 and 2009 involved 28 nerve lesions from 23 patients who constituted a population aged 39.35 years in average. Subjective results revealed mean pain score was 2.17/10 with range of 0–8. Cold intolerance was observed in 15 patients out of 23, and mean Quick DASH (Disabilities of the arm, shoulder, and hand in which 0—no disability and 100—extreme disability) score was 35.37/100 with range of 2.27–79.55. As for objective results, mean grip strength was 64.62% of contralateral side with range 0–130 (Chiriac et al., 2012). Investigators observed eight complications of the Neurolac™ device, being two fistulizations close to a joint and a neuroma.

Avance Nerve Graft, AxoGen®, Inc. is a commercially available nerve allograft, since 2007. The tissue is uniquely sterilized and detergent processed to decellularize the material while retaining the physical microstructures including endoneurial tubes, basal lamina, and laminin; along with vital protein elements found in native nerve tissue (Brooks et al., 2012; Lundborg, 2003). These characteristics facilitate in axonal regeneration. A multisite clinical study evaluating the safety and efficacy of the *Avance* nerve graft enrolled 108 subjects who collectively contributed with 68 injuries consisting of (45 sensory, 15 mixed, and 8 motor nerves). With the majority of repairs being digital nerves of the hand, those that qualified were assessed via quantitative and qualitative measures. These included a Medical Research Council grading system (MRCC) and subjective measurements of pain and function assessments (Brooks et al., 2012). Of all 108 patients treated, only 59 provided sufficient follow-up assessments, and of those 89.5% reported positive results. The MRCC assessed meaningful recovery by nerve type, gap length, time to repair, age, and mechanism of injury. The criteria for determining full return of motor or sensory recovery was to obtain a value of M3/S3 or greater according to quantitative data. 87.3% of repairs reported a return of motor and sensory function, while nerve gaps ranging from 5 to 50 mm all reported full to satisfactory recovery of function. Time of recovery was divided into three groups: acute (3 weeks after repair), delayed (3 weeks to 3 months), and chronic (post 3 months); respectively, meaningful recovery was rated at 87%, 100%, and 83%. In the age assessment, young, middle, and older subgroups, respectively, demonstrated 100%, 88%, and 93% of meaningful recovery. All injures were isolated to the upper extremities and consisted of lacerations, complex reconstructions, and neuroma; 89%, 88%, and 82%, respectively, exhibited meaningful recovery (Brooks et al., 2012). This clinical analysis proved that the *Avance* biomechanical conduit compares favorably to the gold standard nerve autograph and is both efficacious and safe.

PNI is a debilitating process that requires early attention to prevent demyelination (neuropraxia) and/or axonal degeneration. Both complicate the nerve repair cascade and lead to impaired electrical conduction, deficits of sensory and mechanical function, and pain. Autologous nerve grafts are considered a gold standard for bridging nerve gaps; however, numerous tissue-engineered nerve grafts are currently being used as an alternative. The poly(dl-lactide-ε-caprolactone) Neurolac yielded positive results during clinical trials, and its transparency, biodegradability, and flexibility makes it an adventitious option. However, serious side effects and high cost of the scaffold may overshadow Neurolac's benefits hinder neurosurgeons from utilizing the synthetic nerve guide scaffold. The decellularized allograft *Avance* has shown to provide safe and effective nerve regeneration through many randomized clinical studies. The allograft provided functional recovery in sensory, mixed, and motor nerve injuries in gaps up to 50 mm. No complications were noted in patients treated with *Avance*.

All considered, further research in the field of tissue-engineered nerve scaffold is necessary to change the culture of current operational trends. The trend of research in regards to nerve regeneration is currently focused on utilizing conductive polymer matrices and conduits. Taking advantage of the electrical nature of neurons and the nervous system, electrically conductive polymers such as polyaniline, polypyrrole, and poly(3,4-ethylenedioxythiophene) are being investigated for use as NGCs. Electrically conducting polymers as NGCs could lead to more efficient axonal outgrowth and muscle reinnervation. Next-generation studies could focus on the use of ionically conducting polymers for greater electrical conductivity in physiological environments. Ionically conducting polymers could overcome the shortcomings of inconsistent conduction of electrically conducting polymers, as well as address issues with polymer biodegradability (James et al., 2014; Anderson et al., 2015; Shelke et al., 2016). Such advanced, next-generation research efforts could lead to faster, more effective, regeneration of neural tissue, particularly effective for segmental nerve defects resulting from severe PNI.

13.8 Conclusions

Tissue-engineered devices are viable methods for regeneration and repair of native tissue defects. Their properties include suitable biocompatibility and native responses that allow the tissue-engineered device to heal defects. Extensive research has been conducted on the science behind these devices over the past couple of decades and continues to be improved on to this day. New devices are being created that use various cost-effective polymers and natural materials that foster a suitable environment for new tissue growth and development. Concepts for devices are even further improved through surface modification that allows for even greater biocompatibility and cellular attachment. In addition, tissue-engineered devices are able to work with a wide range of native tissue types in the human body and thus can have near boundless capability in what physicians can work with. Products are able to be applied for a wide variety of tissue types, including bone, ligaments, nerves, and skin. These tissue-engineered devices can be used to great benefit in treating future patients for a large variety of both chronic and acute tissue defects and the use of which will improve the lives of patients for years to come.

Acknowledgments

The authors gratefully acknowledge funding from the Connecticut Regenerative Medicine Research Fund (Grant number: 15-RMB-UCHC-08), National Science Foundation Award (Grant numbers: IIP-1311907, IIP-1355327, EFRI-1332329), and Department of Defense (Grant number: OR120140). The Raymond and Beverly Sackler Center for Biomedical, Biological, Physical and Engineering Sciences.

References

Adam, C., Eckstein, F., Milz, S., Schulte, E., Becker, C., Putz, R. 1998. The distribution of cartilage thickness in the knee-joints of old-aged individuals—Measurement by A-mode ultrasound. *Clin Biomech.* 13: 1–10.

Anderson, M., Shelke, N.B., Manoukian, O., Yu, X., McCullough, L., Kumbar, S.G. 2015. Peripheral nerve regeneration strategies: Electrically stimulating polymer based nerve growth conduits. *Crit Rev Biomed Eng.* 43(2–3): 131–159.

Antonova, E., Le, T.K., Burge, R., Mershon, J.E. 2013. Tibia shaft fractures: Costly burden of non-unions. *BMC Musculoskelet Disord.* 14: 42.

Arasteh, S., Kazemnejad, S., Khanjani, S., Heidari-Vala, H., Akhondi, M.M., Mobini, S. 2015. Fabrication and characterization of nano-fibrous bilayer composite for skin regeneration application. *Methods.* pii: S1046–2023(15)30060–8.

Badhe, S.P., Lawrence, T.M., Smith, F.D., Lunn, P.G. 2008. An assessment of porcine dermal xenograft as an augmentation graft in the treatment of extensive rotator cuff tears. *J Shoulder Elbow Surg.* 17: 35S–39S.

Balint, R., Cassidy, N.J., Cartmell, S.H. 2014. Conductive polymers: Towards a smart biomaterial for tissue engineering. *Acta Biomater.* 10: 2341–53.

Barber, F.A., Burns, J.P., Deutsch, A., Labbe, M.R., Litchfield, R.B. 2012. A prospective, randomized evaluation of acellular human dermal matrix augmentation for arthroscopic rotator cuff repair. *Arthroscopy.* 28: 8–15.

Berta, A., Duska, Z., Tóth, F., Hangody, L. 2015. Clinical experiences with cartilage repair techniques: Outcomes, indications, contraindications and rehabilitation. *Jt Dis Relat Surg.* 26: 84.

Bertleff, M.J., Meek, M.F., Nicolai, J.P. 2005. A prospective clinical evaluation of biodegradable Neurolac nerve guides for sensory nerve repair in the hand. *J Hand Surg Am.* 30: 513–8.

Bishop, G.B., Einhorn, T.A. 2007. Current and future clinical applications of bone morphogenetic proteins in orthopaedic trauma surgery. *Int Orthop.* 31: 721–7.

Bond, J.L., Dopirak, R.M., Higgins, J., Burns, J., Snyder, S.J. 2008. Arthroscopic replacement of massive, irreparable rotator cuff tears using a GraftJacket allograft: Technique and preliminary results. *Arthroscopy.* 24: 403–9.

Boskey, A.L., Coleman, R. 2010. Aging and bone. *J Dent Res.* 89: 1333–48.

Brooks, D.N., Weber, R.V., Chao, J.D., Rinker, B.D., Zoldos, J., Robichaux, M.R. 2012. Processed nerve allografts for peripheral nerve reconstruction: A multicenter study of utilization and outcomes in sensory, mixed, and motor nerve reconstructions. *Microsurgery.* 32: 1–14.

Burke, J.F., Yannas, I.V., Quinby, W.C. Jr., Bondoc, C.C., Jung, W.K. 1981. Successful use of a physiologically acceptable artificial skin in the treatment of extensive burn injury. *Ann Surg.* 194: 413–28.

Burkus, J.K., Transfeldt, E.E., Kitchel, S.H., Watkins, R.G., Balderston, R.A. 2002. Clinical and radiographic outcomes of anterior lumbar interbody fusion using recombinant human bone morphogenetic protein-2. *Spine.* 27: 2396–408.

Calori, G.M., Tagliabue, L., Gala, L., d'Imporzano, M., Peretti, G., Albisetti, W. 2008. Application of rhBMP-7 and platelet-rich plasma in the treatment of long bone non-unions: A prospective randomised clinical study on 120 patients. *Injury* 39(12): 1391–402.

Cecchi, S., Bennet, S., Arora, M. 2016. Bone morphogenetic protein-7: Review of signalling and efficacy in fracture healing. *J Orthop Translat.* 4: 28–34.

Chandika, P., Ko, S.-C., Oh, G.-W., Heo, S.-Y., Nguyen, V.-T., Jeon, Y.-J. et al. 2015. Fish collagen/alginate/chitooligosaccharides integrated scaffold for skin tissue regeneration application. *Int J Biol Macromol.* 81: 504–13.

Chiriac, S., Facca, S., Diaconu, M., Gouzou, S., Liverneaux, P. 2012. Experience of using the bioresorbable copolyester poly(DL-lactide-epsilon-caprolactone) nerve conduit guide Neurolac for nerve repair in peripheral nerve defects: Report on a series of 28 lesions. *J Hand Surg Eur.* 37: 342–9.

Ciampi, P., Scotti, C., Nonis, A., Vitali, M., Di Serio, C., Peretti, G.M. 2014. The benefit of synthetic versus biological patch augmentation in the repair of posterosuperior massive rotator cuff tears: A 3-year follow-up study. *Am J Sports Med.* 42: 1169–75.

Ciardelli, G., Chiono, V., Vozzi, G., Pracella, M., Ahluwalia, A., Barbani, N. 2005. Blends of poly-(εε-caprolactone) and polysaccharides in tissue engineering applications. *Biomacromolecules.* 6: 1961–76.

Clarke, B. 2008. Normal bone anatomy and physiology. *Clin J Am Soc Nephrol.* 3: S131–9.

Colvin, A.C., Egorova, N., Harrison, A.K., Moskowitz, A., Flatow, E.L. 2012. National trends in rotator cuff repair. *J Bone Joint Surg Am.* 94: 227–33.

Cooper, J.A., Lu, H.H., Ko, F.K., Freeman, J.W., Laurencin, C.T. 2005. Fiber-based tissue-engineered scaffold for ligament replacement: Design considerations and *in vitro* evaluation. *Biomaterials.* 26: 1523–32.

Crawford, D.C., DeBerardino, T.M., Williams, R.J. 2012. NeoCart, an autologous cartilage tissue implant, compared with microfracture for treatment of distal femoral cartilage lesions. *J Bone Joint Surg Br.* 94: 979–89.

Dahabreh, Z., Calori, G.M., Kanakaris, N.K., Nikolaou, V.S., Giannoudis, P.V. 2009. A cost analysis of treatment of tibial fracture nonunion by bone grafting or bone morphogenetic protein-7. *Int Orthop.* 33: 1407–14.

De Long, W.G. Jr., Einhorn, T.A., Koval, K., McKee, M., Smith, W., Sanders, R., Watson, T.W.G. 2007. Bone grafts and bone graft substitutes in orthopaedic trauma surgery: A critical analysis. *J Bone Joint Surg.* 89: 649–58.

Derwin, K.A., Baker, A.R., Spragg, R.K., Leigh, D.R., Iannotti, J.P. 2006. Commercial extracellular matrix scaffolds for rotator cuff tendon repair. Biomechanical, biochemical, and cellular properties. *J Bone Joint Surg Am.* 88: 2665–72.

Derwin, K.A., Codsi, M.J., Milks, R.A., Baker, A.R., McCarron, J.A., Iannotti, J.P. 2009. Rotator cuff repair augmentation in a canine model with use of a woven poly-L-lactide device. *J Bone Joint Surg Am.* 91: 1159–71.

Desai, B.M. 2007. Osteobiologics. *Am J Orthop.* 36: 8–11.

Desmyter, S., Goubau, Y., Benahmed, N., Wever, A., Verdonk, R. 2008. The role of Bone Morphogenetic Protein-7 (Osteogenic Protein-1 (R)) in the treatment of tibial fracture non-unions an overview of the use in Belgium. *Acta Orthopædica Belgica* 74(4): 534.

Dimitriou, R., Tsiridis, E., Giannoudis, P.V. 2005. Current concepts of molecular aspects of bone healing. *Injury* 36(12): 1392–1404.

Dua, R., Centeno, J., Ramaswamy, S. 2014. Augmentation of engineered cartilage to bone integration using hydroxyapatite. *J Biomed Mater Res B Appl Biomater*. 102: 922–32.

Flood, J. 2010. The role of acetaminophen in the treatment of osteoarthritis. *Am J Manag Care*. 16: S48–54.

Freeman, J.W., Woods, M.D., Laurencin, C.T. 2007. Tissue engineering of the anterior cruciate ligament using a braid–twist scaffold design. *J Biomech*. 40: 2029–36.

Friedlaender, G.E., Perry, C.R., Cole, J.D., Cook, S.D., Cierny, G., Muschler, G.F., Zych, G.A., Calhoun, J.H., LaForte, A.J., Yin, S. 2001. Osteogenic protein-1 (bone morphogenetic protein-7) in the treatment of tibial nonunions. *J Bone Joint Surg Am*. 83-A(Suppl 1): S151–8.

Gadjanski, I., Vunjak-Novakovic, G. 2015. Challenges in engineering osteochondral tissue grafts with hierarchical structures. *Expert Opin Biol Ther*. 15: 1583–99.

Garrison, K.R., Donell, S., Ryder, J., Shemilt, I., Mugford, M., Harvey, I., Song, F. 2007. Clinical effectiveness and cost-effectiveness of bone morphogenetic proteins in the non-healing of fractures and spinal fusion: A systematic review. *Technol Assess*. 11: 1–150.

Ghasemi-Mobarakeh, L., Prabhakaran, M.P., Morshed, M., Nasr-Esfahani, M.H., Baharvand, H., Kiani, S. 2011. Application of conductive polymers, scaffolds and electrical stimulation for nerve tissue engineering. *J Tissue Eng Regen Med*. 5: e17–35.

Giannoudis, P.V., Tzioupis, C. 2005. Clinical applications of BMP-7: The UK perspective. *Injury* 36(3): S47–S50.

Giannoudis, P.V., Dinopoulos, H., Tsiridis, E.P.V. 2005. Bone substitutes: An update. *Injury*. 36: S20–7.

Gobbi, A., Karnatzikos, G., Kumar, A. 2014. Long-term results after microfracture treatment for full-thickness knee chondral lesions in athletes. *Knee Surg Sports Traumatol Arthrosc*. 22: 1986–96.

Griffin, J.W., Hogan, M.V., Chhabra, A.B., Deal, D.N. 2013. Peripheral nerve repair and reconstruction. *J. Bone Joint Surg*. 95: 2144–51.

Grinsell, D., Keating, C.P. 2014. Peripheral nerve reconstruction after injury: A review of clinical and experimental therapies. *Biomed Res Int*. 2014: 698256.

Gupta, A.K., Hug, K., Berkoff, D.J., Boggess, B.R., Gavigan, M., Malley, P.C. 2012. Dermal tissue allograft for the repair of massive irreparable rotator cuff tears. *Am J Sports Med*. 40: 141–7.

Gupta, A.K., Hug, K., Boggess, B., Gavigan, M., Toth, A.P. 2013. Massive or 2-tendon rotator cuff tears in active patients with minimal glenohumeral arthritis: Clinical and radiographic outcomes of reconstruction using dermal tissue matrix xenograft. *Am J Sports Med*. 41: 872–9.

Han, L.H., Suri, S., Schmidt, C.E., Chen, S. 2010. Fabrication of three-dimensional scaffolds for heterogeneous tissue engineering. *Biomed Microdevices*. 12: 721–5.

Heineken, F., Skalak, R. 1991. Tissue engineering: A brief overview. *J Biomech Eng*. 113: 111–2.

Iannotti, J.P., Codsi, M.J., Kwon, Y.W., Derwin, K., Ciccone, J., Brems, J.J. 2006. Porcine small intestine submucosa augmentation of surgical repair of chronic two-tendon rotator cuff tears. *J Bone Joint Surg Am* 88(6): 1238–44.

James, R., Nagarale, R.K., Sachan, V.K., Badalucco, C., Bhattacharya, P.K., Kumbar, S.G. 2014. Synthesis and characterization of electrically conducting polymers for regenerative engineering applications: Sulfonated ionic membranes. *Polym. Adv. Technol*. 25: 1439–45.

Jiang, X., Lim, S.H., Mao, H.Q., Chew, S.Y. 2010. Current applications and future perspectives of artificial nerve conduits. *Exp Neurol*. 223: 86–101.

Jiang, Y.G., Zhang, S.F., Qi, Y.Y., Wang, L.L., Ouyang, H.W. 2011. Cell transplantation for articular cartilage defects: Principles of past, present, and future practice. *Cell Transplant*. 20: 593–607.

Johnson, E.O., Soucacos, P.N. 2008. Nerve repair: Experimental and clinical evaluation of biodegradable artificial nerve guides. *Injury*. 39(Suppl 3): S30–6.

Jung, H.J., Fisher, M.B., Woo, S.L. 2009. Role of biomechanics in the understanding of normal, injured, and healing ligaments and tendons. *Sports Med Arthrosc Rehabil Ther Technol*. 1: 9.

Jungebluth, P., Moll, G., Baiguera, S., Macchiarini, P. 2012. Tissue-engineered airway: A regenerative solution. *Clin Pharmacol Ther.* 91: 81–93.

Kanakaris, N. K., Lasanianos, N., Calori, G.M., Verdonk, R., Blokhuis, T.J., Cherubino, P., De Biase, P., Giannoudis, P.V. et al. 2009. Application of bone morphogenetic proteins to femoral non-unions: A 4-year multicentre experience. *Injury* 40: S54–S61.

Kim, B.S., Mooney, D.J. 1998. Development of biocompatible synthetic extracellular matrices for tissue engineering. *Trends Biotechnol.* 16: 224–30.

Kimura, Y., Hokugo, A., Takamoto, T., Tabata, Y., Kurosawa, H. 2008. Regeneration of anterior cruciate ligament by biodegradable scaffold combined with local controlled release of basic fibroblast growth factor and collagen wrapping. *Tissue Eng.* 14: 47–57.

Kon, E., Delcogliano, M., Filardo, G., Fini, M., Giavaresi, G., Francioli, S. 2010. Orderly osteochondral regeneration in a sheep model using a novel nano-composite multilayered biomaterial. *J Orthop Res.* 28: 116–24.

Lambers Heerspink, F.O., van Raay, J.J., Koorevaar, R.C., van Eerden, P.J., Westerbeek, R.E., van 't Riet, E. 2015. Comparing surgical repair with conservative treatment for degenerative rotator cuff tears: A randomized controlled trial. *J Shoulder Elbow Surg.* 24: 1274–81.

Lenart, B.A., Martens, K.A., Kearns, K.A., Gillespie, R.J., Zoga, A.C., Williams, G.R. 2015.Treatment of massive and recurrent rotator cuff tears augmented with a poly-l-lactide graft, a preliminary study. *J Shoulder Elbow Surg.* 24: 915–21.

Lissenberg-Thunnissen, S.N., de Gorter, D.J., Sier, C.F., Schipper, I.B. 2011. Use and efficacy of bone morphogenetic proteins in fracture healing. *Int Orthop.* 35: 1271–80.

Longo, U.G., Lamberti, A., Maffulli, N., Denaro, V. 2010. Tendon augmentation grafts: A systematic review. *Br Med Bull.* 94: 165–88.

Lundborg, G. 2003. Richard P. Bunge memorial lecture. Nerve injury and repair—A challenge to the plastic brain. *J Peripher Nerv Syst.* 8: 209–26.

Ma, X., Sun, Y., Cheng, X., Gao, Y., Hu, B., Wen, G. 2015. Repair of osteochondral defects by mosaicplasty and allogeneic BMSCs transplantation. *Int J Clin Exp Med.* 8: 6053.

Marston, W.A., Hanft, J., Norwood, P., Pollak, R. 2003. The efficacy and safety of dermagraft in improving the healing of chronic diabetic foot ulcers results of a prospective randomized trial. *Diabetes Care.* 26: 1701–5.

Matsiko, A., Levingstone, T.J., O'Brien, F.J. 2013. Advanced strategies for articular cartilage defect repair. *Materials.* 6: 637–68.

McCarron, J.A., Milks, R.A., Mesiha, M., Aurora, A., Walker, E., Iannotti, J.P. 2012. Reinforced fascia patch limits cyclic gapping of rotator cuff repairs in a human cadaveric model. *J Shoulder Elbow Surg.* 21: 1680–6.

Meek, M.F., Den Dunnen, W.F. 2009. Porosity of the wall of a Neurolac nerve conduit hampers nerve regeneration. *Microsurgery.* 29: 473–8.

Meyer, F., Wardale, J., Best, S., Cameron, R., Rushton, N., Brooks, R. 2012. Effects of lactic acid and glycolic acid on human osteoblasts: A way to understand PLGA involvement in PLGA/calcium phosphate composite failure. *J Orthop Res.* 30: 864–71.

Miller, N.C., Askew, A.E. 2007. Tibia fractures: An overview of evaluation and treatment. *Orthop Nurs.* 26: 216–23.

Nirmal, R.S., Nair, P.D. 2013. Significance of soluble growth factors in the chondrogenic response of human umbilical cord matrix stem cells in a porous three dimensional scaffold. *Eur Cell Mater.* 26: 234–51.

Omae, H., Steinmann, S.P., Zhao, C., Zobitz, M.E., Wongtriratanachai, P., Sperling, J.W. 2012. Biomechanical effect of rotator cuff augmentation with an acellular dermal matrix graft: A cadaver study. *Clin Biomech.* 27: 789–92.

Ouzzine, M., Venkatesan, N., Fournel-Gigleux, S. 2012. Proteoglycans and cartilage repair. *Methods Mol Biol.* 836: 339–55.

Park, J.H., Hong, J.M., Ju, Y.M., Jung, J.W., Kang, H.W., Lee, S.J. 2015. A novel tissue-engineered trachea with a mechanical behavior similar to native trachea. *Biomaterials.* 62: 106–15.

Paul, M., Kaur, P., Herson, M.R., Cheshire, P., Cleland, H., Akbarzadeh, S. 2015. Use of clotted human plasma and aprotinin in skin tissue engineering—A novel approach to engineering composite skin on a porous scaffold. *Tissue Eng C: Methods.* 21(10): 1098–1104.

Persidis, A. 1999. Tissue engineering. *Nat Biotechnol.* 17: 508–10.

Pfister, B.J., Gordon, T., Loverde, J.R., Kochar, A.S., Mackinnon, S.E., Cullen, D.K. 2011. Biomedical engineering strategies for peripheral nerve repair: Surgical applications, state of the art, and future challenges. *Crit Rev Biomed Eng.* 39: 81–124.

Pham, Q.P., Sharma, U., Mikos, A.G. 2006. Electrospinning of polymeric nanofibers for tissue engineering applications: A review. *Tissue Eng.* 12: 1197–1211.

Phipatanakul, W.P., Petersen, S.A. 2009. Porcine small intestine submucosa xenograft augmentation in repair of massive rotator cuff tears. *Am J Orthop.* 38: 572–5.

Proctor, C.S. 2014. Long-term successful arthroscopic repair of large and massive rotator cuff tears with a functional and degradable reinforcement device. *J Shoulder Elbow Surg.* 23: 1508–13.

Qu, D., Mosher, C., Boushell, M., Lu, H. 2015. Engineering complex orthopaedic tissues via strategic biomimicry. *Ann Biomed Eng.* 43: 697–717.

Ravindran, S., Kotecha, M., Huang, C.C., Ye, A., Pothirajan, P., Yin, Z. 2015. Biological and MRI characterization of biomimetic ECM scaffolds for cartilage tissue regeneration. *Biomaterials.* 71: 58–70.

Roberts, T.T., Rosenbaum, A.J. 2012. Bone grafts, bone substitutes and orthobiologics: The bridge between basic science and clinical advancements in fracture healing. *Organogenesis.* 8: 114–24.

Sampath, T.K., Maliakal, J.C., Hauschka, P.V., Jones, W.K., Sasak, H., Tucker, R.F. 1992. Recombinant human osteogenic protein-1 (hOP-1) induces new bone formation *in vivo* with a specific activity comparable with natural bovine osteogenic protein and stimulates osteoblast proliferation and differentiation *in vitro*. *J Biol Chem.* 267: 20352–62.

Scherman, P., Kanje, M., Dahlin, L.B. 2004. Bridging short nerve defects by direct repair under tension, nerve grafts or longitudinal sutures. *Restor Neurol Neurosci.* 22: 65–72.

Schwartz, J.A., Wang, W., Goldstein, T., Grande, D.A. 2014. Tissue engineered meniscus repair influence of cell passage number, tissue origin, and biomaterial carrier. *Cartilage.* doi:1947603514526038.

Selmi, T., Verdonk, P., Chambat, P., Dubrana, F., Potel, J.F., Barnouin, L. 2008. Autologous chondrocyte implantation in a novel alginate–agarose hydrogel: Outcome at two years. *J Bone Joint Surg Br.* 90: 597–604.

Shelke, N.B., Lee, P., Anderson, M., Mistry, N., Nagarale, R.K., Ma, X.M. 2016. Neural tissue engineering: Nanofiber-hydrogel based composite scaffolds. *Polym. Adv. Technol.* 27(1): 42–51.

Siemionow, M., Sonmez, E. 2007. Nerve allograft transplantation: A review. *J Reconstr Microsurg.* 23: 511–20.

Singh, K., Nandyala, S.V., Marquez-Lara, A., Fineberg, S.J. 2014. Epidemiological trends in the utilization of bone morphogenetic protein in spinal fusions from 2002 to 2011. *Spine (Phila Pa 1976)* 39: 491–6.

Spalazzi, J.P., Dagher, E., Doty, S.B., Guo, X.E., Rodeo, S.A., Lu, H.H. 2008. *In vivo* evaluation of a multiphased scaffold designed for orthopaedic interface tissue engineering and soft tissue-to-bone integration. *J Biomed Mater Res A.* 86: 1–12.

Taylor, C.A., Braza, D., Rice, J.B., Dillingham, T. 2008. The incidence of peripheral nerve injury in extremity trauma. *Am J Phys Med Rehabil.* 87: 381–5.

Temenoff, S.J., Mikos, G.A. 2000. Review: Tissue engineering for regeneration of articular cartilage. *Biomaterials* 21: 431–40.

Termaat, M.F., Den Boer, F.C., Bakker, F.C., Patka, P., Haarman, H.J. 2005. Bone morphogenetic proteins. Development and clinical efficacy in the treatment of fractures and bone defects. *J Bone Joint Surg Am,* 87: 1367–78.

Thangarajah, T., Pendegrass, C.J., Shahbazi, S., Lambert, S., Alexander, S., Blunn, G.W. 2015. Augmentation of rotator cuff repair with soft tissue scaffolds. *Orthop J Sports Med.* 3: 2325967115587495.

Toolan, B.C. 2006. Current concepts review: Orthobiologics. *Foot Ankle Int.* 27: 561–6.

Topp, K.S., Boyd, B.S. 2006. Structure and biomechanics of peripheral nerves: Nerve responses to physical stresses and implications for physical therapist practice. *Phys Ther.* 86: 92–109.

Varkey, M., Ding, J., Tredget, E.E. 2015. Advances in skin substitutes—Potential of tissue engineered skin for facilitating anti-fibrotic healing. *J Funct Biomater.* 6: 547–63.

Vukicevic, S., Oppermann, H., Verbanac, D., Jankolija, M., Popek, I., Curak, J. et al. 2014. The clinical use of bone morphogenetic proteins revisited: A novel biocompatible carrier device OSTEOGROW for bone healing. *Int Orthop.* 38: 635–47.

Walton, J.R., Bowman, N.K., Khatib, Y., Linklater, J., Murrell, G.A.C. 2007. Restore orthobiologic implant: Not recommended for augmentation of rotator cuff repairs. *J Bone Joint Surg.* 89: 786–91.

Wang, H., Li, Y., Zuo, Y., Li, J., Ma, S., Cheng, L. 2007. Biocompatibility and osteogenesis of biomimetic nano-hydroxyapatite/polyamide composite scaffolds for bone tissue engineering. *Biomaterials.* 28: 3338–48.

Wong, I., Burns, J., Snyder, S. 2010. Arthroscopic GraftJacket repair of rotator cuff tears. *J Shoulder Elbow Surg.* 19: 104–9.

Xiong, Y., Ren, C., Zhang, B., Yang, H., Lang, Y., Min, L. et al. 2014. Analyzing the behavior of a porous nano-hydroxyapatite/polyamide 66 (n-HA/PA66) composite for healing of bone defects. *Int J Nanomed.* 9: 485–94.

Xu, H., Wang, Y., Su, X., Zhang, X., Zhang, X. 2014. Safety and efficiency of biomimetic nanohydroxy-apatite/polyamide 66 composite in rabbits and primary use in anterior cervical discectomy and fusion. *Int J Polym Sci.* 2014: 6.

Xu, Q., Lu, H., Zhang, J., Lu, G., Deng, Z., Mo, A. 2010. Tissue engineering scaffold material of porous nanohydroxyapatite/polyamide 66. *Int J Nanomed.* 5: 331–5.

Yamamoto, A., Takagishi, K., Osawa, T., Yanagawa, T., Nakajima, D., Shitara, H. 2010. Prevalence and risk factors of a rotator cuff tear in the general population. *J Shoulder Elbow Surg.* 19: 116–20.

Yang, W., Both, S.K., van Osch, G.J., Wang, J., Jansen, J.A., Yang, F. 2015. Effects of *in vitro* chondrogenic priming time of bone-marrow-derived mesenchymal stromal cells on *in vivo* endochondral bone formation. *Acta Biomater.* 13: 254–65.

Zelen, C.M., Gould, L., Serena, T.E., Carter, M.J., Keller, J., Li, W.W. 2014. A prospective, randomised, controlled, multi-centre comparative effectiveness study of healing using dehydrated human amnion/chorion membrane allograft, bioengineered skin substitute or standard of care for treatment of chronic lower extremity diabetic ulcers. *Int Wound J.* 12: 724–32.

Zhang, X., Bogdanowicz, D., Erisken, C., Lee, N.M., Lu, H.H. 2012. Biomimetic scaffold design for functional and integrative tendon repair. *J Shoulder Elbow Surg.* 21: 266–77.

Zhang, X., Lu, M., Wang, Y., Su, X., Zhang, X. 2014. The development of biomimetic spherical hydroxyapatite/polyamide 66 biocomposites as bone repair materials. *Int J Polym Sci.* 2014: 6.

Zhu, W., Castro, N.J., Cheng, X., Keidar, M., Zhang, L.G. 2015. Cold atmospheric plasma modified electrospun scaffolds with embedded microspheres for improved cartilage regeneration. *PloS One.* 10: e0134729.

14

Evaluation of Toxicity and Safety of Nanomaterials: The Challenges Ahead

Y. K. Gupta and Amit Dinda

CONTENTS

14.1 Introduction

Application of nanoscience and nanotechnology in medicine is projected to revolutionize the practice of medicine in near future. It has evolved into a new area of research and development designated as nanomedicine. However, these nano-enabled systems need better characterization of end point for their therapeutic efficacy and safety. Regulatory research for *in vitro* and *in vivo* toxicity testing as well as novel methods for assessment of multifunctional nanosystems is of critical importance for evaluation of safety of different therapeutic application of nanomaterials.

The application of nanomaterials in therapeutics is size-dependent in nanoscale dimensions. Due to the nanoscale dimension, the materials acquire novel physiochemical properties with a high surface-to-mass ratio.

The examples of nano-therapeutics and nanodiagnostics include drugs, vaccine, implantable medical devices, sensors, and hybrid multifunctional products. These novel nanosystems acquire unique diagnostic and therapeutic functions, which is not possible with larger macro or micro scale. The most popular application of nanotechnology in medicine is development of new drug delivery systems, which accounts for about 80% of sale and 60% of patent filing worldwide.

14.2 Human Exposure to Nanomaterials

14.2.1 Nanomedicine

These nano-enabled systems contain the drug or other active biomolecules along with the nanomaterials that are biologically active. They are capable of producing interactions depending on biological triggers such as pH and temperature variation. Nanocarrier can improve the bioavailability of insoluble drugs. It can target the drug to the site of action like cancer cells with a capability of development of targeted therapy sparing the normal tissue. Nanoformulation can be made for crossing the biologic barriers such as blood–brain barrier (BBB) and biofilm. Nanomaterials can be used for functional and molecular imaging as well as simultaneous therapeutic intervention (theragnosis). Nanosystems are being used for coating implantable medical devices such as stents and wound dressing. Nanotechnology also plays an important role in regenerative medicine and cell-based therapy (Kubik et al., 2005; Wagner et al., 2006).

Hundreds of companies are involved in nanomedicine research and development leading to large number of products in the pipeline for market. The application area of these products includes drugs, cosmetics, diagnostics, imaging, tissue engineering, wound dressing, and many other areas related to health and medical practice. Commercial investment for R&D in nanotechnology is one of the highest when compared with other fields in biomedical sciences (Resnik and Tinkle, 2007). The nanocarrier system can deliver drug to the target site of action. The classical example is delivery of cytotoxic anticancer drug to the cancer area. It will increase the bioavailability of the drug in the cancer tissue sparing other organs, thus reducing the systemic toxicity of the drugs. Due to targeting, the total requirement of drug will be much less than the current conventional chemotherapy (Al-Abd et al., 2015). Also, this technology can help to develop oral delivery system for drugs that are now only available in injectable forms. Therefore, nanotechnology can provide low-cost, low-toxic, simple, and more effective treatment for many diseases (Fredolini et al., 2009; Dinda and Prashant, 2010; Gartiser et al., 2014; Prashant et al., 2014; Chen et al., 2015; Islam et al., 2015; Kang et al., 2015, Lee et al., 2015; Vishinkin and Haick 2015; Ashraf et al., 2016; Davachi et al., 2016, Kaushik et al., 2016).

While the advances in application of nanotechnology in medicine have opened a new horizon for cutting-edge cost-effective medical therapy, it has raised concern about its potential hazard and safety for humans and environment. Thus, it needs the development of new safety assessment strategy with ethical, social, and legal consequences (Fatehi et al., 2012).

14.2.2 Nano-Cosmetics

The interesting properties of nanosystem have a huge potential application in cosmetics industry. The most important example is the use of TiO_2 nanoparticle (NP) for protection of ultraviolet rays in sunlight. Though it is widely used in many sunscreen lotions and cream, its long-term safety is a question according to recent literature (Zhang et al., 2015). NPs are being used for eye liners, nail polish, lipsticks, soap, shampoo, and many other products. These nano-cosmetics need proper evaluation for transdermal absorption and toxicity as well as their potential for contamination of water in environment.

14.2.3 Nanotechnology Application in Agriculture, Animal Husbandry, and Food Chain

Another important mode of human exposure is through food chain—the ever-increasing application of nanomaterials and nanotechnology for increased agricultural productivity through sustained localized release of nutrients for plants, nanopesticide for enhanced crop protection (Kookana et al., 2014; Melanie et al., 2014), nanomedicine for animal farming, and veterinary practices (Pradhan et al., 2015). Nondegradable nanomaterials may enter into complex food-chain pathway. Through fodder it can enter in the systemic circulation of cow and be secreted in milk, which can enter human system especially with potential adverse effect on pregnant women and fetus. Nanosystems are also used for food fortification as well as food packaging (Underwood and van Eps, 2012).

14.2.4 Environmental Exposure

The NP may contaminate air generated through emission of motor vehicles, industries, explosives used for war and mining activities. Their entry into human system through respiratory route may be a health hazard. Similarly, any nonbiodegradable nanomaterial contaminating surface water may enter into human system through gastrointestinal tract as well as skin during bathing and swimming (Sajid et al., 2015).

14.2.5 Occupational Exposure

All persons engaged in laboratory and industry involved in fabricating and handling of NP systems have the potential for exposure. Special precautions are essential during manufacturing, storage, transportation, and disposal of the nanomaterials especially for nondegradable systems. Industry may be a potential source of environmental contamination (Bergamaschi et al., 2015).

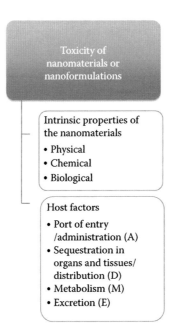

FIGURE 14.1
Factors responsible for toxicity of nanomaterials.

Although extensive research is being conducted in the area of nanomaterials for different therapeutic intervention, there is lack of understanding and paucity of critical information regarding their safety as well as toxicity. The assay procedure, tool, and techniques for evaluation of the toxicity of these materials need more uniformity and standardization. The need for the development of guideline as well as methods for the assessment of safety of nanomaterials for therapeutic use is still being debated in the scientific community (see Figure 14.1).

14.3 Intrinsic Properties of Nanomaterial

14.3.1 Physical Characteristics

14.3.1.1 Size

Size of the nanomaterial/NP is one of the key factors for its ability to pass through intracellular and paracellular pathways, internalization kinetics in the cells, mode of internalization such as micropinocytosis, macropinocytosis, and different forms of phagocytosis. Arbitrarily, the NPs can be subclassified according to their size into four classes: Ultrafine (≤5 nm), fine (>5 and ≤50 nm), small (>50 and ≤100 nm), and large (>100 and <1000 nm). According to the glomerular filtration barrier, the ultrafine NPs are most suitable to pass through glomerular filtration and be excreted in urine. Ultrafine and fine NPs are most likely to enter in the cell by micropinocytosis, and the large one by phagocytosis. The size of the phagolysosomal vacuole inside the cells is dependent on the size of the endocytosed NP, which in turn can affect cellular metabolism. The hemorrheology (homing and traveling in the circulating blood) of NPs is also size-dependent. Therefore, endothelial cell contacts will be more if NPs travel through more peripheral column of the circulating blood (Marquis et al., 2009).

14.3.1.2 Shape

Shape of the NP is an important factor for its interaction with the cellular and subcellular membranes as well as ability to penetrate through different barriers. If one compares a round NP (three dimension), a flat NP like graphene (two dimension), and a long nanotube/nanowire (one dimension), then this difference will be evident. *In vivo* use of nondegradable nanotube has a potential danger of unpredictable penetration into intracellular organelles such as mitochondria and causing cellular dysfunction. Similarly, in the circulating blood the nanotube and graphene-like structure may cause injury to the cellular elements including endothelial cells. Platelet activation and tissue injury associated release of procoagulant factors may induce intravascular coagulation enhancing the thromboembolism (Almeida et al., 2011).

14.3.1.3 Surface Property

Surface property, especially the surface charge, is very important for interaction of the particle with other cell membrane and glomerular filtration barrier. This is also an important determinant for its tendency to absorb other molecules like different components of plasmaproteins on the surface as well as aggregability. Modification of surface like pegylation can decrease the reticuloendothelial sequestration and increase the circulation time of NPs. Excessive cationic charge may be more disruptive to the cellular systems (Nam et al., 2013).

14.3.2 Chemical Properties

14.3.2.1 Composition

Biodegradability, which is the most important determinant of life cycle of NP, depends on the composition. Materials such as metal and ceramics will be nondegradable, whereas protein, lipid, carbohydrate, and many biopolymers are biodegradable. The degradability of polymers is variable. High molecular weight polymer such as polycaprolactone (PCL), which is used in many *in vivo* implants, are nondegradable whereas low molecular weight PCL degrades slowly. Composition of NP determines its intracellular metabolism *in vivo* (Møller et al., 2011; Nam et al., 2013).

14.3.2.2 Properties of Degradation Products

Composite NPs containing several different materials should be studied for their degradation kinetics and the degradation products.

14.3.3 Biological Property

Before assessing the safety for *in vivo* use of any NP, it is very important to study its biological properties with *in vitro* experiments. Several standard assays such as hemolysis, platelet aggregation, 3-(4,5-dimethylthiazol-2-yl)-2,5-diphenyltetrazolium bromide (MTT), and enzyme lactate dehydrogenase (LDH) assay can be performed (Napierska et al., 2010). However, depending on the nonbiodegradability and intended *in vivo* use certain special tests may be carried out such as mutagenesis assay, assay for protein corona formation for intravenous use, assay of degradability in simulated gastric juice for oral delivery system, and so on. Certain molecules such as surfactant poloxamer acts as biological response modifier (BRM) (Khan et al., 2015). Safe concentration of these molecules is important to avoid unpredictable behavior of NPs (Kang et al., 2015).

14.4 Host Factors

14.4.1 Port of Entry/Administration (A)

14.4.1.1 Oral

There is a great deal of research going on to develop nanocarrier or nanoformulation of drugs, which currently can be administered only by parental route. Oral delivery of anti-cancer drugs by nanocarrier is the classical example. Certain composition of NP like lipid NPs has shown considerable success for developing oral delivery system. Excessive sequa-tion of NPs in the mucus layer of the intestine should be excluded. After absorption, if the NPs enter mesenteric circulation then high sequestration of NP in the liver is a possibility and in that case it may cause excessive accumulation of the drug in the organ. Oral deliv-ery may be targeted to lymphatic pathway and in that situation it may bypass liver. Oral route of entry may be a health hazard in case of contamination of drinking water or food chain with NPs as discussed earlier (Ojer et al., 2015).

14.4.1.2 Intravenous

The nanoformulation developed for intravenous administration needs special attention for safety evaluation. The potential for surface absorption of proteins and other molecules in blood, interaction with red and white blood cell, platelets, activation of coagulation fac-tors, and endothelial cell interaction should be explored (Wacker, 2013).

14.4.1.3 Intramuscular

This route may be used for nanoadjuvant-based vaccination or localized slow release sys-tem of drugs or other biomolecules. The possibility of inflammatory reaction and foreign body granuloma formation should be excluded (Wissing et al., 2004).

14.4.1.4 Respiratory

All respiratory delivery of nanoformulation has an issue of size-dependent distribution in the bronchial tree, bronchiole, alveolar duct, and alveoli. Possibility of trapping and sequestration of NPs in alveolar macrophages is a possibility. Although the lungs have a huge absorptive surface area for entry of NPs into the circulation, chronic lung diseases may alter the property of air–blood barrier in the alveoli. Air pollution with NPs is a major threat for environmental nanotoxicity through respiratory route (Fattal et al., 2014).

14.4.1.5 Skin or Transdermal Entry

Larger size of NPs (>100 nm) usually do not cross the barrier of keratinized skin epithe-lium, which may be a safety point with nanosystems used in cosmetics with sun screen.

However, its potential absorption through skin of young children and sweat pores in hot and humid environment needs caution. Use of silver NPs for wound dressing and anti-infective cream or solution needs special mention. Silver NPs are toxic and high absorption through wound bed is a point of concern. Therefore, transdermal absorption kinetic should be studied in *ex vivo* model with pig skin or human cadaveric skin (Nafisi et al., 2015).

14.4.2 Sequestration in Organs or Tissue/Distribution (D)

14.4.2.1 Transit Time from Peripheral Circulation

Unlike drug or other biomolecules the NPs are a particulate system that cannot freely pass from intravascular to extravascular compartment. They exit from circulation over a time depending on the sequestration kinetics in different organs. Hence, for nanodrug delivery system NPs act as the nano-depots of drug and release of the drug depends on degradation kinetics of the carrier. Thus, conventional pharmacokinetics of the drug is altered when incorporated in nanodelivery system (Stockmann et al., 2015; Ulubayram et al., 2015).

14.4.2.2 Sequestration of NPs in Reticuloendothelial Organs (Liver and Spleen)

Depending on physical characteristics, NPs can be rapidly phagocytosed by the macrophage system and accumulate in liver as well as spleen. The potential of hepatic sequestration should be evaluated for all drugs to exclude hepatotoxicity. Excessive sequestration in liver and spleen may interfere with targeting of nanoformulation to cancer, or other organ like lungs (Qi et al., 2012).

14.4.2.3 Sequestration in Vital Organs (Lungs, Heart, Kidney, and Brain)

Sequestration in lungs will be advantageous for diseases localized in lungs. It can be achieved easily by optimizing respiratory route of delivery. However, translocation of nondegradable NPs to lungs from their initial sequestration in reticuloendothelial organ has been observed, which may cause adverse effect. Kidney is the main excretory organ and involved with filtration of blood. The NPs can be sequestrated in the mesangial cells in the glomeruli. The ultrafine NPs may pass through glomerular filtration barrier. Nephrotoxicity is a major concern with all heavy metals. Hence, all metallic NPs should be investigated for their renal sequestration and potential nephrotoxicity. Usually muscle cells are nonphagocytic cells. Thus sequestration into cardiac muscle of NPs is a relatively rare phenomenon. However, if multifunctional NPs are being used, which may interfere with conduction system of the heart, then necessary experiments should be done to determine its cardiotoxicity. Sequestration in brain should be excluded for any nondegradable as well as multifunctional NP, which has a potential to disrupt BBB. For any brain targeted nanodrug delivery system, the sequestration kinetics in the brain and consequence of disruption of BBB should also be studied (Bennewitz and Saltzman, 2009; Beck-Broichsitter et al., 2015).

The sequestration kinetics of the NPs in different organs can be studied with fluorescent dye loaded or radiolabeled NPs. Use of *in vivo* imaging, fluorometry or radioactivity detecting systems may be utilized for sequestration study of NPs in different organs. In case of drug-loaded NPs, analytical systems such as high performance liquid chromatography (HPLC) and liquid chromatography–mass spectrometry (LCMS) should be used for estimating the sequestration kinetics of drug in different organs, and blood. For metallic NPs, atomic absorption spectrophotometry (AAS) or inductively coupled plasma (ICP) should be used (Marquis et al., 2009; Naqvi et al., 2009).

14.4.3 Metabolism (M)

Following sequestration in different organs, the degradation and metabolism of the NP should be studied. *In vivo* degradation may be different from *in vitro* degradation in many NP systems. Effect of intermediate metabolic products of the NPs should be explored if significant amount of materials need to be administered (Kumar et al., 2012).

14.4.4 Excretion (E)

In case of all nondegradable NPs such as gold NPs, it is very important to know how they are being excreted from the body. The gold NP (GNP) cannot be metabolized inside the body. According to the literature and our study, the ultrafine GNP with diameter around 5 nm can easily pass through urine across glomerular filtration barrier. However, larger GNPs are suggested to be slowly excreted through the bile. For biodegradable polymeric NPs also it is important to evaluate excretion of the products of metabolism of NPs (Vinluan and Zheng J. 2015).

Alternative test strategy is essential for safety assessment of multifunctional composite NP system (Wolfram et al., 2015). The following issues need to be addressed:

1. Nanoformulation for drug delivery system is a heterogenous system consisting of the nanocarrier and the drug or biomolecules.
2. Nanoformulation may be a combination product consisting of different functional components: Drug and device, drug and biologic, device and biologic, and drug and device with biologic.
3. Justification is needed for all components of the nanoformulation for therapeutic and/or diagnostic efficacy of the system.
4. How to evaluate safety issue for nanomaterials used in tissue engineering and cell-based therapy is also a major challenge.

With progressive advancement of nanoscience, there is a need for continuous upgrading, modification, and introduction of alternative test strategy for safety evaluation of nanoformulation. The routine toxicity tests may not be helpful for assessing safety issues in many of these advanced systems.

References

Al-Abd AM, Aljehani ZK, Gazzaz RW, Fakhri SH, Jabbad AH, Alahdal AM, Torchilin VP. 2015. Pharmacokinetic strategies to improve drug penetration and entrapment within solid tumors. *J Control Release.* 219: 269–77.

Almeida JP, Chen AL, Foster A, Drezek R. 2011. *In vivo* biodistribution of nanoparticles. *Nanomedicine (Lond).* 6: 815–835.

Ashraf S, Pelaz B, Del Pino P, Carril M, Escudero A, Parak WJ, Soliman MG, Zhang Q, Carrillo-Carrion C. 2016. Gold-based nanomaterials for applications in nanomedicine. *Top Curr Chem.* 370: 169–202.

Beck-Broichsitter M, Nicolas J, Couvreur P. 2015. Design attributes of long-circulating polymeric drug delivery vehicles. *Eur J Pharm Biopharm.* 97: 304–17.

Bennewitz MF, Saltzman WM. 2009. Nanotechnology for delivery of drugs to the brain for epilepsy. *Neurotherapeutics.* 6: 323–36.

Bergamaschi E, Murphy F, Poland CA, Mullins M, Costa AL, McAlea E, Tran L, Tofail SA. 2015. Impact and effectiveness of risk mitigation strategies on the insurability of nanomaterial production: Evidences from industrial case studies. *Wiley Interdiscip Rev Nanomed Nanobiotechnol.* 7: 839–55.

Chen W, Fu L, Chen X. 2015. Improving cell-based therapies by nanomodification. *J Control Release.* 219: 560–575.

Davachi SM, Kaffashi B, Zamanian A, Torabinejad B, Ziaeirad Z. 2016. Investigating composite systems based on poly l-lactide and poly l-lactide/triclosan nanoparticles for tissue engineering and medical applications. *Mater Sci Eng C Mater Biol Appl.* 58: 294–309.

Dinda A, Prashant CK. 2010. Novel biomaterials and nano-biotechnology approaches in tumor diagnosis. *Adv Sci Technology.* 76: 78–89.

Fatehi L, Wolf SM, McCullough J et al. 2012. Recommendations for nanomedicine human subjects research oversight: An evolutionary approach for an emerging field. *J Law Med Ethics.* 40: 716–50.

Fattal E, Grabowski N, Mura S, Vergnaud J, Tsapis N, Hillaireau H. 2014. Lung toxicity of biodegradable nanoparticles. *J Biomed Nanotechnol.* 10: 2852–64.

Fredolini C, Tamburro D, Gambara G, Lepene BS, Espina V, Petricoin EF 3rd, Liotta LA, Luchini A. 2009. Nanoparticle technology: Amplifying the effective sensitivity of biomarker detection to create a urine test for hGH. *Drug Test Anal.* 1: 447–54.

Gartiser S, Flach F, Nickel C, Stintz M, Damme S, Schaeffer A, Erdinger L, Kuhlbusch TA. 2014. Behavior of nanoscale titanium dioxide in laboratory wastewater treatment plants according to OECD 303 A. *Chemosphere.* 104: 197–204.

Islam MA, Reesor EK, Xu Y, Zope HR, Zetter BR, Shi J. 2015. Biomaterials for mRNA delivery. *Biomater Sci.* 3: 1519–33.

Kang H, Mintri S, Menon AV, Lee HY, Choi HS, Kim J. 2015. Pharmacokinetics, pharmacodynamics and toxicology of theranostic nanoparticles. *Nanoscale.* 7: 18848–62.

Kaushik A, Tiwari S, Dev Jayant R, Marty A, Nair M. 2016. Towards detection and diagnosis of Ebola virus disease at point-of-care. *Biosens Bioelectron.* 75: 254–72.

Khan TA, Mahler HC, Kishore RS. 2015. Key interactions of surfactants in therapeutic protein formulations: A review. *Eur J Pharm Biopharm.* 97: 60–7.

Kookana RS, Boxall AB, Reeves PT et al. 2014. Nanopesticides: Guiding principles for regulatory evaluation of environmental risks. *J Agric Food Chem.* 62: 4227 – 4240.

Kubik T, Bogunia-Kubik K, Sugisaka M. 2005. Nanotechnology on duty in medical applications. *Curr Pharm Biotechnol.* 6: 17–33.

Kumar M, Singh G, Arora V, Mewar S, Sharma U, Jagannathan NR, Sapra S, Dinda AK, Kharbanda S, Singh H. 2012. Cellular interaction of folic acid conjugated superparamagnetic iron oxide nanoparticles and its use as contrast agent for targeted magnetic imaging of tumor cells. *Int J Nanomed.* 7: 3503–16.

Lee DS, Im HJ, Lee YS. 2015. Radionanomedicine: Widened perspectives of molecular theragnosis. *Nanomedicine.* 11: 795–810.

Marquis BJ, Love SA, Braun KL, Haynes CL. 2009. Analytical methods to assess nanoparticle toxicity. *Analyst.* 134(3): 425–39.

Melanie K, Thilo H. 2014. Nanopesticide research: Current trends and future priorities. *Environ Int.* 63: 224–235.

Møller P, Mikkelsen L, Vesterdal LK, Folkmann JK, Forchhammer L, Roursgaard M, Danielsen PH, Loft S. 2011. Hazard identification of particulate matter on vasomotor dysfunction and progression of atherosclerosis. *Crit Rev Toxicol.* 41: 339–68.

Nafisi S, Schäfer-Korting M, Maibach HI. 2015. Perspectives on percutaneous penetration: Silica nanoparticles. *Nanotoxicology.* 9: 643–57.

Nam J, Won N, Bang J, Jin H, Park J, Jung S, Jung S, Park Y, Kim S. 2013. Surface engineering of inorganic nanoparticles for imaging and therapy. *Adv Drug Deliv Rev.* 65: 622–48.

Napierska D, Thomassen LC, Lison D, Martens JA, Hoet PH. 2010. The nanosilica hazard: Another variable entity. *Part Fibre Toxicol.* 7: 39.

Naqvi S, Samim M, Dinda AK, Iqbal Z, Telagoanker S, Ahmed FJ, Maitra A. 2009. Impact of magnetic nanoparticles in biomedical applications. *Recent Pat Drug Deliv Formul.* 3: 153–61.

Ojer P, Iglesias T, Azqueta A, Irache JM, López de Cerain A. 2015. Toxicity evaluation of nanocarriers for the oral delivery of macromolecular drugs. *Eur J Pharm Biopharm.* 97: 206–17.

Pradhan N, Singh S, Ojha N, Shrivastava A, Barla A, Rai V, Bose S. 2015. Facets of nanotechnology as seen in food processing, packaging, and preservation industry. *Biomed Res Int.* 2015: 17 pages, Article ID 365672.

Prashant CK, Bhat M, Srivastava SK, Saxena A, Kumar M, Singh A, Samim M4, Ahmad FJ, Dinda AK. 2014. Fabrication of nanoadjuvant with poly-ε-caprolactone (PCL) for developing a single-shot vaccine providing prolonged immunity. *Int J Nanomed.* 9: 937–50.

Prashant CK, Kumar M, Dinda AK. 2014. Nanoparticle based tailoring of adjuvant function: The role in vaccine development. *J Biomed Nanotechnol.* 10: 2317–31.

Qi J, Lu Y, Wu W. 2012. Absorption, disposition and pharmacokinetics of solid lipid nanoparticles. *Curr Drug Metab.* 13: 418–28.

Resnik DB, Tinkle SS. 2007. Ethics in nanomedicine. *Nanomedicine (Lond).* 2: 345–50.

Sajid M, Ilyas M, Basheer C, Tariq M, Daud M, Baig N, Shehzad F. 2015. Impact of nanoparticles on human and environment: Review of toxicity factors, exposures, control strategies, and future prospects. *Environ Sci Pollut Res Int.* 22: 4122–43.

Stockmann C, Roberts JK, Yellepeddi VK, Sherwin CM. 2015. Clinical pharmacokinetics of inhaled antimicrobials. *Clin Pharmaco Kinet.* 54: 473–92.

Ulubayram K, Calamak S, Shahbazi R, Eroglu I. 2015. Nanofibers based antibacterial drug design, delivery and applications. *Curr Pharm Des.* 21: 1930–43.

Underwood C, van Eps AW. 2012. Nanomedicine and veterinary science: The reality and the practicality. *Vet J.* 193: 12–23.

Vinluan RD 3rd, Zheng J. 2015. Serum protein adsorption and excretion pathways of metal nanoparticles. *Nanomedicine (Lond).* 10: 2781–94.

Vishinkin R, Haick H. 2015. Nanoscale sensor technologies for disease detection via volatolomics. *Small.* 11: 6142–64.

Wacker M. 2013. Nanocarriers for intravenous injection—the long hard road to the market. *Int J Pharm.* 457: 50–62.

Wagner V, Dullaart A, Bock AK, Zweck A. 2006. The emerging nanomedicine landscape. *Nat Biotechnol.* 24: 1211–7.

Wissing SA, Kayser O, Müller RH. 2004. Solid lipid nanoparticles for parenteral drug delivery. *Adv Drug Deliv Rev.* 56: 1257–72.

Wolfram J, Zhu M, Yang Y et al. 2015. Safety of nanoparticles in medicine. *Curr Drug Targets.* 16: 1671–81.

Zhang X, Li W, Yang Z. 2015. Toxicology of nanosized titanium dioxide: An update. *Arch Toxicol.* 89: 2207–17.

Index